D0786864

*Medicare Prospective Payment and
the Shaping of U.S. Health Care*

Medicare Prospective Payment and the Shaping of U.S. Health Care

RICK MAYES, PH.D.
Department of Political Science
University of Richmond
Richmond, Virginia

and

ROBERT A. BERENSON, M.D.
The Urban Institute
Washington, D.C.

The Johns Hopkins University Press
Baltimore

The Johns Hopkins University Press
2715 North Charles Street
Baltimore, Maryland 21218-4363
www.press.jhu.edu

Library of Congress Cataloging-in-Publication Data
Mayes, Rick, 1969–
Medicare prospective payment and the shaping of U.S. health care /
Rick Mayes and Robert A. Berenson.
p. ; cm.
Includes bibliographical references and index.
ISBN 0-8018-8454-3 (hardcover : alk. paper)
1. Medicare. 2. Medicare—Claims administration. 3. Medical care, Cost of.
4. Hospitals—Prospective payment. I. Berenson, Robert A. II. Title.
[DNLM: 1. Medicare—economics. 2. Prospective Payment System—economics—United States.
3. Costs and Cost Analysis—United States. 4. Health Policy—United States.
5. Managed Care Programs—economics—United States. WT 31 M997m 2006]
RA412.3.M39 2006
368.4'2600973—dc22   2006010566

A catalog record for this book is available from the British Library.

For Ben and Ellen Mayes   R. M.

To my mother, Clare Berenson   R. A. B.

CONTENTS

The origins of this book, ironically, are rooted in a rejection. Back in 2001 or early 2002, I submitted a manuscript on Medicare's payment policy for hospitals to the *Journal of Health Politics, Policy, and Law*. Like most manuscript submissions, mine had as many weaknesses as strengths and needed substantial revisions. Fortunately, though, the reviewers' stinging (yet accurate) criticisms came with a very helpful and lengthy letter by the journal's editor at the time, Mark Peterson. All scholars should be so lucky to receive constructive suggestions that create a comprehensive road map for improvement. It took a day or two to digest all of the literature references and recommendations for additional research (namely, personal interviews with key policy makers) that he suggested. But the first few interviews I conducted—with Representative Pete Stark, former House Ways and Means Committee chair Dan Rostenkowski, former Ways and Means Committee staff member David Abernethy, former Senate Finance Committee staff member Lisa Potetz, former ProPAC chair Stuart Altman, and former House Ways and Means Committee ranking minority member Bill Gradison—led to more than sixty additional interviews and the discovery of how and why Medicare payment policy has significantly influenced the delivery, organization, and financing of U.S. health care.

Subsequently, the *Journal of Policy History* accepted a new and improved version of my manuscript, after its reviewers strengthened it even more. And the journal article later became the inspiration for this book-length examination of Medicare payment reforms, which Bob Berenson graciously agreed to help me write after we collaborated on an article on cost shifting for *Health Affairs* in 2003, with Jason Lee and Anne Gauthier at AcademyHealth. My first thanks, therefore, go to Mark Peterson and the editors at the *Journal of Policy History* for their time and patience with my scholarship.

An earlier and truncated version of Chapters 1 and 2 appeared in the *Journal of the History of Medicine and Allied Sciences* (2006) under the title "The Origins, Development, and Passage of Medicare's Revolutionary Prospective Payment System." An older draft of Chapters 3 and 4 appeared in the *Journal of Policy History* (2004) under the title "Causal Chains and Cost Shifting: How Medicare's Rescue Triggered the Managed Care Revolution." Portions of Chapter 6 appeared in *Heath Economics, Policy, and Law* (2006), in an article entitled "Pursuing Cost Containment in a Pluralistic Payer Environment," and portions of Chapter 7 appeared in the *Journal of Health Law* (2005) in an article entitled "Medicare and America's Health Care System in Transition: From the Death of Managed Care to the Medicare Modernization Act of 2003 and Beyond." I am grateful to these journals' editors for allowing me to use these works in this present volume.

This book would not exist were it not for the generosity of numerous policy makers who allowed me to interview them at length. Their names are listed in the appendix. I am indebted to all of them for providing me with an insider's perspective on how Medicare payment reforms were developed, implemented, and adjusted over time, as well as how they interacted with other parts of the U.S health care system. A number of individuals, in particular, shared hours with me or even allowed me to interview them more than once: Jack Ashby, Sheila Burke, Allen Dobson, Paul Ginsburg, Stuart Guterman, William Hsiao, Linda Magno, James Mongan, Jack Owen, Leon Panetta, Julian Pettengill, Rick Pollack, Robert Reischauer, Tom Scully, Bruce Vladeck, and Gail Wilensky.

I have benefited greatly from the friendship, mentoring, and scholarship of a number of individuals, including Henry Abraham, Ed Berkowitz, Farasat Bokhari, Martha Derthick, John Echeverri-Gent, Ken Elzinga, Dan Fox, Dan Gitterman, Colleen Grogan, Jacob Hacker, Allan Horwitz, Bob Hurley, Carol Mershon, Jim Morone, Jon Oberlander, David O'Brien, Tom Oliver, Larry Sabato, Richard Scheffler, Herman Schwartz, and Deborah Stone. My progress in academia has been due, in part, to their support and encouragement. This book began as a research project at the University of California, Berkeley, School of Public Health, under a National Institute of Health postdoctoral traineeship. Since then, it has been supported by generous faculty research grants and a junior research leave from the University of Richmond.

It has been my good fortune to be a member of the Department of Political Science at the University of Richmond, where I have enjoyed the company of a kind and nurturing group of colleagues: Sheila Carapico, Akiba Covitz, Jennifer Erkulwater, Art Gunlicks, Jimmy Kandeh, Melissa Labonte, John Outland, Dan Palazzolo, Tracy Roof, Andrea Simpson, Pat Thiel, Yamina Truda, Vincent Wang, Ellis West, and John Whelan. I have also enjoyed the intellectual stimulation and friendship of numerous students with a significant interest in health care, many of whom have taken my U.S. Health Care Policy and Politics course: Casey Abare, Cecelia Ackerman (who transcribed several interviews), Jon Alpern, Scott Annett, Ryan Babiuch (who transcribed several interviews), Megan Bailey, Amanda Biddle, Kelly Billig, Becky Brenner, Justin Burk, Ruthie Byrne, Drew Callison, Elise Carlin, Nicole Conner, Tom Cosgrove, Randy De Martino, Abbie Emerson (who transcribed several interviews), Emily Fellin, Paul Gardner, Adam Greenblatt, Deborah Hendryx, Matt Hitchcock, Taylor Hubbard, Jake Kayser, Faith Keck, Allison Kirk, Jackie Knupp, Dave Larkin, Marcie Lipper, Christine Livingston, Bill Longley, Emily Newman, Brian Pagels, Justin Polselli, Roger Revell, John Rosato, Andrew Ryan, Kristin Schmidt, Jaime Settle, Lauren Skiles, Matt Summers, Jason Sutton, Meredith Stewart, Jeff Vergales, Chris Wellington, Conrad Williams, Matt Williams, and Kathryn Winslow.

Bob Berenson and I owe enormous debts of gratitude to David Colby, Tim Jost, David Smith, and Tom Weill, and to Joe White, who was the official reviewer for the Johns Hopkins University Press. All of them read either the penultimate or ultimate chapter drafts of our book. Their comments, criticisms, and suggestions for revision took months to address, and they may not agree with all of our final arguments and observations, but their reviews dramatically improved the overall quality of our book. Any errors that remain—particularly after their close critiques—are solely our fault.

I wish to thank the Johns Hopkins University Press for helping us make this book come to fruition. Wendy Harris has been a superb editor. I greatly appreciate and am thankful to her for believing in this project when it was only an idea on a few pages of paper. Special thanks as well to Susan Lantz and Brendan Coyne for working with our final manuscript drafts and for their very helpful recommendations for improvement.

Finally, this book is dedicated to my family. My parents, Ben and Ellen Mayes, are two of the people I admire most in life. I literally cannot thank them enough for their love and support. My brother, David, and his wife, Erika, have been an inspiration to me on many occasions, and I am exceedingly grateful to them. I consider my in-laws, Pat and David Gilpatric, to be two of my best friends. And my wife Jennifer and our two boys Timothy and Benjamin are the biggest joys in my life.

R. M.

I was pleased when Rick Mayes asked me to join in this collaboration to explain the importance of prospective payment in Medicare. After all, he had already done most of the heavy lifting by interviewing scores of individuals who had left important imprints on the Medicare program. He had the history down—all I needed to do, as a policy wonk working at the Urban Institute, was help him make sense of that history.

That I should be in a position to offer up policy remedies for Medicare could be viewed as surprising. Certainly it is to me. For most of my professional career, I practiced medicine and as a general internist saw more than my share of Medicare patients. But learning how to code and bill Medicare for my services (and sometimes complain about inadequate payments) is not the proper preparation for understanding the various elements—fiscal, political, operational, and, yes, clinical—that must be factored into payment policy decisions. Rather, it was the three years I spent in what was then proudly called the Health Care Financing Administration as a senior political appointee in the Clinton administration that I developed my interest in and perspectives about Medicare payment policies.

That opportunity came pretty much out of the blue, so my first acknowledgment must go to Nancy-Ann DeParle, the HCFA administrator who hired me to run the Center for Health Plans and Providers, which was then the place from which all Medicare payment policy flowed. I also thank Mike Hash, Carol Cronin, and Kathy King, who also were political appointees during my HCFA tenure and provided much-appreciated collegiality and support as we collectively fought against Republican efforts to dismantle the traditional Medicare program. That fight continues.

I learned most of what I know about how Medicare works generally, and about prospective payment specifically, from the dedicated and hardworking career civil servants I had the privilege to work with at the center. Here, there is room to acknowledge only the senior leadership, but I benefited from contact with remarkable expertise throughout the agency. In no particular order, I want to thank Kathy Buto, Tom Hoyer, Tom Gustafson, Barbara Wynn, Stuart Streimer, Gary Bailey, Sharon Arnold, and Parashar Patel, most of whom have moved on to other jobs in other places but who gave their best to making Medicare the successful program it is, while helping me get through the day.

I have had three tours of duty working in the federal government—from the bowels of the Parklawn Building with Community Health Centers, to the rarified air of the Old Executive Office Building as a member of the Carter White House Domestic Policy Staff, to riding the I-95 corridor between Baltimore and D.C. while serving in HCFA. These have been the best three jobs I've had. I hope my contribution to Rick's book demonstrates that along the way I've learned the importance of federal government programs and the respect owed to the staff who administer them.

R. A. B.

AAPCC	adjusted average per capita costs
AHA	American Hospital Association
AMA	American Medical Association
ASCs	ambulatory surgery centers
ASIM	American Society of Internal Medicine
BBA	Balanced Budget Act of 1997
CABG	coronary artery bypass grafting
CBO	Congressional Budget Office
CDHC	consumer-directed health care
CHA	Connecticut Hospital Association
CMS	Centers for Medicare and Medicaid Services
COBRA	Consolidated Omnibus Reconciliation Act of 1985
CON	certificate of need
CPR	customary, prevailing, and reasonable
DSH	disproportionate share hospitals
DRGs	diagnosis-related groups
ERISA	Employee Retirement Income Security Act
ESP	Economic Stabilization Program
FAH	Federation of American Hospitals
FEHBP	Federal Employees Health Benefits Program
GAO	Government Accountability Office
GDP	gross domestic product
HCFA	Health Care Financing Administration
HCFPA	Health Care Facilities and Planning Act
HHS	Health and Human Services
HI	Hospital Insurance (trust fund)
HIAA	Health Insurance Association of America

HIPAA	Health Insurance Portability and Accountability Act
HMO	health maintenance organization
ICFs	intermediate care facilities
IPAs	independent practice associations
LPNs	licensed practical nurses
M + C	Medicare + Choice
MAACs	maximum allowable actual charges
MedPAC	Medicare Payment Advisory Commission
MEI	Medicare Economic Index
MMA	Medicare Prescription Drug, Improvement, and Modernization Act
MSAs	medical savings accounts
OASI	Old Age and Survivors Insurance (trust fund)
OMB	Office of Management and Budget
PHOs	physician-hospital organizations
POS	point of service plan
PPO	preferred provider organization
PPRC	Physician Payment Review Commission
PPS	prospective payment system
ProPAC	Prospective Payment Assessment Commission
PSROs	professional standards review organizations
RBRVS	resource-based relative-value scale
RNs	registered nurses
RUC	Relative-Value Scale Update Committee
SCHIP	State Children's Health Insurance Program
SGR	sustainable growth rate
SHARE	Standard Hospital Accounting and Rate Evaluation
SMI	Supplementary Medical Insurance (trust fund)
SNFs	skilled nursing facilities
SSA	Social Security Administration
TEFRA	Tax Equity and Fiscal Responsibility Act
UCR	usual, customary, and reasonable
VE	voluntary effort
VPS	volume performance standard
WHO	World Health Organization

*Medicare Prospective Payment and
the Shaping of U.S. Health Care*

Introduction

While growth rates in private health spending per capita have bounced up and down, federal Medicare expenditures per enrollee have shown a consistent downward trend. Why? Because history shows that government regulation works. Through regulatory efforts—prospective payment of hospitals, volume performance standards for physicians, and the (unpopular but effective) Balanced Budget Act (BBA) of 1997—Medicare has slowed its rate of expenditure growth . . . The not-so-sad history of Medicare cost containment shows that solutions do exist and they do work.

—*Thomas Bodenheimer, M.D., University of California, San Francisco*

I hate this whole G— d— system [Medicare]. I'd blow it up if I could, but I'm stuck with it. If it were up to me, I'd buy everybody private insurance and forget about it. Obviously that's what the Republican view is: We ought to do what we do for federal employees—go out and buy every senior citizen a community-rated, structured, and regulated private insurance plan. Let them all go buy an Aetna product, or a Blue Cross product; that's the Republican philosophy. Why should Tom Scully and his staff fix prices for every doctor and hospital in America? Which is what we do.

—*Tom Scully, Administrator (2001–4), Centers for Medicare and Medicaid Services, President and CEO (1995–2001), Federation of American Hospitals*

Most Americans think of Medicare as a health insurance program for providing medical care to elderly persons. To policy makers, however, Medicare is—and has long been—much more than just an entitlement for senior citizens. For more than three decades, it has operated as the leading vehicle for the federal government's subsidization and massive expansion of the U.S. health care system. This role evolved and grew in the years following Medicare's implementation. Over time, it has become an enormously expensive program, which currently costs the government more than $330 billion a year and serves approximately forty-two million people (up from $1.3 billion and nineteen million people in its first full year of operation, 1967).[1] In addition to financing medical care for millions of senior citizens and people with disabilities, Medicare provides significant funds for medical education, research, and the care of disadvantaged and vulnerable people. It is also the single largest purchaser of hospital and physician services, which makes it "the eight-hundred-pound gorilla" of the U.S. health care system.[2] So when the federal government makes a dramatic change to Medicare's payment methods, it profoundly affects (directly and indirectly) the cost-benefit calculations and policy decisions of medical providers, insurers, employers, and health care administrators across the country.

The biggest and most intense battle within the U.S. health care system during the past two decades has been over two interrelated questions: first, who will control the manner in which medical care is paid for, and second, how much will it cost? The primary argument of this book is that—contrary to conventional wisdom and whole libraries of books and articles that point to managed care as the biggest "change agent" in American medicine in the last twenty years—the private sector neither initiated this battle nor provided the critical innovation that transformed health care in the United States. Instead, it was Medicare's transition to a prospective payment system (PPS) that triggered and repeatedly intensified the economic restructuring of the U.S. health care system. With prospective payment, "Medicare sets prospectively the payment amount (rates) providers will receive for most covered products and services and providers agree to accept them as payment in full," according to the Medicare Payment Advisory Commission (MedPAC). "Thus, in most instances, providers' payments are based on predetermined rates and are unaffected by their costs or posted charges."[3]

Medicare payment reforms have empowered the federal government, making it similar to health care systems in other Western countries.[4] They have given the U.S. government control over the price of most medical care and ended the era—dating back to the 1920s—in which doctors and hospitals' authority over medical prices and decision making went virtually unquestioned.[5] The key to Medicare's role as the leading catalyst for change in the U.S. health care system is the program's immense size and influence.[6] As the single largest individual buyer of health care and the "first mover" in the annual payment game between those who provide medical care and those who pay for it, Medicare invariably drives the behavior of medical providers and private payers.

Medicare's revolutionary transition from traditional cost reimbursement (generally paying hospitals and physicians their costs) to a prospective payment model began in 1983. In that year, Congress changed the program's method of paying hospitals to a system of predetermined payment amounts for individual diagnosis-related groups (DRGs). Following the success of DRGs at restraining the rate of growth in Medicare's hospital expenditures, Congress in 1989 enacted a similar program—a resource-based relative-value scale (RBRVS) with a standardized fee schedule—for Medicare's reimbursement of physicians. It went into effect in 1992, with a volume performance standard (VPS) provision that was designed to operate as an expenditure target (or total limit on how much Medicare would spend on physician services).[7] With the Balanced Budget Act (BBA) of 1997, Congress reformed the reimbursement processes of the remaining cost-based components of Medicare, including outpatient ambulatory services and postacute care (such as skilled nursing facilities and home health agencies). By 2003, twenty years after Medicare started the payment revolution within the U.S. health care system, the program had become fully "prospectivized" in its reimbursement of all medical providers.

Each time Congress and the Health Care Financing Administration (HCFA, later renamed the Centers for Medicare and Medicaid Services, or CMS) changed one part of Medicare from cost reimbursement to prospective rate setting, the overall growth of the program's expenditures slowed. Yet these spending reductions often came at the expense of providers compensating by increasing their revenues from private payers. "When Medicare slows its rate of expenditure growth," explains David Abernethy, former senior Medicare specialist and staff director of the House Ways and Means Health Subcommittee, "hospitals' overall rate of revenue growth slows and that, in the end, puts the final pressure on private payers."[8] This use of cost shifting (or, if one prefers, "cross subsidization" or "differential pricing") by medical providers in which, as Paul Ginsburg, president of the Center for Studying Health System Change, explains, "changes in administered prices of one payer lead to compensating changes in prices charged to other payers for care," propelled the growth of private sector efforts (namely, managed care) to achieve similar cost control. Chapter 4 explores this issue in greater detail.

Ultimately, the change in Medicare's reimbursement policy temporarily altered the balance of power between the federal government and medical providers. By increasing the scope and extent of Medicare's regulation through prospective payment, Congress for the first time gained the upper hand in its financial relationship with hospitals and then with physicians in terms of setting medical *prices*. Yet, apart from Medicare's VPS (later replaced by a sustainable growth rate, or SGR) for Part B—which has fallen apart since 2000—the federal government has done relatively little to effectively extend Medicare's success in controlling prices to controlling the *volume* of services provided.[9] So although Medicare's PPS has been more responsible than anything else for rationalizing health care prices in America, the program has done much less to control utilization. Thus, Medicare's rate of expenditure growth remains an issue of enormous political concern.[10]

Policy Feedback and Causal Chains

Social scientists often take a "snapshot" view of political life, explains political scientist Paul Pierson. "How does the distribution of public opinion affect policy outcomes? How do individual social characteristics influence propensities to vote? . . . Disputes among competing theories center on which factors ("variables") in the current environment generate important political outcomes."[11] But the significance of such factors, he points out, is "frequently distorted when they are taken from their temporal context."[12] So there is a strong case to be made for shifting from snapshots to "moving pictures," especially for studying events or phenomena that unfold over longer periods of time (often years).[13] Pierson quotes sociologist James Mahoney, who argues that this is particularly true for studying sequences in which "an event may trigger a chain of causally-linked events that, once itself in motion, occurs independently of the institutions that initially trigger it. This sequence of events, while ultimately linked to a critical juncture period, may culminate in an outcome that is far removed from the original juncture."[14] The trick is to trace the chain of events and test how strong the links are. [15]

This study of Medicare's role as the leading change agent of the U.S. health care system contributes to a growing body of research that focuses on how public policies can be as much of an influence (an independent variable) on political and private actors—through the political and economic feedback they generate—as they are an outcome of them (a dependent variable).[16] The goal is to try to separate the specific order of cause and effect, because sequence analysis is critical for causal analysis.[17] A parallel goal with this type of inquiry is to try to account for how individuals and institutions respond to changes in public policy, recognizing that government reforms often reconfigure incentives other than those originally intended. For example, Jacob Hacker has shown that the parallel growth of public welfare programs (Social Security) and private welfare (health insurance) is a classic example of how "private social benefits have 'policy feedback' effects that are not all that different from the policy feedback effects that are created by public social programs."[18] In both instances, "major public policies constitute important rules, influencing the allocation of economic and political resources, modifying the costs and benefits associated with alternative political strategies, and consequently altering ensuing political development."[19]

Organization

This book is designed to explain how and why Medicare's transition to prospective payment radically transformed the economic orientation of American health care. We argue that the development and major changes in the organization of health care in the United States over the last thirty years have been significantly influenced by major changes to Medicare payment policy. The first several chapters survey the origins, development, and short-term consequences of Medicare's prospective payment system for hospitals.

Chapter 1 focuses on how rampant medical inflation in the 1970s forced policy makers to search for ways to control Medicare's rapidly escalating costs. With doctors and hospital executives in control of the U.S. health care system for decades, virtually unrestricted cost reimbursement had become the dominant model for financing public and private medical care. Independent not-for-profit hospitals and physicians practicing alone or in small groups dominated the medical landscape, notes Bradford Gray, principal research associate at the Urban Institute. "Third-party payers (both private and public) played their financing role passively, reluctant to interfere with medical decision making and the doctor-patient relationship. They paid for medical care by reimbursing for costs incurred or charges billed by health care providers and did little to control which services were provided or how much they cost."[20] The medical inflation that grew directly out of these delivery structures and payment systems became unsustainable.

Out of financial necessity, therefore, Congress and a handful of state governments commissioned experiments in alternative reimbursement systems. The most promising conceptual innovation—prospective payment with predetermined reimbursement rates—was the product of pioneering research at the University of Michigan and, particularly, Yale University. Using data from Connecticut's hospitals, Yale professors John Thompson and Robert Fetter demonstrated that medical care could be standardized and measured. As a result, policy makers and administrators were able, for the first time, to compare prices across different hospitals for the same services. They found an enormous amount of unjustifiable variation, which called into question medical providers' authority to regulate their own affairs. By the late 1970s, solving the problem of hospital cost inflation had become one of the leading domestic policy priorities. But no real progress was achieved in either the public or private sector. The failure of President Jimmy Carter's proposals for hospital price controls and of the hospital industry's voluntary efforts at reducing inflation opened a window of opportunity for a drastic change of Medicare's system for reimbursing hospitals.

Chapter 2 examines how Medicare's new system for hospital payment did not come from the private sector or at the urging of a Democratic president. Instead, it came from government-sponsored (and government-tested) health services research. And it was advocated by a new Republican administration that professed a disdain for government regulation. Congressional leaders and members of President Ronald Reagan's administration settled on a variant of New Jersey's alternative hospital reimbursement model—prospective payment using diagnosis-related groups (DRGs)—that came from Thompson and Fetter's research at Yale. Instead of simply paying hospitals their costs, the new model established predetermined (or "prospective") hospital payment rates for hundreds of distinct diagnostic groups. Thus, if a hospital could treat a Medicare patient for less than the standard DRG payment, it was rewarded by being allowed to keep the savings as a profit. If it cost more, it took a loss that policy makers assumed would encourage the hospital's executives to make improvements in efficiency and productivity.

The new and vastly increased amount of government regulation that Medicare's PPS represented was paradoxical in that it purported to mimic the dynamic forces of the free market. By realigning financial incentives, policy makers designed the new system to bring Medicare's rate of cost growth under control. A financial crisis affecting Social Security in 1982–83 provided the Reagan administration and leading members of Congress with the necessary legislative opportunity to pass Medicare's PPS as part of a larger and even more urgent package of welfare state reforms.

Chapter 3 explains how Medicare's new payment model changed hospital administration during its four-year phase-in period. During this time, the hospital industry's financial view of Medicare patients changed significantly. Instead of providing as much care as could be medically justified, hospitals shifted their focus to increasing efficiency and shortening Medicare patients' length-of-stay. The PPS operated as a huge shock to the nation's hospital industry, because it completely reengineered the billing structure accounting for approximately 40 percent of every hospital's total revenue. The rate of growth in Medicare's hospital expenditures slowed considerably. No change in the private sector could ever have effected so much change in the U.S. health care system in so short a time. The Medicare payment reforms "were the most drastic and far-reaching changes in federal health policy since the passage of Medicare itself," notes political scientist David Smith. They were "remarkable for the comprehensiveness and sophistication of their design—indeed, the sheer technical achievement was astonishing."[21]

Medicare's PPS made hospital executives think for the first time about how to become more productive. Previously, hospital executives had no incentive to use their personnel more efficiently, to control their costs on a per-case basis, or to try to figure out what it actually cost to do a specific medical procedure or service. They rarely kept accurate patient records or paid attention to diagnostic coding. Medicare's PPS, therefore, represented a very different way of doing business and an assault on the status quo. Under Medicare's new method of reimbursement, hospitals could make unprecedented profits, but they could also be left with unprecedented financial losses. Hospital executives responded by adopting a more corporate orientation and reaped windfall profits in the early years of Medicare's new payment system.

Hospitals did so well financially that the industry failed to grasp how Medicare's PPS had temporarily shifted the balance of political and financial power from the hospitals to the government. They eventually realized the significant implications involved when Congress began to use Medicare's PPS in the mid-1980s as a major deficit reduction device. Mounting budget deficits led policy makers to change the focus of prospective payment. They manipulated Medicare payment rates in order to generate substantial budgetary savings and financially subsidize specific segments of the hospital industry (teaching, rural, and inner-city hospitals). As a result, instead of becoming more simple and technocratic, Medicare payment policy became more complicated and political.

Chapter 4 outlines how Congress and successive administrations expanded their use of Medicare's PPS in the late 1980s and early 1990s to reduce budget deficits and increase spending in other areas of the federal budget (particularly Medicaid). In addition to mounting fiscal pressures, congressional leaders were responding to the hospital industry's enormous profits in the early years of Medicare's PPS. "By 1987," notes the chairman of the Prospective Payment Assessment Commission (ProPAC), Stuart Altman, "we realized what was going on and so then it became a 'whittling down' or 'taking back' phase."[22] Congress repeatedly adjusted Medicare's payment rates at levels below annual increases in medical inflation, which would not have been enormously consequential had the hospital industry as a whole restrained its cost growth. But it didn't. In the late 1980s and early 1990s, hospitals' costs continued to increase at their pre-PPS rates.

As Congress tightened Medicare's reimbursement policies, hospitals responded by increasing their charges to privately insured payers (the majority of Americans who receive health insurance from their employers). "Why it took private payers until the early 1990s before they began to marshal even a modicum of countervailing market power" is perplexing, notes health economist Uwe Reinhardt.[23] But eventually employers found their paradigmatic response: managed care. The term managed care is problematic, because it conflates and confuses two separate forms of organizational behavior: selective contracting to drive down prices, which became the source of most managed care savings, and actual management of treatment, which became the subject of most of the managed care hype and hysteria.[24] For the purposes of this book, however, we mean by managed care a payment model that is distinct from traditional indemnity health insurance by virtue of the fact that it attempts to influence the way health care is provided and often even restricts patients' access to and choice of medical provider. Prepaid group practice, a form of managed care, did precede Medicare's PPS. But organized medicine's traditional opposition to any form of reimbursement other than the fee-for-service model associated with indemnity insurance kept managed care marginalized for decades.

What ultimately played the biggest role in making market incentives sufficient to induce a paradigm shift in the private sector away from indemnity insurance and toward managed care was the success of Medicare's PPS in controlling health care costs in the public sector. What is ironic about the rapid shift in the U.S. health care system from a predominantly not-for-profit ethos to a more corporate orientation is that it was largely the incidental byproduct of federal policy initiatives designed to control Medicare's costs.[25] In other words, before business behavior triggered the managed care revolution, it largely responded to and was an unintended consequence of government policy making: in this instance, Medicare payment reforms.

Chapter 5 analyzes how the success of Medicare's DRGs for hospitals led policy makers to rationalize the program's reimbursement of physicians. They adopted a resource-based relative-value scale (RBRVS) with a standardized fee schedule. One goal was to reduce payments to surgeons and specialists and increase them to internists and general practitioners. The main goal of the RBRVS and fee schedule, however, was to slow the rate of cost growth of Medicare Part B. After the new payment system went into effect in 1992, the growth in volume and intensity of Medicare's spending on physician services slowed dramatically. Thus, the federal government succeeded in temporarily shifting another balance of power arrangement: in this instance, from physicians to Medicare.

The last two chapters examine the economic transformation of health care in the private sector, the promise of "market competition" and its ultimate failure. Chapter 6 focuses on the ascendancy of managed care in the mid-1990s and the backlash it eventually spawned. During these years, employers experienced minimal to no growth in their health insurance costs, largely because managed care clamped down on medical spending and decreased hospitals' ability to charge privately insured patients more. The United States spent almost $120 billion less on health care in 1996 than the Congressional Budget Office (CBO) had predicted in its 1993 forecast.[26] With declining private payments from managed care, the hospital industry finally achieved significant cost control.

Meanwhile, Republican and Democratic leaders struggled to reach a political consensus on the future direction of Medicare policy. The resulting impasse that developed between President Clinton and congressional Republicans—led by House Speaker Newt Gingrich—became the focal point of bitter budget conflicts in 1995 and a partial federal government shutdown. Following this political debacle and President Bill Clinton's landslide reelection in 1996, leading representatives from both parties returned to using Medicare as a huge "cash cow," passing the Balanced Budget Act (BBA) of 1997. The BBA constituted the ultimate subordination of Medicare to larger fiscal policy goals; it achieved approximately 73 percent of its total budgetary savings ($224 billion) from reductions in Medicare spending.[27] The BBA also attempted to more widely disseminate the supposed virtues of managed care (particularly for coverage of supplemental benefits such as prescription drug coverage) by encouraging millions of Medicare beneficiaries to enroll in private health plans as part of a new Medicare + Choice program.

Chapter 7 documents the economic reckoning the U.S. health care system experienced in the late 1990s and its consequences in the early 2000s. The BBA's major Medicare cuts and the final death throes of restrictive managed care left medical providers with declining payments from both public and private payers in 1998–99. Hospitals and the home health industry were particularly hard hit. When increasing cost pressures returned in the late 1990s, growing numbers of medical providers and managed care organizations found profitability difficult to achieve and bankruptcy a growing threat. In response, hospitals led the way among medical providers in increasing revenues where they could, which was from private payers. Their goal was to negotiate more favorable contracts with private payers and employers. Managed care organizations followed suit and—in reaction to the vehement backlash against them—dropped most of the business practices that had (at least temporarily) restrained health care inflation in the U.S. Many of them also dropped their participation in Medicare + Choice, after years of overreaching for "easy" Medicare profits, which left millions of the program's beneficiaries scurrying to reestablish their coverage under the program's traditional fee-for-service arrangements.

This increased consolidation and the declining effectiveness of market forces triggered a return to rampant medical inflation in the early 2000s. Health plans and hospitals successfully negotiated significant payment increases after years of minimal or no revenue growth. These increases restored most of them to solid financial health. But skyrocketing health insurance costs and a sluggish economy left an additional five million Americans without health insurance coverage by 2004, bringing the nation's total number of uninsured to forty-five million (or 15.6 percent of the population).[28] Medical-related bankruptcies increased substantially, as did the costs of, and enrollment in, Medicaid. In the midst of these and other deteriorating health care trends, President George Bush and Congress passed the largest expansion of Medicare since the program's enactment in 1965. The 2003 Medicare Prescription Drug, Improvement, and Modernization Act (MMA) differed from the pattern established between the 1983 Social Security reforms and the 1997 BBA. It added a hugely expensive (roughly $700 billion) drug benefit, yet with major coverage gaps for millions of people who spend moderate to high amounts on prescription drugs.[29] It injected the first elements of means-testing into Medicare, by which wealthier beneficiaries will pay more than poor beneficiaries for both their Part B (physician and outpatient) services and Part D (drug) benefits. And it pushed the program toward increased privatization with a financial overcommitment to private health plans that enroll Medicare beneficiaries. Nevertheless, it did not provide for true market competition, nor did it increase Medicare's ability to control costs. This fact helps to explain why so many Democrats and Republicans have intensely criticized the MMA.

The conclusion summarizes our analysis and discusses the major issues facing Medicare in the future. With the costs associated with ever-increasing medical innovation and the "baby boom" generation approaching retirement, policy makers will eventually have to confront the growing gap between Medicare's expected expenditures and its available revenue.[30] With the federal budget on an "unsustainable path," according to former Federal Reserve chairman Alan Greenspan, "Congress has promised more than it can continue to deliver and must quickly make major changes in how it manages its finances, especially as it prepares to shoulder the cost of new programs like the prescription drug benefit and growing demands on Social Security and Medicare."[31] Severe financial pressures are likely to force a new chapter of innovative Medicare policy making in the not-to-distant future.

This book is not a comprehensive history or survey of Medicare.[32] Many significant topics and events related to the program are not addressed. Instead, the book's goal is to analyze the origins, evolution, and long-term consequences of Medicare's transition to prospective payment. Our primary focus is on hospitals and physicians, because their payment systems have an extensive history and because they represent the bulk of Medicare spending. Our analysis relies extensively on oral history interviews, data from medical provider organizations, annual reports from government commissions and agencies, and other primary and secondary sources.

We wrote this book to accomplish two major objectives. First, we wanted to explain how and why Medicare, not the private sector, has played the largest role in shaping U.S. health care. And, second, we believe that the 2003 MMA has expedited the necessity of another major reassessment of the program's future. The MMA expanded "an entitlement that is already the fastest growing part of the federal budget," notes Eric Cohen, director of the Bioethics and American Democracy program at the Ethics and Public Policy Center. "It leaves middle-class citizens with significant drug bills to pay, and thus invites future demands to 'sweeten the benefits.' And it punts on the hardest social questions down the road—not only about the economics of Medicare, but about the intersection of modern medicine, an aging society, and the character of American society as a whole. These deeper questions are what lie at the core of the Medicare 'crisis.'"[33] Thus, we want this book to influence both current and future political debates over Medicare's programmatic and financial future.

One of our more ironic findings is that Medicare payment policy has become more political and technically complicated since the advent of prospective payment rather than less, as its designers and advocates intended.[34] The increased use of Medicare as a deficit-reduction device by several administrations and Congresses explains much of this critical development. The key, according to Lisa Potetz—a senior Medicare specialist on ProPAC and the House Ways and Means and Senate Finance Committees between 1984 and 1995—is that the PPS offered a means for achieving enormous budgetary savings that Congress could, and did, use for a variety of other purposes and programs.[35]

What adds another wrinkle of complexity to Medicare payment policy is that not all medical providers are the same. Teaching and rural hospitals, for example, have fundamentally different cost structures than for-profit suburban hospitals. Physicians who perform specialized surgeries have practices that, in terms of resource utilization, training, and even the nature of their professional activities are dramatically different from physicians who practice family or general medicine.

Thus, as payment policy becomes increasingly subordinated to fiscal policy, Congress has tried to ensure that the "rough justice" of Medicare's PPS remains as financially fair as possible for America's medical providers. But the criteria for fairness have always been open to competing definitions. Consequently, much of the increased politicization of Medicare payment policy stems from the inevitable conflict over what constitutes fairness when paying medical providers. Should all hospitals be able to cover all of their costs every year? How much more should Medicare pay specialist physicians than general practitioners? How much more should Medicare pay teaching hospitals—as compared to regular community hospitals—for the same care, given teaching hospitals' unique mission and cost structures? These are inherently, if not primarily, political questions. And they are only going to become more intense as actuarial and fiscal trends continue along their worrisome trajectories.[36] The aging of the population, together with the seemingly inexorable annual increases in medical inflation and health care spending, will create fiscal problems requiring immense political remedies.[37] In sum, the same kind of financial pressures that led to the development and adoption of prospective payment will force future policy makers to seek a broader set of innovative reforms.

CHAPTER ONE

Origins and Policy Gestation

For growing numbers of Americans, the cost of care is becoming
prohibitive . . . Costs have skyrocketed but values have not kept pace.
We are investing more of our nation's resources in the health of our
people, but we are not getting a full return on our investment.

—*President Richard Nixon, 1971*

In the 1970s there was a cost crisis in health care, a rapid escalation of
costs. But there was no political stomach yet for a regulatory strategy
of any kind for Medicare. There was still much more pressure to spend
than not to spend. That was the whole culture surrounding Medicare
at the time.

—*Judith Feder, Dean, Georgetown Public Policy Institute*

The 1970s marked a period of enormous change within the U.S. health care system. Rapidly increasing medical inflation forced those who paid for patients' care—employers and the government—to begin pursuing limits on cost increases. They had no choice: Medicare's expenditures were doubling at the unsustainable rate of every five years, and employers' health insurance premiums were increasing by more than 15–20 percent a year.[1] "In a short time, American medicine seemed to pass from stubborn shortages to irresponsible excess," as medical historian and sociologist Paul Starr has noted. "Rising costs brought medical care under more critical scrutiny, and the federal government, as a major buyer of health services, intervened in unprecedented ways."[2]

The assault by policy makers on the medical profession's authority took different forms and involved shifting tactics over the course of the decade. It began with crude wage and price controls imposed by President Nixon in 1972, and included seminal changes enacted by Congress to Social Security and Medicare that placed the first ever limits on what hospitals could charge for Medicare patients' routine or "hotel" costs (room and board). Meanwhile, innovative researchers at Yale and the University of Michigan pioneered new systems for measuring and categorizing what hospitals actually did to patients and how much it cost hospitals. For the first time, policy makers could compare prices across different hospitals for the same services. And when they did, they found significant and inexplicable variation, which contributed to a stunning loss of confidence in the ability of doctors and hospitals to regulate their own affairs. The situation became so severe in some areas of the country that several states received permission from the federal government to act as "policy laboratories" by implementing their own payment reforms.

Toward the end of the decade, unrelenting medical inflation forced President Jimmy Carter to subordinate his national health insurance priority to an ambitious plan for containing hospital costs. The goal that had guided policy makers for years, expanding medical care and insurance coverage, became eclipsed by (and then contingent on) the urgent need to control health care costs.

The Pinnacle of Providers' Power

When the decade began, doctors ruled the U.S. health care system. Their efforts at accumulating economic, professional, and political power, dating back to at least the 1920s, had met with extraordinary success. Even the first political "defeat" that the American Medical Association (AMA) suffered—the passage of Medicare and Medicaid in 1965—turned out to be to doctors' (and hospitals') enormous financial benefit. With doctors in control of medicine in the United States, those who paid the bills they charged had little to no means of questioning the necessity of the care patients received. The not-for-profit Blue Cross (hospital) and Blue Shield (physician) systems, along with commercial insurers, essentially served as efficient payment operations. Originally developed in the 1940s, with the cooperation of several state hospital and medical associations, they made the practice of medicine significantly more lucrative for doctors and hospitals.

The federal government had become deeply involved in expanding the country's patchwork system of health care.[3] It built up the *supply* of hospitals and doctors through increased funding of medical research and federal subsidies for hospital construction. It also greatly expanded the *demand* for, and access to, medical providers' services through Medicare and Medicaid. Medicare, in particular, strengthened hospitals' and doctors' power by paying the former on a "cost +" and the latter on a "customary, prevailing, and reasonable" basis.[4] (Blue Shield had originally developed and referred to this payment method as "usual, customary, and reasonable."[5]) Thus, Medicare adopted the same third-party, fee-for-service reimbursement model developed by Blue Cross/

Blue Shield, and then incorporated them as "primary intermediaries" to perform the bulk of Medicare's day-to-day work of receiving bills from doctors and hospitals and making payments to them. [6] Consequently, professional power was cemented through a reimbursement system that neither imposed limits nor required outside approval. Instead, the system "insulated the doctor-patient relationship from lay interference, and preserved the physician's right to untrammeled use of his own and the hospital's resources to resolve the patient's medical problem," explains Jeff Goldsmith.[7]

Policy makers did try to influence or improve physician practice patterns with modest regulatory initiatives, but their influence was minimal at most. Professional standards review organizations (PSROs)—established by the federal government in the early 1970s to monitor patients' quality of care—became dominated by physicians and lacked any power or authority to fundamentally change health care delivery to improve quality. The 1974 National Health Planning and Resources Development Act contained a provision for states to impose certificate of need (CON) laws that required health care providers to obtain state approval to make substantial capital investments in new equipment or hospital facilities.[8] Subsequent studies found that the manner in which the CON laws were implemented led to their general ineffectiveness.[9] The legislation also established 205 small agencies across the country equipped with the authority to say no to hospitals' requests for expansion. But they lacked the tools to make hospitals restrain their costs and become more efficient.[10]

With medical providers in control of the health care system, unrestricted cost reimbursement became the modus operandi for financing American medical care. Not surprisingly, health care spending skyrocketed. When hospitals increased their costs, they received more revenue and could expand their operations. If they lowered their costs, they received less revenue and ran the risk of falling behind their competitors. Thus, there was no incentive whatsoever to lower costs.[11] William Hsiao, who later spearheaded the development of Medicare's fee schedule for physicians in the 1980s, began his career in 1969 by examining hospitals for the Social Security Administration (SSA). He remembers the hospital industry's opposition to even adopting standard accounting procedures:

> The first question I asked was: "Why do we pay hospitals 2 percent extra on top of their costs?" The answer was that they had bad debts, that hospitals had to grow, and so on and so forth. So I then asked: "Alright, how do the hospitals calculate their costs?" And we discovered that there was no uniform accounting system or anything close to it . . . So I was deputized by the SSA to meet with the AHA's [American Hospital Association's] leaders in Chicago and raise these issues with them . . . This eventually led me to Blue Cross, because the govern-

ment paid the hospitals based on what Blue Cross was paying on a cost-basis to the hospitals. I came to realize that the AHA really did not know that much and that the rules were set by Blue Cross. Although I and others pushed, we could not make the hospitals adopt uniform accounting systems.[12]

With little to no constraints, hospital costs soared. The financial temptations to expand resources became literally irresistible. In retrospect, "cost reimbursement was just stupid," admits Michael Bromberg, former executive director of the Federation of American Hospitals (FAH), which represents the nation's for-profit, investor-owned hospitals. "I mean, it was just stupid. The Pentagon learned this lesson; you don't give people their costs, because you just give them an incentive to spend more,"[13] which is what hospitals did. One result was that Medicare's financial health became a subject of intense debate among leading policy makers.

Medicare's Cost Problems

The politics of Medicare policy have often been waged under the auspices of "crisis-oriented" concerns over the solvency of the program's trust funds.[14] When Congress passed Medicare in 1965, the public health insurance program was comprised of two parts with separate financing arrangements. Part A, the Hospital Insurance (HI) trust fund, pays for beneficiaries' hospital costs. It is currently financed from a 2.9 percent payroll tax. Part B, the Supplementary Medical Insurance (SMI) trust fund, pays for beneficiaries' physician and outpatient expenses. It is financed by general tax revenues and monthly premiums paid by beneficiaries. Because Part A is financed by a payroll tax, it can conceivably approach insolvency by paying out more in expenditures than it receives in tax revenue. Part B, however, is immune to such threats, for all intents and purposes, because its partial funding from general tax revenues operates as an "open pipeline" to the federal Treasury.

Scholars disagree over whether policy makers, particularly the influential House Ways and Means Committee chairman Wilbur Mills, designed Medicare to be insulated from regular political debate or, rather, to encourage it. Theodore Marmor and Jonathan Oberlander argue that the "bankruptcy crises" that have repeatedly erupted over Medicare are a perverse outcome, unintended by those who designed the program to be a vehicle for smoothly and effectively achieving national health insurance via incremental steps.[15] Conversely, Eric Patashnik and Julian Zelizer see a certain institutional logic to Medicare's design that, they argue, has "served a valuable social purpose by periodically forcing policy makers to engage in a healthy examination of one of the nation's largest and most expensive social programs."[16]

Either way, Medicare spending has increased dramatically over the decades. Policy makers knew when it was implemented that Medicare lacked adequate cost controls. Wilbur Cohen, undersecretary of the Department of Health, Education, and Welfare at the time, has admitted as much: "'The sponsors of Medicare, including myself, had to concede in 1965 that there would be no real controls over hospitals and physicians. I was required to promise before the final vote in the Executive Session of the House Ways and Means Committee that the Federal agency would exercise no control.'"[17] Lacking sufficient cost-control mechanisms, Medicare's expenditures quickly became a major political problem.[18] President Lyndon Johnson fumed in 1967 that Wilbur Mills was "all over the ticker" in his attempt to explain Medicare's increased costs.[19] In 1974, Mills maintained that Medicare's costs had increased far beyond the original estimates, largely because no provisions for cost containment existed.[20] Testimony by Mills before Congress in 1980, four years after he left Congress, reveals that Medicare's rapid cost escalation surprised him: "You know, when you author a program, you expect it to be perfect. I thought Medicare was. I thought it would take care of the costs of the medical problems that older citizens would encounter. We never envisioned anything such as we are hearing today of the . . . total costs that are being paid by this program."[21]

The manner in which Congress inaugurated the program partly explains why Medicare's expenditures exploded so quickly.[22] Basically, it immediately "blanketed in" nineteen million beneficiaries on July 1, 1966, without any of them ever having paid into the program. Medicare's financing structure precluded it from experiencing a grace period in which its trust funds could build up some measure of reserves from annual surpluses.[23] Instead, Medicare began operation as a genuine "pay-as-you-go" system, in which payroll tax revenues from workers went (and continue to go) directly to providing Part A hospital benefits for retirees.[24] Retirees' monthly contributions helped finance Part B, but over time they covered less and less of the program's costs.[25]

Medicare's cost control problems were also the result of what Marmor and Starr have both referred to as the program's "politics of accommodation."[26] In attempting to gain the cooperation of doctors and hospitals, the Social Security Administration's approach to running Medicare demonstrated three accommodating characteristics: (1) a commitment to remaining primarily a distributor of popular entitlement benefits, (2) a desire to avoid controversy and have operations run smoothly, and (3) an effort to secure exclusive administration of Medicare.[27] The SSA's strategy was eminently successful in getting Medicare up and running, notes Judith Feder, "but in the process, maintaining the compromises through which the goal was achieved became an end in itself."[28]

One result of the SSA's desire to have the medical community embrace Medicare was that doctors' "customary, prevailing, and reasonable" fees—the criteria by which the program based its reimbursement—rose precipitously. Newly established doctors, who had no charge profiles yet, naturally began billing at unprecedented levels, and the SSA paid them. When older doctors saw the behavior of their younger associates, they too raised their fees.[29]

While doctors' demands became a major cause of Medicare's profligacy, increased physician costs paled in comparison to those of hospitals (see table 1.1).[30] "Medicare gave hospitals a license to spend," according to Rosemary Stevens. "The more expenditures they incurred, the more income they received. Medicare tax funds flowed into hospitals in a golden stream, more than doubling between 1970 and 1975, and doubling again by 1980."[31] Medicare's formula for hospital reimbursement invited abuse, because it operated on a "cost + 2 percent basis" for all services. Since the 2 percent was a percentage of costs (and was added by Congress to reflect, among other things, the added nursing costs for Medicare patients),[32] it offered hospitals a small bonus for each and every cost increase. While the Consumer Price Index increased 89 percent between 1966 and 1976, hospital costs grew a staggering 345 percent.[33]

In effect, medical providers took advantage of the unique economic dynamics surrounding medical care: Although the occurrence of illness usually exists beyond one's control, the demand for care constitutes essentially a discretionary decision. Insurance against the financial costs of health services, such as Medicare, allows the consumption of those services to vastly increase.[34] Moreover, as Nobel laureate Kenneth Arrow famously argued in December 1963 in the *American Economic Review*, patients are uniquely dependent on physicians to make informed decisions on their behalf, due to patients' lack of medical knowledge and the inherent uncertainty underlying much medical decision making.[35] Therefore, if physicians decided that some form of medical care was needed, it was promptly provided and paid for without question by third-party insurers.[36]

Because Medicare lacked sufficient financial restraint, cost estimates soon fell glaringly short of initial predictions.[37] When Congress passed Medicare in 1965, the House Ways and Means Committee projected annual expenditures of $238 million. Assuming that 95 percent of elderly people might enroll in Part B (this prediction proved accurate), the committee estimated that, at most, total Medicare expenditures would be $1.3 billion in 1967, the first full year of operation.[38] The figure, instead, came in at $4.6 billion. The committee also predicted hospital spending to be $3.1 billion for 1970 and $4.2 billion for 1975, with money left over in the hospital trust fund. Actual expenditures were $7.1 billion and $15.6 billion, respectively.[39] Medicare spending was doubling every five years (see table 1.1). Consequently, as Oberlander explains, Medicare "quickly acquired a reputation, as chairman of the Senate Finance Committee Russell Long put it, as a 'runaway program.'"[40]

TABLE 1.1
Medicare Expenditures in Billions, Parts A and B, 1967–80

Year	Total Costs	Part A (Hospital)	Increase	Part B (Physician)	Increase
1967	$4.6	$3.4	—	$1.2	—
1970	7.1	5.1	50%	2.0	67%
1975	15.6	11.3	123	4.3	115
1980	35.7	25.1	122	10.6	147

SOURCE: Medicare Board of Trustees, Federal Hospital Insurance Trust Fund, 1996.

The 1972 Social Security Amendments

As more and more policy makers became concerned about Medicare's finances, they began looking for ways to control the program's costs. The process began with an admission by some leading government officials, who had championed the program and pushed for its passage, that Medicare's design was inherently inflationary. At the end of his service as Social Security Administrator in 1972, Robert Ball stated that Medicare had "simply accepted the going system of the delivery of care" by modeling its reimbursement patterns on Blue Cross plans for hospitals and private insurance policies for doctors. Seven years after Medicare's passage, he argued, attitudes had changed significantly. The public was beginning to favor reforms in the basic system of health care financing and looked to Medicare "to help provide the leverage to bring about change." According to Ball, "the program no longer received criticism for interfering too much in the health care system but rather for interfering too little."[41]

Policy makers' first effort at restraining medical inflation came as part of a larger campaign to combat inflation. In late 1971, the Nixon administration introduced its Economic Stabilization Program (ESP). The ESP was a broad-based system of wage and price controls, which was absolutely anathema to Republican free market principles and made Nixon the target of widespread conservative criticism.[42] The ESP was designed to deal with inflation that policy makers believed came from rapid increases in wages and other input costs. There was special concern for the health care sector (especially hospitals), in which prices and expenditures were rising much faster than those in the economy overall.[43] Nixon's ESP helped to dampen the annual growth in hospital cost inflation to approximately 6 percent until May 1974, when the program expired. Afterward, hospital cost inflation jumped back up to 15 percent per year.[44]

Another effort by policy makers to control Medicare's cost growth culminated in Section 223 of the 1972 Social Security Amendments. Stuart Altman, one of the Nixon administration's chief health care policy advisors, explains the legislation's background and intent:

Now that's a fascinating piece of legislation, because it's a combination of half cost controls and half expanded spending. It included new Medicare coverage for "end stage renal" patients, the disabled, nursing homes, and so on. But it also included Section 223, which said that even though Medicare is obligated to pay for whatever a hospital's costs are in treating Medicare beneficiaries, there are certain costs that can be deemed "unreasonable." There was a lot of controversy over what was "unreasonable." But ultimately what they implemented were limits that differentiated two kinds of hospital costs: (a) routine and (b) ancillary. The argument was that if a cost was ancillary and if it was related to how sick the patients were or if it was new technology, then Medicare should and would pay for it. But if the cost was routine, then there should be limits to it.[45]

In short, Section 223 attempted to define what allowable costs were and then constrain the variability in these costs across hospitals.[46] Or as James Mongan, a staff member of the Senate Finance Committee at the time, puts it: "We understood that people might be sicker and have different ancillary costs, but by God the routine or 'hotel' costs ought to bear some similarity to all other hospitals."[47] The limits began operation in 1975, soon after Nixon's ESP ended. Over time, they had a modest effect in restraining hospital cost inflation.

As occurs with virtually all inflexible payment formulas, though, hospital administrators eventually learned how to maximize reimbursement. "Now if you look over the course of the 1970s, the hospitals kept modifying the definitions and extending the line beyond which costs were considered 'unreasonable'. In other words, the hospitals kept redefining what was 'routine' and what was 'ancillary'," explains Altman. "For example, they would take nurses and change them into 'respiratory nurses', which made them a fully reimbursed ancillary cost. In other words, what were previously considered routine costs became ancillary by category and fully reimbursed."[48]

In addition to setting the first limits on what Medicare would pay hospitals, the 1972 Social Security Amendments also authorized the government to begin experiments with alternative forms of hospital reimbursement (Section 222).[49] Responsibility for implementing the demonstration projects was split between the SSA's Bureau of Health Insurance, headed by Tom Tierney, and the Office of Research and Statistics, headed by Clif Gaus. Both men reported to Arthur Hess, deputy administrator of the SSA.

Fortunately for the SSA, it did not have to construct its own experiments in new forms of hospital payment from scratch. After the 1972 Social Security Amendments passed with Section 222 included, several states approached the SSA with requests to conduct payment experiments. Maryland was the first state to seek a waiver from the

SSA in order to set its own Medicare payment rates. As part of an "all-payer" system, Medicare, Medicaid, and private insurers would all pay the same rates for the same hospitals' services and would cover hospitals' uncompensated costs ("charity care"). One purpose of the "all-payer" model was to make sure no patients became viewed as "second class" due to their status as lower payers.

The states that chose to experiment with their own plans had little to lose financially. Under the terms of the demonstration projects, the federal government agreed to absorb any losses a state might incur if the experiments failed and their actual costs proved to be higher than they would have been under the standard cost reimbursement model.[50] The states' hospitals, however, could be harmed financially if the new systems did not work. Hence, elected state leaders faced the possibility of a politically disastrous situation if the experiments went awry.

A major disagreement erupted within the SSA over whether or not to grant states the waivers they wanted to determine their own Medicare hospital rates. Many within the Bureau of Health Insurance, in particular, were concerned that this could lead to runaway costs and loss of control over Medicare as a national program. They also feared that the states might try to make Medicare overpay in order to subsidize other payers, particularly Medicaid. Ultimately, Arthur Hess unilaterally decided to allow the states to experiment with alternative forms of hospital payment. Over the vehement opposition of Tom Tierney and many others within the SSA, he became convinced of the need for a transformation of Medicare from the traditional cost-based reimbursement system. "This may not be the way the nation goes," he told Gaus, "But we're going to learn a hell of a lot."[51]

In the long run, political scientist Robert Hackey has observed, Section 222 had a tremendous impact on health care regulation and reimbursement politics. It encouraged the proliferation of state rate-setting experiments that redefined the relationship between payers, providers, and government regulatory agencies. In addition to strengthening the power of state health care bureaucracies, the demonstration projects funded under Section 222 provided federal officials with unique opportunities for extensive policy learning at the state level that would otherwise have been impossible.[52]

Conceptual Innovation at the University of Michigan and Yale University

The same year that the SSA gave the approval for state Medicare waivers saw the first scholarly article on the topic of what became known as *prospective payment*. In September 1974, *Inquiry* published William Dowling's article "Prospective Payment of

Hospitals." It was the first conceptual description of the significant transformation and shifting of financial risk that Medicare would initiate a decade later. According to Dowling, a professor at the University of Michigan at the time:

> Prospective reimbursement—or more accurately, prospective budget- or rate-setting and reimbursement—is a method of paying hospitals in which 1) amounts or rates of payment are established in advance for the coming year; and 2) hospitals are paid these amounts or rates regardless of the costs they actually incur . . .
>
> Prospective rate setting differs from retrospective cost reimbursement in that payment rates are specified in advance rather than determined after the fact and are not based on costs actually incurred during the prospective year . . . Prospective payment systems are designed to introduce market-place-like financial incentives into the provider sector. Providers face firm fixed prices for their services. If they are able to keep their costs below these prices, they will make a surplus; if not, they will suffer a loss. Thus providers are definitely at risk.[53]

The concept of prospective payment was predicated on the controversial and untested theory that the cost of medical care could be predictable and responsive to changing economic incentives. Yet how would the prospective rates be determined, especially if each patient's medical cost varied significantly across and even within hospitals, due to factors such as a patient's age, gender, or the severity of his or her condition? In other words, how predictable could the costs of medical care truly be? Nobody knew for sure.

In order for a system for paying hospitals predetermined rates to be established, patients would first have to be separated into unique "product" categories based on diagnoses or procedures (i.e., pneumonia, hip replacement, congestive heart failure, etc.). Performing the necessary research for establishing product categories and payment rates would require the cooperation of hospitals, which was hard to come by. Moreover, hospital recordkeeping in the 1970s was generally sloppy at best, and occasionally nonexistent. Even if researchers had readily available and comparable hospital data, how would they run their analyses? At the time there were no statistical software systems for analyzing complex medical records. Personal computers did not yet exist. And performing massive statistical analyses was a labor-intensive, arduous activity involving enormous and enormously expensive mainframe computers that only a select number of major institutions could afford.

Serendipitously, as is so often the case in research, the solutions to these formidable obstacles came by way of researchers trying to solve other problems and answer different questions. In the early 1970s, a research team at Yale University headed by

John Thompson—a former nurse who once worked the night shift on Bellevue Hospital's prison ward and a professor of public health and hospital administration—was trying to find out why the costs of maternity, newborn, and nonmaternity medical care among Connecticut's thirty-five hospitals varied by as much as 100 percent.[54] (In other words, care cost twice as much at some hospitals as it did at others.) This striking variation in costs had no obvious explanations, Thompson observed, because "Connecticut is not like other states. There is essentially one labor market [with] people going from town to town. Moreover, all hospitals in Connecticut were accredited, and there were no for-profit hospitals."[55] In other words, all hospitals in Connecticut were public and had roughly the same labor costs. So, as Thompson asked, "What was going on in the most expensive hospitals and in the cheapest hospitals?"[56]

At the time, Yale was uniquely positioned to generate the kind of conceptual innovation necessary for developing prospective payment. It had some of the brightest researchers and small departments that provided for far more interdisciplinary collaboration than is usually the case at most major research universities. According to Richard Averill, who became the lead project manager for Thompson's research team:

> It all began when Thompson said that studying the significant variation in hospital costs "sounds like an industrial control problem. But I don't necessarily know all that much about industrial control, so I'll find out whoever the guru is at the School of Administrative Sciences in this area." So he went over and spoke with Bob Fetter—a professor at the School of Organization and Management—and he said, "Well, tell me what your products are." And John said something like, "We treat patients." And Bob would say something like, "and Ford makes cars, but there's a big difference between," in those days, "a Pinto and a Lincoln."
>
> And so this started the genesis of essentially saying, "In order to do any analysis of real statistical quality with controls, you need a product definition in a hospital." But then you kind of start working backwards and say, "Okay, in order to come up with a product definition, we first need some data."[57]

In order to categorize all of the different products that hospitals produced and how much it cost them to produce each one, Thompson and Fetter needed a significant amount of hospital data. Fortunately, the thirty-five hospitals in Connecticut had by law reported audited costs to the state legislature since 1948, using a uniform chart of accounts. From 1960 on, the Connecticut Hospital Association (CHA) had collected the standardized financial information, broken down between maternity, newborn, and nonmaternity patients, from all thirty-five hospitals.[58] In addition, recalls Thompson, "We had the Connecticut Hospital Association and Connecticut Blue

Cross who were very close to our program and who gave us a lot of data."[59] Given the unprecedented amount of claims data from multiple Connecticut hospitals, Thompson and Fetter could perform the first major analysis of substantial variation in costs between hospitals.

With the assistance of their colleagues, Fetter and Averill created an interactive computer program designed to facilitate the rapid analysis of complex medical information.[60] "You could sit doctors down and say, 'Now here's a diagnosis. What factors do you think are going to affect the use of resources treating this diagnosis? Is it age? Is it certain complications? Is it the patient's sex? What is it?'" explains Thompson. "We could sit there and test it on this interactive program, which was called AUTOGRP."[61]

Thompson and Fetter's goal was to group all patients into a limited number of distinct and medically meaningful diagnostic categories (DRGs), and then measure each individual patient's consumption of hospital resources. Ironically, the primary purpose of prospective payment with DRGs was not cost control, which is what it became later at the state (New Jersey) and federal level. Rather, the researchers envisioned their work serving as a basis for quality assessment to improve care for patients and for the better use of limited and expensive medical resources. Thompson and Fetter were surprised at the hospital community's total lack of interest in their findings:

> There we were with what we thought was a major management breakthrough. In other words, hospital administrators could now begin to see how much it was costing them to produce these "products" [DRGs] and whether the medical staff was treating these patients differently, keeping some patients in too long, ordering too many x-rays or too much lab work . . . This was the first time anybody in hospital management could do this . . . We went all over the United States to preach the gospel of hospital product lines, and it was absolutely amazing how little attention anybody paid to this idea.[62]

Thompson and Fetter had demonstrated for the first time that hospitals could separate their patients into distinct categories, based on diagnosis, and then measure how much each category cost the hospital financially. Hospital administrators were slow to realize the extent to which Thompson and Fetter's innovation could transform American medicine, but a handful of progressive health officials were ready for a revolution.

New Jersey as a "Policy Laboratory" for Experimentation

Following their "discovery" of prospective payment, as Thompson later described it, he and Fetter grew increasingly eager to test their new system of hospital reimbursement. "Then one of those serendipitous things happened," according to Thompson. "The health officer of New Haven was a young physician by the name of Joanne Finley, and she was called down to New Jersey by a candidate for governor by the name of Brendan Byrne who said that hospitals had become a big issue in his campaign . . . She knew all about DRGs, because, as health officer in New Haven, she was on the Yale faculty and had come to the various research symposiums on the new system. She said yes and Byrne was elected."[63]

New Jersey's state government had technically been responsible as far back as the late 1930s for regulating the health insurance premiums charged by the state's Blue Cross organization (they must be "reasonable"), as well as the payments made from Blue Cross to hospitals (neither "excessive" nor "inadequate").[64] Ostensibly, the state's commissioner of insurance was the final arbiter of what Blue Cross premiums and payments should be. In reality, though, the New Jersey Hospital Association reviewed itself and then received the public stamp of state approval on its decisions.[65] This left Blue Cross "caught between the political pressures that limited its premiums, and a rate review system that failed to limit its payments to hospitals," note political scientists James Morone and Andrew Dunham. "By 1969, Blue Cross was reporting a $13 million deficit."[66]

In response to the hospital industry's demands for protection against the incursion of new, aggressive for-profit hospital chains (such as Humana) and the anguished pleas of Blue Cross to limit the steady annual increases in hospital payment rates, New Jersey passed the Health Care Facilities and Planning Act (HCFPA) in May 1971.[67] The legislation heralded great change. The act gave the New Jersey Department of Health increased regulatory power to review hospital payments and to increase the roadblocks facing for-profit hospital chains through more demanding "certificate of need" requirements.[68] In actuality, little changed in terms of hospital rate setting. Nevertheless, the insular world of the New Jersey hospitals had been quietly penetrated by the state and, in the process, the seeds of enormous change had been planted.[69]

In February 1974, one month after the newly elected Governor Brendan Byrne was inaugurated, the Center for the Analysis of Public Issues—a public interest group inspired by Ralph Nader—published an exposé report entitled *Bureaucratic Malpractice*.[70] It strongly criticized the state's Department of Health for failing to implement HCFPA appropriately. The report charged that the hospital industry was essentially regulating itself and that cost control was not likely to result from a system based on asking hospitals how much they wanted to spend next year.[71] *Bureaucratic Malpractice* was that rare research report that actually found a ready audience. The country had just been through Watergate. Reforming the political system and eliminating corruption were enormously popular campaign pledges. And health care costs were a growing concern just as a new system was in place that allowed the state to take significant authority over skyrocketing hospital budgets.[72]

Joanne Finley and her Department of Health set about transforming the traditional relationships between hospitals and payers. They moved to a new rate review model known as the Standard Hospital Accounting and Rate Evaluation (SHARE) system.[73] SHARE was designed to have all hospitals report their expenditures in a standardized way to allow for meaningful comparisons between hospitals. The essential feature of the SHARE system was "peer grouping" hospitals within different categories (e.g., small, large, urban, suburban). The unit of payment to hospitals under the new system was a per diem (a flat payment per day) and the basis of payment was the hospital's costs.[74] If any hospital's proposed budget for the following year exceeded the median increase of its peers, it had to negotiate for an exception.[75] Moreover, the state established a target percentage increase in per-diem payment rates for each year. In the system's first year, 1975, the target rate was 2 percent, which was laughable given the state's 11 percent overall rate of economic inflation. The state quickly had to compromise on a 9 percent annual increase.[76]

SHARE was an initial but modest attempt to both rationalize hospital payments and challenge the hospital industry's power in New Jersey.[77] The program only regulated Blue Cross and Medicaid payment rates (roughly 40 percent of total hospital payments), which led hospitals to shift more of their costs to their unregulated payers, mostly commercial insurers. Within five years, payments from commercial insurers were 30 percent higher than payments from Blue Cross for the same services.[78] Many urban hospitals, which served a disproportionate share of Medicaid and uninsured patients, were experiencing serious budget deficits under the new SHARE system. Due to their location, they did not have enough commercially insured patients to whom they could shift their costs. Eighteen of the state's hospitals were pushed to the verge of financial collapse.[79]

Dissatisfied with a system that regulated hospitals on a per-diem rate and only for Medicaid and Blue Cross payers, Finley and her colleagues in the Department of Health entered into negotiations with the New Jersey Hospital Association and Blue Cross for the purposes of moving to a new system.[80] They wanted a statewide prospective payment system. In order to regulate prices for *all* payers in the state—which constituted far more governmental control over the hospital industry than had ever existed—Finley and her colleagues found an ingenious way to neutralize the hospital industry's otherwise unified and formidable political power.[81] They proposed that the state's new regulatory system for all payers should set hospital payment rates in such a way as to cover hospitals' uncompensated charity care (or bad debt). Because both would benefit financially, the state's inner-city hospitals—often headed by charismatic and articulate nuns—became aligned with the state's commercial insurers in favor of the state's new proposal.[82] Finley was reported to have told Jack Owen, president of the New Jersey Hospital Association, "If you don't come along on this plan, I'll split your damned association."[83]

This clever mixture of crosscutting politics enabled Finley and her allies to push their reform legislation (S 446) into an advantageous political position. Urban hospitals desired financial assistance for providing care to their disproportionately poor patients; commercial insurers wanted relief from increased cost shifting imposed on them by all hospitals; state legislators desired an increased measure of cost control to address Medicaid's cost escalation; and the federal government wanted states to experiment with different forms of hospital reimbursement in order to develop a national model of reform for Medicare. As a result, S 446 passed easily in 1978.[84] The legislation outlined a timetable for a new, prospective system of reimbursement to begin in early 1980.

It is ironic that the new legislation never specifically mentioned DRGs, because they were the basis for the original waiver that New Jersey had received in 1976 to experiment with prospective payment.[85] The hospital industry in New Jersey complained to the legislature that policy makers were exceeding their authority. But the legislation had already been passed. The industry's complaints were to no avail. Moreover, during this period hospitals were consumed with a bigger battle at the federal level against President Jimmy Carter and his bold new plan for controlling hospital costs.

President Carter and Hospital Cost-Containment Battles

The late 1970s were marked by a continuing national preoccupation with inflation, particularly in the area of health care. In 1977, Medicare and Medicaid expenditures were double what they had been only three years earlier.[86] From 1974 to 1977, hospital costs increased at an annual rate of approximately 15 percent, more than double the economy's overall rate of inflation.[87] It is interesting to note that ostensibly unsustainable health care cost inflation is a frequently reoccurring phenomenon in the United States. In the late 1970s, public opinion polls showed that health care costs were among Americans' top three domestic policy concerns.[88] Consequently, hospital cost containment emerged as the leading health policy initiative for President Carter and his administration, particularly for secretary of health, education, and welfare Joseph Califano. With medical inflation growing rapidly, Carter's campaign pledge of achieving national health insurance became linked to the goal of first trying to control hospital costs.

Carter's initial proposal in April 1977 marked the first major attempt by the federal government to aggressively regulate the hospital industry. The president actively campaigned for his proposal, arguing that its passage would "slow a devastating inflation trend, which doubles health costs every five years."[89] Carter's plan entailed a formula that set a 9 percent cap on the annual growth in hospital expenditures (consistent with the underlying rate of inflation); it also imposed strict limits on the construction of new health care facilities.[90] The plan would have placed limits on all hospital payment rates, public and private. Urban Democrats generally favored the president's plan, but Sun Belt and southern Democrats from areas with growing populations were less enthusiastic. Many of them thought that Carter's plan would restrain the growth of hospital revenues in an inequitable manner that would lock southern hospitals into an inferior quality level relative to their northern counterparts (the "fat will get fatter" critics charged).[91] Califano claimed that hospitals had abused the cost reimbursement model for too long. Rather than being "institutions of last resort," he argued, hospitals had become "settings of first choice for treating too many minor ailments, especially when the insurance coverage was good."[92]

Carter's proposal galvanized the hospital industry. "Califano helped us achieve unanimity when he talked about hospitals making obscene profits," says Alex McMahon, president of the AHA at the time. "Nothing drives you together better than a very visible enemy, and Califano became one by his own choice."[93] The industry responded by vigorously opposing Carter's proposal and offering a voluntary effort (VE) in its place.[94]

Carter's 1977 and 1979 proposals failed in large part because congressional Democrats, notably representatives Dan Rostenkowski (chair of the House Ways and Means Health Subcommittee) and future House majority leader Richard Gephardt, favored trying the hospitals' voluntary approach first. "I've got commitments from the hospital associations that if I let them come up with a voluntary program, they will embrace cost containment," Rostenkowski recalls telling President Carter in one highly charged conversation. "And I told the hospital representatives, as I stuck my index finger in their nose, Mr. President, 'You screw me and I'll be around for a long time and you better watch out'."[95] The hospitals' VE did have a salutary effect in 1978, bringing the rate of hospital cost inflation down to 12.8 percent (these were days when general inflation was approaching double digits), but it proved to be short lived.[96]

In 1979, hospital spending increased 14.5 percent after Carter reintroduced a modified version of his original cost-containment plan.[97] This time his proposal advanced farther than his 1977 proposal had. It was voted out of committee and onto the House floor. Carter's new plan would impose controls on hospitals only if their cost increases exceeded a limit of approximately 13 percent.[98] Again, though, the hospital associations—together with the help of the American Medical Association—were able to defeat Carter's proposal.[99] Virtually all Republicans opposed Carter's plan as excessively complex and an overly intrusive violation of the private sector by the government at a time when deregulation was rapidly gaining popularity. Democrats were split. On November 15, 1979, the president's proposal was defeated in the House by a vote of 234 to 166.[100]

The onus now was squarely on the hospital industry to deliver results. Caps and price controls were rejected in favor of renewed pledges from hospital representatives that they would "clean up their act." Yet their voluntary effort failed. With the demise of Carter's proposal, hospital cost inflation jumped 17 percent in 1980 and 18 percent in 1981.[101] The hospital industry's political credibility plummeted as the failure of its second VE embarrassed even its closest political allies.[102] The VE "was tremendously successful in its first year," argues the AHA's McMahon, "partially successful the second year, and then really fell apart in about its third year when nobody paid attention" anymore.[103] Looking back on this period as one of "treading water," McMahon notes that the hospital industry "began to hear a message from the federal and state governments and, increasingly, from business, a thoroughly powerful message that said, 'Okay, if you don't like government price controls, figure out something to do.' The pressures were there, and so 'treading water' pretty soon turned into a movement toward finding a new system of incentives."[104] The stage was set for a radical transition in hospital reimbursement. Yet it did not come from the private sector. Ironically, it came from a Republican president who professed a love for the free market and inveighed against government intrusions in private commerce.

At the close of the Carter administration, hospital cost inflation was outstripping even the double-digit inflation afflicting the rest of the economy. Medicare's expenditures were increasing at an unsustainable rate that threatened the solvency of the program's trust funds. It had become clear that hospitals could not be paid under the traditional cost reimbursement model indefinitely. It was also obvious that the hospital industry could not reform itself. Because Carter's efforts at passing an "all payer" form of hospital cost control proved overly ambitious and politically unfeasible, federal policy makers gradually turned their attention to reforming the single largest purchaser of hospital care: Medicare. Financial necessity became the mother of payment innovation.

CHAPTER TWO

Development, Growing Appeal, and Passage of Prospective Payment

The CEO of one of the companies in my federation, who shall remain nameless, said to me, "The day this becomes law"—he told me this as the Medicare legislation was going through in '83—he said, "I'm selling the company the day this [prospective payment] law passes." I said, "Why?" He said, "Because you could be an idiot and make a fortune on Medicare reimbursement. Any mistake you made you got reimbursed." I suppose that was true, but on the other hand if you want to do the right thing and reward efficiency, then the law was good.

—*Michael Bromberg, Executive Director,*
Federation of American Hospitals

The traditional model of cost reimbursement was insanity. On the face of it, it encouraged people to do more; it paid them to do more and not in any particularly rational way. Going to prospective payment with DRGs, therefore, had all the right things going for it politically and conceptually . . .

—*Sheila Burke, Deputy Staff Director (1982–85),*
Senate Finance Committee

The 1980s began with a continuation and worsening of medical inflation from the previous decade. Hospital spending grew 16.4 percent, and the nation's total health care expenditures reached $230 billion in 1980, a threefold increase from $69 billion in 1970.[1] Ronald Reagan, the Republican Party's presidential nominee, won a decisive victory over the Democrat incumbent, Jimmy Carter, by, among other things, arguing for the expansion of the free market and reduced government regulation. Yet the free market was not solving the problem of medical inflation. In Reagan's first full year in office, hospital spending increased 17.5 percent.[2] The following year the country slipped into the worst recession in half a century, with the unemployment rate reaching almost 11 percent, which led to a sizeable decrease in payroll tax revenue used to finance Medicare and Social Security.

This deadly combination of inexorably rising medical inflation and deep economic deterioration forced policy makers to pursue radical reform of Medicare to keep the program from insolvency. Federal policy makers—led primarily by President Reagan's health and human services secretary, Richard Schweiker—eventually turned to the one alternative reimbursement system that analysts and academics had studied more than any other and even tested with apparent success in New Jersey: prospective payment with diagnosis-related groups. Rather than simply reimbursing hospitals whatever costs they incurred treating Medicare patients, the new model would pay hospitals a predetermined set rate based on the patient's diagnosis. The payment would be unrelated to any specific hospital's costs. Instead, it would be a national payment based on the average costs of a general hospital. Thus, if a hospital could treat a patient for less than the standard DRG payment, it could keep the savings as a profit. If it cost the hospital more, it had to absorb the difference as a financial loss. Once Republican leaders became convinced that prospective payment could be used to reduce federal budget deficits—as well as create new profit and efficiency incentives for hospitals—the political obstacles to radically transforming Medicare finally dissolved.

Ironically, the biggest change in health policy since Medicare and Medicaid's passage in 1965 went virtually unnoticed by the general public. Nevertheless, the change was significant. For the first time in U.S. history, the federal government acquired a sizeable measure of power in its financial relationship with the hospital industry. Together with Congress's development and use of the budget reconciliation process, Medicare's new prospective payment system with DRGs infringed upon the hospital industry's long-standing control over its rate of spending. The biggest problem, though, was that nobody knew for sure if and how exactly Medicare's new payment system would work.

New Political Landscape amid Mounting Fiscal Pressures

The early 1980s witnessed a unique convergence of political and economic developments that opened a window for a major reform of Medicare. The Republicans' takeover of the White House and Senate in 1981 coincided with a deep recession, as well as a growing conviction among policy makers of both political parties that

Medicare's rate of expenditure growth was unsustainable. The hospital industry had been given two opportunities to voluntarily contain its cost growth and markedly failed at both. It appeared that the forces that drove hospital inflation were beyond hospital administrators' control. Thus, by 1981, even leading representatives of the hospital industry were convinced of the political inevitability of major reform to Medicare's payment system.[3]

Paradoxically, Republican control of the White House and Senate created a more favorable political environment for a Medicare reform plan—one involving *increased* government regulation—than had previously existed. With Republicans in power, the onus fell squarely on them to find a way to avoid Medicare's approaching insolvency. Given the administration's short-term goals for reducing domestic spending, however, a free market approach to reforming Medicare was not possible, notes Jonathan Oberlander.[4] As a result, fiscal necessity overwhelmed political ideology.[5] Republicans would have to increase the government's authority over medical providers, because the federal government needed budgetary savings immediately and the hospital industry had shown it was unable to reform itself. "We basically concluded that we had to fix the hospitals because there are fewer of them, they're less political, there's a lot of money there, and we thought we could beat them up a lot easier than three to four hundred thousand doctors," recalls Allen Dobson, head of the Health Care Financing Administration's Office of Research.[6]

Reagan's choice for secretary of Health and human services, former Republican Senator from Pennsylvania Richard Schweiker, proved particularly auspicious for Medicare reform. In contrast to Carter's HHS secretary, Joseph Califano, Schweiker was a more conciliatory policy maker. He also had years of experience handling health care policy in Congress as a senior member of the Senate Finance Committee. The failure of the hospital industry's two voluntary efforts had persuaded him that the government would have to initiate payment reform.[7] In fact, restraining the escalation in health care costs became his highest legislative priority as secretary of HHS.[8] As a regular summer visitor to the New Jersey Shore, Schweiker formed close personal relationships with health care representatives and policy makers who were initiating the state's experiment in using prospective payment for hospitals.[9] He had read the two existing books on DRGs and grew convinced that prospective payment was the way to go.[10] Transitioning Medicare to a prospective payment system emerged as his primary goal, "sort of his crowning achievement as secretary of HHS," according to Julian Pettengill, a senior HCFA analyst at the time.[11]

Before Schweiker could convince leading members of Congress and other health policy leaders of the superiority of prospective payment, he first had to convince his own subordinates. The political appointees who headed HCFA, administrator Carolyne Davis and associate administrator Patrice Feinstein, did not initially share their boss's enthusiasm for prospective payment. Schweiker "was a conservative Republican," Davis notes, "but many of his political instincts were true Wilbur Cohen [a liberal Democrat]."[12] Consistent with the larger themes and guiding principles of Reagan's new administration, Davis and Feinstein favored a "procompetitive," market-based approach to reforming Medicare that emphasized health maintenance organizations and moving beneficiaries into various forms of private insurance.[13] "They really didn't like this idea of prospective payment; they decided it was terribly regulatory," recalls Pettengill.[14] Nevertheless, Schweiker's insistence that a prospective payment proposal be ready for legislative consideration in 1982, together with a lack of alternative proposals that were thoroughly researched and tested, forced Davis and her colleagues to change their minds.

Political and economic events in the early 1980s made Medicare reform seem increasingly necessary. The Republicans' takeover of the Senate in 1981 coincided with the highest recorded rates of hospital cost inflation. Bob Dole became chair of the powerful Senate Finance Committee, which along with the House Ways and Means Committee controlled Medicare policy. Recognized at the time as the most important figure on Capitol Hill for health-financing legislation,[15] Dole saw the failure of the hospital industry's voluntary efforts as evidence of the need for radical reform to safeguard Medicare's financial solvency.[16]

Dole's chief of staff, Sheila Burke, became the key staff member on the Senate side in leading the effort for Medicare payment reform. A former nurse, she viewed the traditional model of cost reimbursement as "insanity. On the face of it, it encouraged people to do more; it *paid* them to do more and not in any particularly rational way," she explains. "Going to DRGs, therefore, had all the right things going for it politically and conceptually . . . In effect, you could say to the average member of Congress—who tended to not want to get into the minutiae of Medicare policy because it was one of the more boring aspects of their lives—'Why should it [a specific hospital service or procedure] cost anything different between L.A. and San Francisco, or San Francisco and Chicago, or Chicago and Detroit?'"[17]

Dan Rostenkowski, who became chair of the House Ways and Means Committee in 1981, similarly concluded that the private sector was incapable of reforming itself. Paul Rettig, who worked for Rostenkowski, observed that most members of the Ways and Means Committee shared Rostenkowski's opinion that cost reimbursement had to be gotten rid of as soon as possible.[18] The key to a prospective payment model according to select members of Congress, Rettig added, was that it could fundamentally change the decision-making habits of doctors and hospitals.[19] Previous efforts had failed to do this, but it was necessary if Medicare's rate of expenditure growth was ever to be brought under control. Conveniently, federal policy makers could turn to some of their colleagues at the state level, especially in New Jersey, to learn from their experiments with different forms of prospective payment.

New Jersey's Experiment with DRGs

When President Carter's proposals for hospital cost containment failed to pass in Congress, a number of state initiatives began operation. New Jersey's plan seemed particularly promising.[20] The state's new prospective payment system sought to significantly transform the financial incentives for hospital administrators. Again, with traditional cost reimbursement, the more a hospital did for a patient, the more money it received in payments. Under New Jersey's DRGs, policy makers established a standard price in advance for each and every case that a patient could present. If a hospital could treat the patient for less than the standard DRG payment, it could keep the difference as a profit. If the hospital spent more than the standard DRG payment, it had to absorb the difference as a loss.

Conspicuously absent from the political negotiations that led up to both the passage and implementation of DRGs in New Jersey were physicians. This was especially ironic, given that policy makers designed the new prospective payment system in part to change physician behavior. John Thompson points to the political tactics of Joanne Finley, the state's commissioner of health and ardent champion of prospective payment reform, as a big part of the explanation: "She played politics. The first thing she did was to neutralize the doctors by keeping them busy and distracted on issues of medical quality," he explains. "She'd say to them, 'You and I are concerned about quality, and that's all you have to worry about. We're going to . . . look at every case, every hospital admission and its length of stay, and the New Jersey Medical Society is going to be authoring a report.'"[21]

The state's innovative system for regulating hospital payments encouraged greater efficiency and cost control, but it seemed to have as many detractors as supporters. The state's Department of Health experienced a number of trials and tribulations in getting prospective payment up and running, according to Richard Averill, project manager for the Yale research team that designed the plan. Some hospital industry representatives argued that "Grandma was going to be thrown out on the street" and that "prospective payment was akin to communism or cookbook medicine."[22] Averill maintains that Jack Owen (head of the New Jersey Hospital Association) was instrumental in persuading the majority of his member hospitals to ignore the criticisms and cooperate with the state's Department of Health: "Jack was a pretty open and progressive kind of leader and so I think in no small part the system came into being because he was just open-minded." Averill also credits the New Jersey Department of Health: "They really got a bunch of very bright people who were really committed to moving to prospective payment. It became sort of a religious exercise with people who had intense 'New York/New Jersey' personalities squared."[23]

Starting in May 1980, twenty-five hospitals began billing patients on a DRG-specific rate per case. By October 1982, all New Jersey hospitals were operating under the DRG system.[24] Although the change was momentous, it was far from instantaneous. Only a minority (about one-quarter to one-third) of the state's hospitals began the experiment in 1982, and their participation was voluntary, which made them initially unrepresentative. Hence, evidence of change early on was anecdotal and occasionally even embarrassing. (In one anomalous case, a payment of $6,000 was made for a broken finger.)[25]

A major problem with evaluating the new program's performance was the considerable lag in hospital data that researchers could analyze. Bruce Vladeck, who later served as administrator of HCFA from 1993 to 1997, was assistant commissioner for health planning and resources development under Joanne Finley from 1979 to 1982. As the principal investigator of New Jersey's DRG experiment, Vladeck had the responsibility to assess the DRGs' performance. He explains how technology limitations hindered the process of evaluating the state's experiments:

> The most amazing thing about this experience was that all of the time we were doing this, until when I left the department in early 1982 and even after we had set the 1982 [hospital payment] rates, the New Jersey Department of Health did *not* own a computer . . . The Yale people did some of the work on their computers and then we had to time-share with one of the three or four state mainframe computers in those days, which were controlled by New Jersey's Department of Transportation. But it was always very frustrating. We also bought time through the time-sharing system at Rutgers University. But we could only afford, given our budget constraints, to run our stuff at night. It was all mainframe stuff and all the data entry was still pretty much done manually, so it took us quite a while. And the data submissions from the hospitals themselves were manual, so we had to get them all keypunched in before we could do anything with them.[26]

Analyzing the data years later, researchers discovered that New Jersey's experiment with DRGs did restrain hospital cost inflation.[27] The change that hospitals experienced varied depending on their financial status.[28] Poorer hospitals profited the most from the new system, because uncompensated care was now factored into the state's DRG payment rates.[29] The net result was a strengthening of the financial position of hospitals that had previously experienced deficits and struggled financially. Access for New Jersey's uninsured population was improved.[30]

Commercial insurers also benefited from the new DRG system, because other payers began picking up more of the uncompensated care burden. Prior to the introduction of DRGs, there was a "hidden tax" paid by patients with commercial insurance (that is, insurance other than Blue Cross), to cover the cost of care that New Jersey hospitals rendered to people who were under- or uninsured.[31] Patients with commercial insurance were charged more by the hospitals for all services and procedures, while Blue Cross, Medicare, and Medicaid insulated themselves from paying this hidden tax. But due to the fact that this cross-subsidy between payers became factored into the state's new DRG system, the twenty-five hospitals that began the experiment in 1980 reduced their charges to commercially insured patients (on average) by 10 percent from what they had been in 1979.[32]

In effect, hospitals no longer had to play Robin Hood, rescuing under- and uninsured patients by charging more to commercially insured patients. The state took over this responsibility. The change did not generate additional revenues for hospitals; it simply redistributed the burden more equitably across privately insured patients. Employers who provided commercial for-profit insurance no longer paid substantially more than employers who provided Blue Cross insurance (which at the time was tax-exempt and not-for-profit).[33]

The state's new DRG system also appeared to change the behavior of many hospital administrators. They cut hospital inventories, reduced administrative overhead, and did not replace staff as quickly as vacancies occurred. Not all hospitals, though, made extensive changes. According to Hsiao and colleagues, the hospitals with large operating deficits made the greatest effort to reduce costs, while those with surpluses made minimal changes.[34] In short, those hospitals that were doing the worst financially made the most changes and benefited significantly.

The extent of change in hospital administration varied across the state, but virtually all hospital administrators were unsuccessful in fundamentally changing physician behavior. The most administrators were able to do in the realm of medical decision making was reduce patients' average length-of-stay.[35] When hospital budgets were in balance, administrators viewed physicians as indispensable professionals who supplied their institutions with revenue-generating patients and medical prestige. If budgets became tight, it was still easier and preferable for administrators to look for spending reductions that did not involve personal confrontations with physicians.[36]

Ultimately, the New Jersey experiment, as much as anything, provided a feasible alternative to traditional cost reimbursement. "Over time we clearly demonstrated that at the barest minimum, you could get such a system off the ground and the hospitals kept functioning and, lo and behold, they seemed to be responding to the incentives in the system," recalls Averill. "Hospitals got paid, Grandma was not thrown out onto the street prematurely by hospitals, and so it was generally viewed as a positive change despite all the predictions to the contrary."[37] Federal policy makers were especially encouraged that an alternative reimbursement system existed, and it was just in time, because Medicare's financial health was deteriorating rapidly.

Social Security and Medicare's Trust Fund Crises

By 1982, federal policy makers' concerns about the financial stability of Medicare were escalating and becoming part of even larger worries about growing federal budget imbalances. Mushrooming budget deficits (stemming from Reagan's major tax cuts passed the previous year), together with the highest unemployment rate and the worst recession since the Great Depression, created a sense of fiscal and economic crisis. The immediate concern of leading members of Congress was the fact that declining payroll taxes threatened to exhaust Social Security and Medicare's trust funds. When the Social Security boards of trustees released their annual reports on April 1, 1982, they noted "that unless action was taken soon, the Social Security system would be unable to pay cash benefits on time to retirees and survivors, beginning in July 1983."[38] Medicare's trust funds were in better shape, they reported, but the program still "faces very serious financial problems—indeed, bankruptcy—in the late 1980s or early 1990s unless taxes are increased considerably or expenditures are greatly reduced."[39]

The short-term solution to Social Security's crisis that policy makers adopted only exacerbated Medicare's financial problems. They borrowed from Medicare's Hospital Insurance trust fund to shore up Social Security's Old Age and Survivors Insurance (OASI) trust fund.[40] Carolyne Davis, HCFA's administrator, recalls that inter-fund borrowing became a leading catalyst for forcing a major reform of Medicare:

> I remember when Secretary Schweiker called and he said, "I really need to borrow $14 billion." That sounded very odd, and I remember saying to him, "Mr. Secretary, I would really like to *not* give it to you, because our [Medicare] trust fund is going to be bankrupt in 1995." And he said, "I can appreciate that, but you don't understand that I have to send Treasury checks out next month to Social Security beneficiaries and we don't have the money. So I have to borrow it from you even though I am sympathetic to the fact that you've got a problem with that. But we'll fix it." That was my first acknowledgement that they were going to fix Medicare . . .[41]

Inter-fund borrowing and the recession's effect on payroll tax revenue combined to move up the projected insolvency date of Medicare's HI trust fund to 1988.[42] It also did not help that hospital costs in 1982 increased at three times the general rate of inflation.[43]

Congress responded to the mounting fiscal crises by passing the Tax Equity and Fiscal Responsibility Act (TEFRA) in August 1982.[44] Signed into law on September 3 by President Reagan, TEFRA predominantly dealt with closing tax loopholes and other revenue provisions entirely unrelated to Medicare.[45] But it also included various measures aimed at curtailing Medicare's cost growth. These measures effectively sounded the official death knell for retrospective cost-based reimbursement, the system that the hospital industry had painstakingly fought for and solidified over decades.[46] As a result, TEFRA became a key stepping-stone to passing prospective payment legislation the following year.

TEFRA represented a major political and strategic shift in policy makers' focus on containing hospital costs. Whereas the Carter administration's proposals had sought to cap hospital prices for all payers, public and private, the Reagan administration narrowed its attention to the "problems" of government programs. "The focus turned very much to, 'We're running these public programs. We have to run them better, more efficiently. We have to economize our expenses,'" says Paul Ginsburg, deputy assistant director of the Congressional Budget Office at the time.[47] In contrast to Carter's efforts, which were derailed by intense partisanship, Congress approved the new Medicare constraints with little disagreement between politicians of widely divergent political views. Regulating prices for just Medicare was far less threatening to the hospital industry than Carter's "all-payer" proposal. Republicans in general, and Senator Dole in particular, led the attack on behalf of tough new constraints on hospital spending. Representatives of the hospital industry were reduced to a strategy of damage control.[48]

TEFRA imposed the most significant restrictions on Medicare payments to hospitals in the program's history. By extending the existing limits on hospital payment to also include patients' ancillary costs—those above and beyond the basic "hotel" costs of room, food, and nursing services—it essentially paid hospitals an average payment per case. Generally speaking, the more acutely ill the patient, the greater the percentage of the hospital bill attributable to ancillary services. Moreover, hospitals would only be reimbursed up to a maximum of 120 percent of their average cost per case *within* their own hospital class or "peer group" (based on a hospital's number of beds and geographic location).[49] If a hospital could treat a patient for less than the average of the other hospitals in its peer group, it could keep 50 percent of the difference as a profit. If it cost the same hospital more than the average within its peer group, it had to absorb 75 percent of the difference as a loss in the first two years of TEFRA's operation, and all of the loss thereafter.[50] Putting hospitals in the position of sharing both profits and losses on each case was intended by policy makers to encourage them to behave more efficiently and scrutinize everything they did for a patient.

TEFRA's other main cost-containment device came in the form of a cap on the annual increase in hospitals' average payment per case. Hospitals would have a "target" rate of growth based on the general rate of wage and price inflation in that region, notes political scientist David Smith. Policy makers intended to use the cap to "ratchet down the annual rate of inflation in hospital costs, eventually to no more than 10 percent—a grim prospect for the hospitals considering their past and recent history of relatively unconstrained cost increases."[51] And by allowing policy makers to "score" the future reductions in Medicare spending as budgetary savings,[52] TEFRA represented a harbinger of things to come. Medicare policy would be increasingly subordinated by Congress to budgetary policy and, specifically, the need for deficit reduction.

TEFRA was a preliminary but strategically effective measure. The fact that it set per-diem limits on Medicare reimbursement, which hospitals loathed because TEFRA also included the prospect of an annual growth limit for total expenditures, "was not coincidental," according to several observers.[53] Moving to a payment system that hospitals hated and feared provided Congress with political leverage and a superior bargaining position when DRGs were introduced for consideration the following year.[54] As something of a "doomsday device," TEFRA signaled to the hospital industry that systemic change was inevitable and imminent. The not-so-subtle implication was that the hospital industry should "come to the bargaining table" to support the transition to a prospective payment system.[55] It worked, according to John Iglehart: "Addressing upwards of 3,000 hospital administrators during a special televised conference [in August 1982], Alexander McMahon, president of the AHA, said, "hospitals that keep costs low with be rewarded. After 16 years of cost reimbursement, we're moving to a prospective basis." McMahon urged administrators not to despair. "We still have more money in 1983 than we did in 1982. There will be 14 percent more dollars available for Medicare, but there will not be 17 percent as projected."[56]

To show that the American Hospital Association was willing to cooperate in a transition to prospective payment, McMahon and a number of state hospital association executives asked Jack Owen, president of the New Jersey Hospital Association, to become their Washington representative in the spring of 1982.[57] His experience of having worked successfully with policy makers in New Jersey gave him a unique credibility in representing the nation's largest hospital organization. The AHA was especially eager to cooperate with policy makers to change Medicare if it meant getting rid of TEFRA's new payment policies. "People really wanted to create a better set of incentives," says Rick Pollack, current executive vice president of the AHA, who joined the organization in 1982. "TEFRA was kind of a stopgap to put the tourniquet on Medicare spending, but it wasn't anything that people wanted to see go beyond a stopgap kind of approach. So, yes, we were very much 'on board.'"[58]

Developing a Prospective Payment Proposal with or without DRGs

TEFRA called for the Secretary of HHS to develop, in consultation with the Senate Finance and House Ways and Means Committees, a proposal for prospective reimbursement by December 31, 1982.[59] Had there not been almost a decade of research and demonstrations by HCFA,[60] it literally would have been impossible to meet the four-month deadline. But policy makers were able to draw upon years of research by HCFA's Office of Research and Development and New Jersey's experience with DRGs. "The DRG prospective payment system moved forward as rapidly as it did because it basically was a wrinkle on all the work that had been done for the implementation of the Section 223 cost limits," argues Judith Lave, director of HCFA's Office of Research and Development from 1977 to 1982. "Basically, how you do DRGs, how you weight them, what you should take into consideration, how you should analyze them, so many of the technical issues—not all of them, of course, but much of the analytical groundwork had already been laid."[61]

Although they later became the centerpiece of prospective payment, DRGs were not popular among a number of high-ranking HCFA political appointees, many of whom viewed them as "too technical" or as an ungainly "administered price system" from New Jersey.[62] In fact, "when they first implemented the task force to work on a prospective payment system for Medicare," explains Lave, "DRGs were off the table."[63] Patrice Feinstein, HCFA's associate administrator for policy, was particularly opposed to them, which is noteworthy because she later became a key figure in the political passage and implementation of Medicare's system of DRGs.[64]

In July of 1982, members of the HCFA task force that Schweiker had organized back in 1981 met with him to discuss the two prospective payment models that had emerged from their research and negotiations with the hospital industry.[65] HCFA's technical staff and appointees had decided not to simply adopt New Jersey's model. They considered it "too impure," as the model was operated on a hospital-by-hospital basis and had complicated policies for "outlier" payments (for patients that had unusually long hospital stays or higher costs than the norm).[66] The New Jersey experiment basically showed that the concept of payment for hospital admissions was viable, explains

TABLE 2.1
Annual Increase in Inpatient Hospital Costs:
Demonstration States versus United States

	1979	1980	1981
Connecticut	8.1%	11.4%	15.9%
Maryland	12.1	9.8	15.6
Massachusetts	7.6	14.1	14.1
New Jersey	**11.2**	**10.7**	**11.4**
New York	8.5	10.8	14.1
Rhode Island	10.9	12.4	16.3
Washington	11.2	10.9	18.9
Wisconsin	10.7	12.6	17.6
United States	11.3	12.7	17.3

SOURCE: Adapted and modified from U.S. Department of Health and Human Services, *Report to the Congress: Hospital Prospective Payment for Medicare*, 21, table 3.

Robert Rubin, Schweiker's assistant secretary for planning and evaluation. "But one could say that we advanced from where they were, which may also have been appropriate since we were dealing with a national system and they were dealing with a reasonably homogenous set of hospitals in a small state."[67]

The two models the task force ultimately proposed to Schweiker both included DRGs, but in different ways. The model the task force preferred entailed a flat-rate payment per hospital discharge (in which a hospital would be paid an amount based on number of patients and that hospital's historic cost experience) and only used DRGs to establish total cost limits for individual hospitals. The second model used DRGs as the central price-setting device. It bore a greater resemblance to New Jersey's system, which, at the time, appeared to be working better than any of the other state experiments (see table 2.1).[68] According to David Smith, Schweiker was "flabbergasted at their final recommendation."[69] The flat rate approach was "clearly unacceptable" to him, because it encouraged hospitals to "skim off" the healthier patients while offering hospitals minimal incentives to improve their technology and become more efficient. In the end, he overruled the preferences of his task force and instructed its members to design his department's prospective payment proposal with DRGs as the key price-setting device.[70]

The Reagan administration came to view prospective payment with DRGs as "the response of a prudent purchaser concerned with creating incentives for efficiency and reducing the deficit."[71] In short, DRGs would reduce costs by putting the hospitals at financial risk. With the threat of operating losses for those hospitals unable to deliver care at or below DRG payment rates, prospective payment would virtually force hospitals to increase efficiency and productivity and, in the process, lower their costs.[72]

Lower hospitals costs, proponents argued, would translate directly into lower Medicare expenditures.[73]

The hospital industry may have been resigned to the inevitability of Medicare's switch to prospective payment, but its opinion of DRGs was also mixed. On the same day in August 1982 that Secretary Schweiker held a press briefing on prospective payment, AHA president Alexander McMahon "told reporters that payment by diagnostic groupings was too rigid . . . to accommodate complex cases."[74] Michael Bromberg, executive director of the Federation of American Hospitals (representing for-profit, investor-owned hospitals), was more enthusiastic: "At first I thought DRGs were more of a peer-review screening tool than a payment tool, but a fixed-rate, prospective payment system was a policy my board and I supported."[75]

The last four months of 1982 involved almost round-the-clock, seven-day-a-week work schedules for HCFA's staff and appointees in an effort to have their secretary's *Report to the Congress* completed by TEFRA's December 31 deadline. Primary responsibility for the report's initial draft fell to Allen Dobson, head of the Office of Research and Development. "I wrote the first draft in my kitchen," Dobson recalls, "and then my colleagues . . . spent the next three months getting it right with all the details and complexity needed for the final report."[76]

The report is an extraordinary document. It synthesized the extensive research and theoretical underpinnings of prospective payment dating back to the early 1970s, while also including numerous complex statistical analyses of hospital payment rates, case-mix indices, medical categorizations, and wage indices.[77] It represented the accumulation of more than a decade of academic innovation, state-level experimentation, and research and development by talented technical staff within HCFA. Conceptually, at least, prospective payment with DRGs was ready for a new arena of deliberative conflict: a political debate between and within Congress and the administration.

Piggy-Backing on Social Security's Bailout and Buying Off the Opposition

Financial necessity, particularly the specter of imminent bankruptcy, is the mother of all kinds of major programmatic invention. Policy makers' seminal reform of both Social Security and Medicare in 1983 is a classic example. According to Don Moran, Reagan's associate director for budget and legislation, Social Security's approaching insolvency provided the perfect vehicle for changing Medicare's Part A hospital program to a prospective payment system with DRGs:

Ideas like DRGs have an intellectual life of their own . . . but at some point these ideas hit their nexus to the real-world, tactical-political situation and they either do or do not adhere. So, yes, DRGs had an independent life of their own quite without regard to what anybody in the Reagan administration thought about them per se. But we just pulled them off the shelf as a "plug" to solve the short-term solvency problem with Social Security. Inter-fund borrowing had sprung a temporary leak in Medicare's HI [Hospital Insurance] trust fund, so we needed some kind of magic asterisk to stick in the Social Security deal to say, "Notwithstanding the fact that we are currently bankrupting the HI trust fund, we have a fig leaf [prospective payment] to stick in as a plug when inter-fund borrowing expires on June 30th, so that we can lower the five-year forecast outlays in the HI trust fund and, in so doing, prevent its bankruptcy over the next five years."[78]

There was more momentum and technical development behind prospective payment's ascendancy than Moran's statement suggests. But the truth in his argument that extraordinary political and fiscal circumstances opened a rare window of opportunity for a major policy change is undeniable.

The hospital industry and HCFA's attention may have been on Medicare's hospital payment reform when 1983 began, but "the top legislative priority for Congress and the administration was Social Security and jobs," as the *National Journal* reported that year. "Medicare reform was important, but it was clearly considered a back-burner item."[79] The House Ways and Means and Senate Finance Committees would expedite only one piece of legislation in early 1983, and that was the Social Security reform bill.[80]

Ironically, the first person to suggest the possibility of strategically attaching Medicare's prospective payment proposal to Social Security's bailout bill was Dan Rostenkowski, chair of Ways and Means, who had played the leading role in defending the hospital industry from Carter's hospital cost-containment plans.[81] Rostenkowski contacted Secretary Schweiker about the idea. Schweiker was initially surprised, but quickly supported it.[82] Shortly thereafter, as John Iglehart has chronicled,[83] Rostenkowski's chief counsel, John Salmon, asked Schweiker's assistant secretary for policy and planning, Robert Rubin, "How fast can you do prospective payment?" Rubin responded, "In six weeks." Salmon said, "How about eleven days?" and then explained to him the merits of "one of the greatest legislative engines we'll ever see—the Social Security bill."[84] Bob Dole, Rostenkowski's counterpart as chair of the Senate Finance Committee, objected to the idea at first but eventually agreed after receiving a personal guarantee from the AHA's Jack Owen that "we will get the hospitals to go for it."[85] According to Owen, "My job was not to stop it, but just to help it and go along with it."[86]

Once senior congressional leaders and administration were in agreement, attention turned to buying off any opposition from the hospital industry. It helped that TEFRA's stringent cost controls were set to begin later that same year. Hospitals were looking for anything to avoid TEFRA.[87] Besides the prevailing sense that reform was unavoidable, a major factor that contributed to the hospital industry's relatively receptive attitude about reform was the unprecedented potential for significant profits. "That was one of the things you could sell, because there was a lot of financial slack in the hospital business," acknowledges Owen. "Once they started pulling back on their slack, the hospitals could really start making some money."[88]

Hospital representatives, however, were still divided in their opinion of prospective payment. The Federation of American Hospitals, which represented for-profit hospitals, was enormously enthusiastic.[89] The AHA was comparatively less so, but eager to avoid the effects of TEFRA.[90] Representatives of the nation's teaching hospitals, however, were strongly opposed to the plan.[91] Due to the fact that they train residents, employ academic physicians, and conduct medical research, academic medical centers are more costly than community hospitals. At the same time, they serve a unique and essential need: they advance medical science. Moving to a national prospective rate system would have put them in the impossible situation of competing financially with hospitals that could and would consistently beat them on price.

Consequently, staff members in HCFA and on the Ways and Means Committee recommended increasing DRG payment rates to teaching hospitals as a "cushion."[92] Different economic simulations of this increase, though, produced different results. The issue was critical, because adjusting the payment rates involved massive swings in the total amount of money that teaching hospitals would receive. Too low an adjustment and teaching hospitals would be severely harmed financially; too high an adjustment and the hospitals would receive absurd financial windfalls at Medicare's actuarial expense. Robert Rubin ultimately pushed for a generous doubling of the "resident-to-bed" adjustment increase in DRG rates to teaching hospitals.[93] "It was a bribe, pure and simple," admits Allen Dobson, one of Rubin's colleagues. "It was a bribe and it worked."[94] Teaching hospitals relented and became supportive of prospective payment with DRGs. As Rubin explains,

> Were we overly generous on the teaching adjustment? Sure. I've said publicly innumerable times that the real number was not two [a doubling]. I mean, any fool would know that two is a totally made-up number, but it was close to two . . . That made the teaching hospitals reasonably happy and it gave us a very

important part of New York's political delegation, including [Pat] Moynihan and Charlie Rangel. That was not a trivial issue. We also got the Mayo Clinic exemption, which made Senator [David] Durenberger [R-MN] happy. And we had exemptions for the cancer hospitals, which made the folks in Texas happy.[95]

The Ways and Means and Senate Finance Committees made a few other important adjustments to account for "outlier" cases and to exclude various items from being factored into the DRGs, namely hospital capital and direct medical education. The latter two items would continue to be reimbursed on a traditional cost basis.[96]

Having bought off the hospital industry's opposition, members of both committees were able to pass the legislation quickly and easily. Attaching Medicare reform to critical Social Security reform was a purely opportunistic, but effective, decision. It produced a veto-proof bill that due to its sheer urgency was immune to any single or collective interest-group veto.[97] "A remarkable reality of the process in both chambers was how few legislators were actually involved in designing the legislation," notes John Iglehart. "For the most part, professional staff members made the key decisions."[98] Members of Congress voted for it, however, because Medicare was approaching insolvency and, even more so, because the Social Security legislation had to pass for recipients' millions of monthly checks to continue uninterrupted.[99] "There was no serious debate [about prospective payment] of any consequence," notes Paul Rettig. "It was so overwhelmed by the Social Security rescue that it received very little political attention."[100]

After roughly two months of legislative consideration, most of it focused on adjustments to the OASI program, Congress passed the Social Security bill on March 24, 1983. President Reagan signed it into law one month later on April 20.[101] The single biggest change to the American health care system since Medicare and Medicaid's passage in 1965 went largely unnoticed outside of a small group of hospital representatives and health policy leaders.

The Social Security Amendments of 1983 set a date of October 1 of that year for commencement of Medicare's new payment system.[102] Fundamentally changing in just five months how Medicare would pay the vast majority of the nation's hospitals was an enormously daunting task. HCFA had never done anything of this scope and magnitude. Many within the organization were skeptical that they could actually pull it off.[103] "I called all the senior staff together," recalls Carolyne Davis, "and I said, 'Let me explain something to you: we *will* get this done this fall. If there's anybody here now who thinks we aren't going to, you should be prepared to leave now and give your place to somebody else, because I'm telling you that we will work weekends, evenings; I'll move cots in so we can work all night if we have to, but we are going to get this done.'"[104] And they did. "We took a $40 billion system and we got it in place between April and October 1," Davis added, "and the claims were right and they were on time."[105]

Following a decade of development, experimentation, and analysis, the passage of Medicare's new prospective payment system with DRGs represented something of an administrative revolution. Key to policy makers' success was the strange political attraction of prospective payment. Hospital industry representatives were already desperate for any alternative to TEFRA, but they quickly became keen on the opportunity to make significant profits under the new reimbursement system—at least initially. Congressional leaders of both parties and Reagan administration officials wanted increased control of Medicare to restrain the program's rate of growth, despite the fact that prospective payment required significantly increased government regulation and control of health care. And with Social Security literally on the verge of bankruptcy in 1983, policy makers finally had a legislative vehicle for comprehensive Medicare reform that was unstoppable.

Following the rapid passage of Medicare's new reimbursement system, another set of concerns arose: Would the system actually work? Would Medicare's rate of expenditure growth subside? How would hospitals respond to the new incentives? Would any particular set of hospitals be wiped out financially by the new system? How would patients be affected, if at all? "There was great sensitivity that we were going down a path none of us had gone down before," notes Sheila Burke.

> There had been some rough sort of testing on the state-level, but nothing on the scale of Medicare. We all knew only too well the impact of any change in Medicare could lead to seismic changes in the industry, because Medicare was such a big purchaser. So we were all enormously sensitive to that, and also enormously sensitive to not really knowing how to defend or describe what appeared to be real differences between hospitals, their costs and their mix of cases. We knew far less than one would have hoped about what would occur after making these changes.[106]

The only thing policy makers did know for sure was that, with a program as immense as Medicare, it was impossible to change just one thing.[107] The ripple effects of moving to a prospective payment system were bound to be extensive.

CHAPTER THREE

The Phase-In Years and Beginning of "Rough Justice" for Hospitals

Over time, these new business managers moved in and took over the hospitals, because the doctors would rather play golf on a Wednesday afternoon than run a hospital. And before they knew it, the doctors were pushed out and you had so-called "professional" hospital managers in there. In the end, doctors abandoned their role in managing hospitals.

—*Representative Pete Stark (D-CA)*

In the first year after the PPS went into effect, the chief executive officer of a big hospital came to me and said, "I've got almost a fifty-million-dollar surplus this year! What do I do?" I remember saying, "Put it in the bank and be awful careful with it because you're not going to have it that long. You're going to get reduced."

—*Jack Owen, Executive Vice President (1982–90),*
American Hospital Association

Medicare's transition to its new prospective payment system had a dramatic effect on the nation's hospital industry during the four years of its phase-in period. Never had so much change in hospital management transpired in so short a period of time. Previously, Medicare paid hospitals whatever costs they incurred, so they had no incentive to control their operating expenses. Higher costs translated into increased payments from Medicare, which administrators could and often did use to expand their hospitals' programs and services.[1] The PPS completely upended this status quo. By categorizing all hospital services and procedures, the PPS enabled policy makers to know what medical care would cost *before* Medicare beneficiaries received it; the new system established predetermined payment amounts for 467 different diagnosis-related groups. (To account for new procedures and services, this number has increased over the years and changes often.) If the hospital managed to treat a Medicare patient for less than the DRG allotted, it kept the "savings" as profit. Conversely, if the hospital incurred more costs than the DRG allotted, it had to absorb the difference as a loss.[2] As a result, the structure of Medicare's financial incentives flipped. By separating an individual hospital's level of reimbursement from its production costs, the PPS triggered a radical change in hospital administration. The focus shifted from providing as much care as possible to maximizing the overall profit from each Medicare patient.[3]

Besides gaining greater control over Medicare spending, policy makers hoped that the PPS would fundamentally change physicians' and health care executives' medical decision making. Their goal was to communicate to the hospital leadership, and through them to the medical staffs: "Maybe it's time to back up and think about what you're doing, how you do it, why you do it that way, and whether there aren't better ways to do it," according to Julian Pettengill, one of HCFA's leading technical designers of Medicare's PPS. It was really about making physicians and hospital managers think more broadly and say to themselves, "Is this the best way to do something, is this the best place to be doing this or that hospital procedure, and how can we organize care so that it is more efficient and more effective?"[4] As it turned out, hospital administrators struggled to change physician behavior.[5] But they did become much more corporate in their orientation and, on average, reaped significant financial profits in the early years of the PPS's operation.

The initial success of Medicare's new reimbursement model encouraged a number of leading congressmen and Health Care Financing Administration staff to make a series of changes that, ironically, resulted in the PPS becoming *more* complex and political rather than less (as originally intended). The process began in the mid-1980s when senior congressional leaders turned to the PPS as a new and hugely effective deficit reduction device. By simply restraining the annual increases in Medicare's hospital payment rates, Congress was able to divert tremendous amounts of government revenue for reducing annual deficits and increasing spending in other areas of the federal budget. But bluntly "squeezing" Medicare payments to all hospitals for larger fiscal objectives struck many policy makers as unfair, since some hospitals were in a much better position than others to absorb a decline in Medicare reimbursement. Therefore, Congress began selectively targeting increased payment rates to specific hospital groups (rural and inner city). Along the way, the original goal of the PPS—to establish one set of national, wage-adjusted payment rates—became eclipsed by the new goal of using the PPS to address major federal budget imbalances. In essence, as Medicare payment policy became increasingly subordinated to fiscal policy, Congress sought ways to try to ensure that the inevitable "rough justice" of moving to a national, standardized payment system would remain as financially "fair" as possible to the nation's hospital industry.

Medicare's PPS Transforms Hospitals' Finances

To ensure both the administrative and political success of Medicare's new PPS, policy makers made it hard for hospitals to do anything but prosper financially under the new reimbursement model. They cushioned the transition from retrospective cost reimbursement to prospective payment by basing first-year payments on each individual hospital's historical costs. This locked in what many observers considered to be generous operating margins.[6] One way that hospitals quickly responded was to reduce their Medicare patients' average length-of-stay;[7] in the process, they reaped huge windfall payments from the PPS.[8] "I was surprised at how easily you could lower the length-of-stay and not have masses of people dying in the streets or revolting or something of that sort," recalls James Mongan, former health policy advisor to President Carter and current president of Partners HealthCare in Boston.[9] Medicare patients' length-of-stay in 1984 was 9 percent lower than the year before, which represented the largest annual decline in the history of the program.[10] But what is especially revealing, notes Bruce Vladeck, is that "the data show that the *real* reduction in length-of-stay began in January 1983—not in October '83 when the new DRG system began—which is stupid!" Rational behavior would have been for hospital administrators to maximize payments under the traditional model of cost reimbursement as long as it was still in existence. "But this says something about the mass psychology of behavioral change in the health care system," adds Vladeck.[11]

In fear and anticipation of the approaching transition, hospitals had already started to change their practices in early 1983.[12] Administrators transformed their medical records departments—where accurate coding of patient records determined how much hospitals got paid or whether they got paid at all—with more personnel and improved technology.[13] The cliché of choice became "Medicare's PPS brought medical records out of the basement."[14]

Traditionally, hospitals had not reported their mix of medical cases accurately, nor had they routinely reported secondary diagnoses. This kind of record keeping was irrelevant under Medicare's previous cost-based payment model, in which billing clerks simply tallied up a bill of total expenses and submitted them to Medicare for reimbursement. Accurate and extensive record keeping was also irrelevant for private insurers. Under the new PPS, hospitals transferred the now hugely important responsibility for patient coding to their medical records department, where their staff often learned how to maximize reimbursement for each and every patient.[15] Many hospital managers developed or purchased computer programs that would automatically assign Medicare patients to the highest paying DRG category allowable.[16] Because the hospital claims data that HCFA used to develop the original 467 individual DRGs and their respective payment rates were pre-DRG data, health care management expert George Whetsell explains, "as hospitals improved their data, their case mix complexity increased and their Medicare payments wound up being higher than HCFA anticipated."[17] This phenomenon became known as "DRG-creep."[18] Key to trying to control the amount of DRG-creep was policy makers' use of physicians as something akin to "watchdogs" over hospitals. The PPS initially required that the diagnosis submitted for reimbursement be attested to by the patient's attending physician.[19] But under assault by physicians, HCFA withdrew this requirement.[20]

Widely conceded "overpayment" in the first year of Medicare's PPS created a situation in which hospitals' profit margins increased as their expenses per case dropped.[21] This not only made the first year under the new reimbursement system an anomaly, it also provided most hospitals with an unexpected surge in net profits.[22] According to Stuart Guterman, a HCFA analyst at the time, this financial development came as a major surprise but one that policy makers accepted for political and technical reasons.

> You have to remember, we weren't 100 percent sure what was going to happen and we didn't want to hurt Medicare beneficiaries. But we were prepared to have hospitals go out of business if we felt the system was fair and they were not able to meet the costs that they had to meet in order to stay in business. Nobody wanted a cataclysmic kind of effect, so the idea was to sort of begin this new system by estimating the parameters with a fairly light hand.
>
> We *were* shocked about the [hospitals'] margins, but it made us feel better in a way and it did come out of a mistake. During the first four years, which was the transition period, payments to hospitals were a blend of hospital-specific and federal payment rates. The hospital-specific rates were based on unaudited cost reports [which contained errors that Medicare would not have reimbursed]. This really inflated the payment rates that hospitals were receiving in the first couple of years. That wasn't intended . . . Part of it was also that hospitals responded very quickly to the new incentives, because there was a lot of fat in the system and they could easily keep some of their costs under control.[23]

In short, substantial change ensued after the PPS began operation. According to a 1984 report by the Department of Health and Human Services, "The findings to date are highly suggestive that, as the PPS is implemented, dramatic changes are occurring far more rapidly than either supporters or detractors of the system had thought pos-

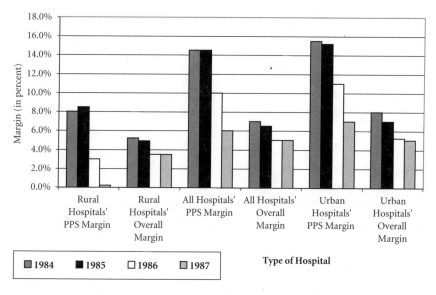

Figure 3.1. Hospitals' Medicare PPS Margins and Overall Margins, 1984–87

Source: Adapted and modified from S. Guterman, S. Altman, D. Young, " Hospitals' Financial Performance," 127–129, exhibits 1, 4.

Note: The PPS margin is best described as the percentage of Medicare PPS payments remaining for hospitals after the costs of treating the program's beneficiaries are accounted for. PPS margin = (*hospitals' total inpatient Medicare payments* − hospitals' total inpatient Medicare costs) / hospitals' total inpatient Medicare payments.

sible."[24] In June of the same year, Michael Bromberg, executive director of the Federation of American Hospitals, said as much in his testimony before Congress: "The Medicare law that brought us prospective payment for the first time has clearly given us incentives 180 degrees different from any we have ever had, and we have responded."[25] In May 1985, Bromberg reiterated his claim that Medicare's "Prospective Payment System is the most effective cost-containment program ever enacted, successful beyond anyone's expectations."[26]

The majority of the nation's hospitals found themselves better off financially in the first couple of years of the PPS than they had ever been.[27] Their positive Medicare PPS margins—which reflected the total amount of Medicare inpatient payments they received relative to the total inpatient costs they incurred treating Medicare patients—were almost 15 percent in 1984 and 1985 (figure 3.1). Hospitals' generous Medicare, Blue Cross, and commercial insurance margins helped to offset their regular losses on both Medicaid and charity care patients, which left them with an average overall profit margin of 6.2 percent (more than double the total increase in the five previous years).[28] The American Hospital Association found that hospitals as a group saw a larger financial gain in 1984 (an $8.3 billion surplus) than in any year since 1963, when their surveys began.[29]

The one negative allegation that arose about the PPS was that it potentially en-couraged hospitals to discharge Medicare patients "quicker and sicker," a term coined by John Rother, who was then staff director of the Senate Special Committee on Ag-ing.[30] The Senate Special Committee on Aging and the late Senator John Heinz (R-PA), in particular, were concerned that hospitals were abusing the new reimburse-ment system by accepting the standard DRG payment and then discharging Medicare patients prematurely in order to maximize profits.[31] Early analyses indicated that, on average, Medicare patients were indeed being discharged earlier and in less stable con-dition compared to before the PPS.[32] But the political fallout from the "quicker and sicker" charge dissipated when researchers were not able to find any discernible differ-ence between Medicare beneficiaries' thirty-day or six-month mortality rates before and after the PPS went into effect.[33] Moreover, as Guterman explains, "The whole idea with the PPS was that you were going to lose money on some patients, make money on most patients, and that it would all come out even in the end. In fact, it worked out *more* than even for the hospitals in the early years of the PPS, so it wasn't like they were taking it on the chin with their sicker patients."[34]

It is not surprising, then, that most everyone was pleased with Medicare's new PPS in its first two years of operation. Medicare's rate of expenditure growth slowed dra-matically, with Part A payments to hospitals providing the bulk of the program's spending reductions (table 3.1). The greatest cost savings for Medicare came from a reduction in the number of hospital admissions.[35] Hospitals still profited hand-somely, so their financial health, on average, was strong.[36] But the pressure was on for hospitals to take maximum advantage of Medicare's new payment incentives.[37]

Increased Hospital Competition and the Rise of Corporate-Oriented Executives

In addition to the radically new financial incentives, hospital managers were quick to change their institutional operations for a more personal but equally motivating reason: their jobs were at stake.[38] "They were terrified," notes Allen Dobson. "The av-erage tenure of a hospital CEO was falling like a rock then."[39] The rate of hospital CEO turnover jumped from 16.9 percent in 1982 to 20.3 percent in 1983 and peaked at 24.2 percent in 1987.[40] A survey in 1985 found that financial managers in the health care industry were experiencing a considerable increase in job tension.[41]

Hospitals were no longer assured of payment at the levels to which they had be-come accustomed. Now they would only do well if they spent less than their peer hospitals.[42] Previous hospital competition came almost exclusively in the form of in-stitutional prestige or, in so many words, a "hospital arms race" with non-price com-

TABLE 3.1
Total Medicare and National Health Expenditures in Billions, 1980–87

Year	National Health Expenditures	Change	All Medicare Expenditures	Change	Medicare Hospital Payments	Change
1980	$249.1	—	$36.4	—	$25.4	—
1981	288.6	15.9%	43.7	20.0%	30.6	20.3%
1982	323.8	12.2	51.2	17.3	35.7	16.5
1983	356.1	10.0	58.1	13.5	39.9	11.8
1984	387.0	8.7	64.8	11.5	44.5	11.7
1985†	420.1	8.5	69.8	7.8	47.1	5.7
1986	452.3	7.7	75.8	8.5	49.2	4.6
1987	492.5	8.9	82.0	8.2	51.3	4.2
1980–83	—	12.7*	—	15.0*	—	16.2*
1984–87	—	8.5*	—	9.0*	—	6.5*

SOURCE: Prospective Payment Assessment Commission, *Medicare and the American Health Care System* (1991), 12, 111.
  *Annual average increase over the four-year period
  †First full year of Medicare's PPS in operation

petition over highly remunerative services to private patients.[43] But the stakes for hospitals' solvency and their managers' survival increased dramatically under the PPS,[44] because for the first time Medicare's method of reimbursement separated hospitals into financial "winners" and "losers."[45] Hospital administrators responded by encouraging their physicians to request fewer diagnostic and laboratory tests for Medicare patients. To improve their bottom lines, hospital executives also reduced their number of full-time hospital employees, particularly nurses.[46] In 1982, hospitals employed 3.1 million workers; by 1985, the number had dropped three percent to 3 million.[47]

The new competition engendered by the PPS also heightened internal divisions within the hospital industry. Each year's average Medicare PPS margin masked an enormous amount of variation around the mean.[48] In other words, with a positive industry average of almost 15 percent Medicare PPS margins in 1984 and 1985, hundreds of hospitals had even higher margins—some much higher.[49] At the same time, nearly a fifth of the nation's hospitals either were so poorly managed or had such an unpredictable and often unfavorable mix of Medicare cases (often small rural hospitals with high fixed and low variable costs) that they still managed to lose money on their Medicare patients.[50] After completing the first (and only) comprehensive analysis of which hospitals emerged as "winners" and "losers" from Medicare's new payment system, Dobson and his colleagues at the analysis research firm Lewin-ICF discovered that there "was essentially a gulf, a divide between the hospitals that figured out how to work and prosper under the PPS and those that did not. It was very systemic."[51]

By necessity, then, hospital administrators became more businesslike.[52] Hospital trustees restructured their institutions' administrative staffs with a growing number of corporate titles.[53] Not-for-profit community hospitals increasingly mimicked their for-profit competitors, notes Rosemary Stevens, by becoming more dependent on tax and bond advisers, corporate lawyers, software specialists, management experts, and politicians.[54] The non-physician administrator became the hospital president, and an increasing number of master's-level vice presidents were appointed, explains Thomas Weil, "who were responsible for major components (some for-profit) within a new organizational chart that often replicated those used in the banking industry."[55]

The one major relationship that the PPS did not change radically was that between hospital executives and physicians.[56] The extent to which Medicare's new payment model transformed physician behavior turned out to be relatively modest.[57] Hospital executives' attempts at reducing the test-ordering practices of their physicians were temporarily successful, but by the end of 1985 these patterns had returned to pre-PPS levels.[58] As physicians continued to practice as they always had, the "creative tension" between hospital executives and physicians—which many policy makers hoped the PPS would engender—failed to materialize.[59] According to James Mongan, "I remember being amused by some of the more aggressive new hospital administrators saying, 'The way we're going to succeed under this new system is to call every doctor in and tell them that we're going to keep track of exactly what every doctor does, his patients' length-of-stay, what his costs are, and that we're going to be all over this because we're going to fire the top third most expensive doctors.'" Not surprisingly, Mongan adds, "that's an easier thing to talk about than to do."[60]

Hospital executives brave enough to broach confrontations with physicians quickly found them unrewarding and even threatening to their own survival.[61] So instead they focused on cost-cutting measures that were more within their realm of unilateral control.[62] Rather than stock, say, fourteen different heart valves and six different prosthetic knees, they often decided to go with just three and two, respectively.[63] And "for the doctor that had an 8 a.m. OR [Operating Room] appointment and always came in at 9 a.m.—which left everyone sitting around for an hour and wasted dollars—the hospitals started giving his slot to other physicians," explains Donald Young, former executive director of Medicare's Prospective Payment Assessment Commission.[64]

Ultimately, most hospital executives encouraged members of their medical staff: (1) to discharge Medicare patients earlier, (2) to transfer them more quickly to less expensive outpatient settings that still operated under traditional cost reimbursement, and (3) to use fewer diagnostic and laboratory tests. The sizeable Medicare profits that resulted from these temporary changes made it seem unnecessary for hospital administrators to cut costs and continue pursuing productivity gains in subsequent years.[65] Instead, most hospitals increased their product and service offerings at the then-unregulated margins of the DRG system: skilled nursing facilities (SNFs), intermediate care facilities (ICFs), and home health agencies.[66] They also invested in new technologies and significantly expanded hospital offerings (e.g., psychiatric, outpatient, and ancillary services).[67] Consequently, Medicare's new inpatient system not only created new incentives for hospitals to become more efficient, it also inadvertently encouraged the locus of hospital care for all patients to shift from inpatient settings to less expensive, yet more generously reimbursed, ambulatory care settings.[68] Improvements in medical technology were already facilitating this shift, but Medicare's new PPS greatly accelerated it.[69] Later, managed care tried to take advantage of the major change in the delivery of care brought about my Medicare.

Hospitals did temporarily become more efficient following the introduction of the PPS.[70] But their gains were rapidly overwhelmed by their subsequent expansion of services and amenities, which led to a decline in the hospital industry's aggregate productivity and a return to the same rapid cost growth that prevailed before the PPS.[71] By 1987, hospital employment had returned to its 1982 level of 3.1 million workers.[72]

The Emergence of Medicare's PPS as a Leading "Deficit-Reduction" Device

The glowing mutual admiration between Congress and the hospital industry over the PPS's success deteriorated rapidly when Congress turned to Medicare in 1986 as a means of addressing the nation's growing budget deficits.[73] The same Michael Bromberg who just a year earlier had effusively praised Congress for its wisdom in changing Medicare's method of reimbursement now accused both the executive and legislative branches of operating in "bad faith" and violating the PPS "contract":

> We were willing to accept our fair share of responsibility in any attempt to reduce the federal deficit. However, the cuts for the Medicare program proposed by the Administration once again go *far* beyond any sense of fairness and proportion. Consequently, health care providers will be asked to absorb much more than their fair share of the reductions. The Administration and Congress should note that the Medicare Hospital Insurance Trust Fund does *not* contribute to the federal deficit. Payments to hospitals under Medicare do not come from general revenues; they are financed by a payroll tax. The pending bankruptcy of Medicare can no longer be held out as a legitimate reason for drastic cuts in the program . . .

Hospitals understood the prospective payment law to be a contract. We have kept our part of the contract, and the system is working. However, if Congress unilaterally changes this contract by freezing or reducing hospital payments, then hospitals can hardly be expected to endorse the program.[74]

Policy makers ignored the hospital industry's complaints[75] and subordinated Medicare payment policy to larger federal budget imperatives by ratcheting down the annual updates (or increases) to Medicare's DRG payment rates.[76] After the first two years of the PPS's operation, in which hospitals received annual net payment increases of 4 percent, Congress directed HCFA to increase DRG rates a mere 0.5 percent in 1986 and 1987.[77] As a result, hospitals' Medicare PPS margins declined considerably (see figure 3.1). According to ProPAC's chairman, Stuart Altman, "We came to realize what was going on with regard to DRG-creep and hospitals' very substantial windfalls in the early years of the DRG system, so in '86 there began a whittling down phase of 'taking it back,' so to speak, from the hospitals."[78]

The key to Congress's ability to extract huge savings from Medicare was the budget reconciliation process. Leon Panetta, chair of the House Budget Committee in the 1980s, observed that the reconciliation process "scared the hell out of" the hospital and other industries.[79] According to Lisa Potetz, a senior hospital analyst on the Senate Finance and House Ways and Means Committee at the time, congressional leaders came to view Medicare's PPS as the most effective tool for simultaneously reducing fiscal deficits and increasing spending in other areas of the budget (particularly Medicaid):

Oh, God, we had these *huge* deficits at the time! And, conveniently, we now had a system in place, the PPS, that had a lot of levers that you could pull in order to generate a tremendous amount of savings. By just reducing the update factor for DRGs or by making small changes to the adjustment for teaching hospitals, you could generate a *tremendous* amount of savings. So, yes, there was this sort of "annual ritual" of tweaking Medicare's update factor.

The other thing to keep in mind was that if you had a pure budget bill that consisted only of tax increases and budget cuts to meet the deficit reduction targets, everyone would have been miserable. But these [reconciliation] bills . . . offered the opportunity to increase spending in other areas as part of a bigger package . . . We did a lot to increase Medicaid coverage in those years. And it was done by saying, "Well, if you have to cut *x* dollars out of Medicare, why not cut *x* + something and do some good things that you'd want to vote *for*."[80]

Using the budget reconciliation process to systematically reduce Medicare spending on hospital care also made for good politics. Hospitals do not vote, but Medicare beneficiaries do. Hence, reducing payments to hospitals has always been viewed by Congress as preferable to making changes that would directly affect Medicare beneficiaries' access to medical care.[81] Manipulating the PPS for larger budgetary purposes became irresistibly attractive to policy makers, because "Medicare was *the* cash cow!" as Robert Reischauer, former head of the Congressional Budget Office, recalls. "There is a very simple reason for this and that is that Congress could get credited for deficit reduction without directly imposing a sacrifice on the public . . . And to the extent that the reduction actually led to a true reduction in Medicare services, it would be difficult to trace back to the Medicare program or to political decision-makers."[82]

Ratcheting down the annual increase in hospital payment rates had a noticeable impact on Medicare's short- and long-term financial condition. The program's average annual increase in hospital spending went from 16.2 percent between 1980 and 1983 to just 6.5 percent between 1984 and 1987 (see table 3.1). Part of this reduction was due to a larger, economy-wide reduction in inflation. But the growth rate of real (inflation-adjusted) Medicare Part A spending still decreased substantially from 5.4 percent annually between 1980 and 1985 to just 1 percent annually between 1985 and 1990.[83] As a result, total expenditures from Medicare's Hospital Insurance Trust Fund were approximately 20 percent lower by the end of the decade than policy makers had expected shortly before the PPS went into effect.[84]

Using the PPS for fiscal purposes fostered an antagonistic relationship between Congress and the hospital industry. Conflict over hospital data escalated and occasionally grew vitriolic.[85] Hospitals increasingly sought to withhold from Congress requested financial information concerning their overall profit margins.[86] They concluded that Congress only meant to use the information to justify further reductions in DRG payment rates.[87] The gamesmanship over hospital data led Congress to rely more and more on ProPAC to provide analysis that would show which parts of the hospital industry could afford lower Medicare reimbursement rates.

ProPAC as Both Independent Analyst and Political Buffer for Federal Legislators

As Congress turned increasingly to Medicare's PPS as a tool in its budget reconciliation process, its need for timely data and analysis grew considerably. The logical organization for providing this kind of information would have been the HCFA, given its role as chief administrator of both Medicare and Medicaid. But by the early 1980s, "HCFA was now somebody Congress doesn't trust," says Paul Rettig, staff director to the House Ways and Means Health Subcommittee from 1976 to 1985.[88] The legislative branch's distrust of the executive branch[89] led many members of Congress to seek out their own independent sources of data analysis and information. (The Congressional Budget Office is another product of this desire for independent data analysis and expert advice.) Furthermore, HCFA was struggling at the time with all of its responsibilities, recalls Sheila Burke.[90]

Consequently, in 1983, Bob Hoyer, a staff member of the Senate Finance Committee, developed a proposal for an independent commission to advise the secretary of HHS and Congress on how to update Medicare's PPS.[91] It became known as the Prospective Payment Assessment Commission.[92] According to David Abernethy, staff director of the House Ways and Means Subcommittee on Health, Congress developed ProPAC in order to have an independent staff with analytic capacity necessary to give Congress better data.[93] ProPAC's rise to prominence rankled some staff members of HCFA, who often felt that their own substantive work on Medicare's PPS was overshadowed by ProPAC. "Our main frustration with ProPAC was that they had a ready venue and ability to get their work out to the public, whereas we didn't," recalls Phil Cotterill, a senior staff member of HCFA's Office of Research. "Our reports to Congress took a long time to get cleared politically within the executive branch, so in fact there were times that our reports were never ultimately sent to Congress because we couldn't get clearance."[94] The frequent delays in obtaining political clearance for its reports contributed to HCFA's declining credibility in Congress.

In addition to providing expert independent advice, both Hoyer and Burke saw ProPAC as meeting another critical need: buffering members of Congress from political pressure.[95] According to Julian Pettengill, "Anytime that you have an organization like ProPAC, it's partly to provide cover to members of Congress. ProPAC can say, 'Here's what we think would be good policy.' That puts the member in a position to say, 'Well, ProPAC says this is good policy. I can take it or leave it. So if I want to do it and I think it's a good idea, I can do it. If I don't want to do it, I can just ignore it.' What a beautiful world that is. ProPAC can be the 'bad guy' and, even better, nobody on ProPAC thought that was a problem."[96] The key to ProPAC was that it was free to be nonpartisan and analytical, which added an element of legitimacy and objectivity to Congress's annual adjustment of Medicare's PPS. "The quality of our staff and our independence were critical," notes Stuart Altman, ProPAC's chairman until 1995. "No one politically bothered us."[97]

ProPAC also became a major political player by virtue of the fact that its annual recommendations to Congress came at key moments of the budget reconciliation process. ProPAC gave Congress many of the recommendations and policy alternatives that Congress wanted at the time and in the form that it needed them.[98] "I don't know how many people on the Hill would be up front in admitting this," recalls the AHA's Rick Pollack. "But they would sort of have a hole in the budget target to reconcilia-

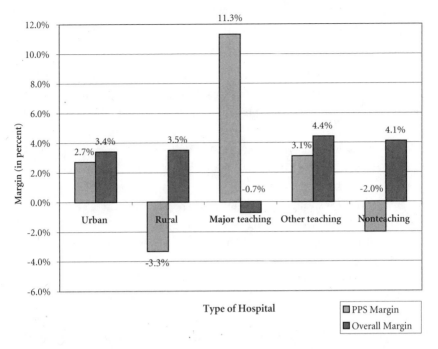

Figure 3.2. Aggregate PPS versus Overall Margins, by Type of Hospital, 1988
Source: Guterman, Altman, Young, "Hospitals' Financial Performance," 132, exhibit 7.

tion . . . and they'd save the PPS update factor to be the last thing to be determined and say, 'Okay, we gotta save a billion bucks over three years, so let's just make this tweak to Medicare's payment system or that tweak.' At the end of the day, it was legislated in the back rooms and it was all a budget number."[99]

ProPAC's initial mandate was to analyze how the PPS should be amended, year by year, to add new DRGs if needed, to change payment rates, and to make suggestions to Congress on how to incrementally improve the system.[100] Its first report came out in 1986, the same year of Congress's contentious hearings with hospital representatives over the industry's "excessive" Medicare profits in the early years of the PPS.[101]

But as Congress began to use Medicare's PPS as a budgetary device, ProPAC's mission broadened to assess "major recent changes in health care of which the PPS is a part but not necessarily the cause."[102] Policy makers wanted to know how the ratcheting down of annual increases in DRG payment rates was affecting specific groups of hospitals (e.g., urban, rural, teaching, for-profit, not-for-profit) within the hospital industry.[103] When they found that hospitals' PPS and overall margins varied wildly across different hospital groups (figure 3.2), ProPAC recommended and Congress initiated a policy of "targeting" Medicare hospital payments more selectively.[104]

Targeting Medicare Payments to Hospitals within a National System of "Rough Justice"

The great weakness in a national payment system like the PPS is the flip side of its great strength: by instituting a prospective model of nationally standardized payment rates, it is not very selective. A for-profit hospital in the affluent suburbs has a fundamentally different cost structure and mix of payers than that of a public, inner-city community hospital. So paying them the same, wage-adjusted price for a given DRG struck many policy makers as unfair,[105] especially when Medicare profits were unevenly distributed during the PPS's phase-in period (see figure 3.2). The gap in profit margins between the wealthiest 5 percent and the poorest 5 percent of all hospitals increased by almost 40 percent during the PPS's first three years of operation.[106]

Policy makers originally designed Medicare's PPS to be a blunt but effective instrument for saving money and changing hospital behavior. Their goal was to move to a single national set of payment rates for all hospital services and procedures that would foster a market-like environment between hospitals that did not previously exist. The "rough justice" inherent in a single national payment system would make hospitals compete under fixed prices, forcing them to lower their costs in order to break even or make a profit. Abolishing the program's tradition of "cost +" payments to hospitals would lead to reduced Medicare expenditures (or increased Medicare savings).[107]

The trick for policy makers, though, was to figure out how to adjust Medicare's payment system at the margins while keeping its fundamental structure and incentives intact. For example, in the original PPS legislation, Congress included an increase in DRG payment rates to teaching hospitals to cover their comparatively larger overhead costs of medical education. It also included a higher payment rate for urban hospitals than rural hospitals based on Medicare cost report data that showed that the average urban hospital's costs per case were approximately 40 percent greater than the average rural hospital's costs per case (reflecting, among other things, different wage rates for nurses and other hospital personnel).[108] Soon thereafter, policy makers enacted other adjustments. In the Consolidated Omnibus Reconciliation Act of 1985 (COBRA), they delayed the PPS's transition to national rates by one year, added an increase in payment rates to hospitals that served a disproportionate share of poor patients (disproportionate share hospitals, or DSH), and reduced, albeit modestly, the system's payments to teaching hospitals.[109]

A congressional requirement that complicated the PPS's task of achieving financial "rough justice" was that of "budget neutrality," which meant that whenever policy makers wanted to financially help one set of hospitals, they had to take funds away from other hospitals.[110] This zero-sum arrangement increased the hospital industry's internal fragmentation and contributed to the PPS's increased politicization.[111] The category of (DSH), in particular, became less of an analytically or geographically justifiable entity and more of a political one.[112] "The rationale for making the DSH adjustment was that urban hospitals with significant low-income populations had a different cost structure from other urban hospitals," observes Linda Magno, former director of HCFA's Division of Hospital Payment Policy (1985–88). "The same thing is *not* true with rural hospitals that treat significant numbers of poor people, but there are a lot of senators from rural areas and they were not going to let this adjustment just be made for urban hospitals."[113] So, in 1986, Congress provided for separate rates of higher Medicare payments for urban *and* rural hospitals that served a disproportionate share of poor patients, as well as for those rural hospitals that acted as large "referral centers" with more than five hundred beds.[114]

Policy makers' categorical adjustments to the PPS adjusted the focus of Medicare's primary mission. The assumption that the program should only pay for its own beneficiaries' care "fell by the wayside pretty fast, and particularly so after the Senate was regained by the Democrats in 1986," notes David Abernethy.[115] Medicare had already evolved into a vehicle for the general subsidization and expansion of America's health care system. But the PPS greatly expanded and increased the program's role in funding medical education, research, and community service (the care of disadvantaged, vulnerable, and geographically remote patients). Serious cost-control efforts did not create Medicare's role in medical education, research, and community service. What they did create, however, were cost constraints on hospitals, which complained and made their concerns visible and explicit.[116] "The larger point is that the PPS created a dynamic or a view among many members of Congress in which Medicare was no longer just a policy for financing health care; it became a form of political pork," says the AHA's Rick Pollack.

> It did so, in part, because there were enormous inequities that quickly developed under the PPS, but also because simplicity was something everyone was trying to achieve. Initially, policy makers were trying to get to a standardized payment rate that would apply to almost every hospital in the country by adjusting for only two things: geographic differences in wages and differences in hospitals' case-mix [the severity of their patients' illnesses], which was really the DRG piece of PPS. But, over time, efforts to achieve equity in good faith complicated everything. You went from a system that was supposed to be relatively

straightforward to a kind of Rube Goldberg thing. So many adjustments were attached to the PPS that the whole notion of fixed prices—as part of a standardized system to promote competition for better or for worse—ceased to exist. It became Balkanized . . . And we were all culpable—the hospital associations, Congress, as well as the administrative agencies—in endlessly tinkering with the PPS, again, in good faith.[117]

Ultimately, as Pollack suggests above, the increased emphasis on "targeting" a greater proportion of Medicare's hospital payments made the PPS far more political than policy makers ever intended. It also made Congress more reliant on ProPAC's analysis to see if the changes were having their desired effect.[118] This elevated ProPAC's profile and vastly increased its influence on policy makers' annual adjustments to Medicare payment policy.[119] ProPAC and Congress became increasingly concerned with how changes in Medicare payment policy would affect, directly and indirectly, the rest of the U.S. health care system. "The key to good health policy rarely involves the simple answer to a simple question," ProPAC's leaders argued. "Understanding the interaction between Medicare and other sources of payment and their relationship to the cost of care is critical to the development of hospital payment policy, because these are forces that affect both the availability and quality of hospital care not only to Medicare beneficiaries but to all Americans."[120]

The advent of Medicare's PPS transformed the U.S. hospital industry. After more than a decade of efforts, policy makers finally succeeded in gaining temporary control of Medicare's spending on hospital care. The pain the hospital industry experienced over the loss of its traditional cost-plus system of billing, however, was easily assuaged by its sizeable Medicare profits in the early years of the PPS. Hospital administrators successfully changed their institutions at the margins and generated unprecedented financial windfalls, which many of them used to expand their operations.

These were the "glory days" to be a hospital administrator, but they came at a price. Increased competition and the rise of corporate-oriented administrators separated the nation's hospitals for the first time into financial "winners" and "losers." Hospitals that were well run and had a favorable mix of well-insured patients made unprecedented profits. Conversely, hospitals that had an unfavorable mix of poorly-insured patients made unprecedented losses, often regardless of how well run they were.[121]

The growing divergence of hospitals' financial performances across the country contributed to the industry's internal fragmentation. Congress exacerbated this trend and also transformed its approach to fiscal policy making, when it turned to Medicare payment policy as a major tool for deficit reduction. By simply ratcheting down the annual increases in Medicare's payment rates to hospitals, Congress found that it could produce enormous budgetary savings and new funds for increased spending on other parts of the federal budget. In the process, the politics of Medicare payment policy became subordinated to the politics of fiscal policy. Medicare payment policy became increasingly political, something the PPS's creators had hoped to avoid.

Medicare Policy's Subordination to Budget Policy, Increased Hospital Cost Shifting, and the Rise of Managed Care

Congress whacks away at the hospital industry financially every time it gets the chance . . . When the hospitals are financially strong—when you look at their financial figures and see how well they're doing— that emboldens policy makers to say, "Hey, you know, they can take a hit."

—David Abernethy, Senior Medicare Analyst and Staff Director (1987–96), House Ways and Means Health Subcommittee

What happened in the late 1980s and early 1990s was that health care costs became such a significant part of corporate budgets that they attracted the very significant scrutiny of CEOs . . . More and more CEOs began saying, "G— d— it, this has to stop!" What was particularly attracting their attention was costs, and they very quickly got animated by their recognition of cost shifting.

—Robert Winters, Chair (1988–94), Health Care Task Force, Business Roundtable

The conventional wisdom on how managed care came to replace traditional indemnity insurance as the nation's dominant form of health coverage is that enlightened businesses led the way in responding to the emergence of market forces in health care in the 1990s.[1] A common textbook treatment of managed care's ascendancy puts it this way: "Transformation of the health care delivery system through managed care has been driven principally by market forces, and reinforced by government."[2] The irony is that the opposite sequence of events is a more accurate portrayal of what actually happened. As this chapter endeavors to show, the transformation of the U.S.

health care system with the rise of managed care was first triggered (albeit indirectly) by government actions and then driven by market forces. In other words, before business behavior was a cause of managed care's extraordinary growth, it was largely a response to, and an *unintended* consequence of, government policy making: in this instance, Congress's increasing use of Medicare's prospective payment system as a deficit-reduction device.

By examining the connections between Medicare's subordination to budget policy and the rise of managed care, we find that government policy makers in the late 1980s increasingly used the PPS as a powerful tool to address federal budget imbalances and increase spending on other government programs at the expense of health care providers (particularly hospitals but also a range of other providers). Instead of increasing the payroll tax for Medicare or making the program's beneficiaries pay more for their medical care, government leaders unintentionally increased less visible tax expenditures—tax revenue forgone—by precipitating a significant increase in health insurance costs for businesses.[3] In short, Congress and the Reagan and George H. W. Bush administrations made it clear that the government was only going to control Medicare's hospital costs; employers were on their own.[4] The hospital industry responded to Congress's systematic reduction in Medicare's generosity by increasing the costs hospitals charged to privately insured patients.[5] This billing behavior, most commonly referred to as "cost shifting," contributed significantly to large annual increases in private health insurance premiums.

Federal tax revenue was forgone in this budgetary process because private businesses simply absorbed the increased costs charged by hospitals. Over time, an increasing number of employers responded to the growing imperative for cost control by discontinuing more expensive indemnity insurance for their workers in favor of cheaper managed care alternatives. Nothing can transform an industry more quickly and profoundly than when the government—if it is an industry's single largest customer—dramatically alters how it pays for goods and services.

Congress and the Hospital Industry's Deteriorating Relationship

By the late 1980s, Medicare's PPS had succeeded, and in ways that policy makers had not originally anticipated. It effectively restrained Medicare's rate of spending increase,[6] and it also helped Congress address growing imbalances in the government's federal budget.[7] Moreover, the hospital industry was not harmed financially by the PPS's emergence as a deficit-reduction device, because Medicare's spending reductions—in the form of annual payment rate updates that were less than the rate of medical inflation—were from a "phony baseline," according to several leading analysts and congressional staff members.[8] In other words, the annual "market basket" inflation updates that the hospitals received were based on projected (rather than actual) increases, explains Linda Magno, HCFA's director of regulatory affairs and hospital payment policy at the time. "So hospital inflation would be forecasted to increase, say, 6.2 percent; but, in reality, for several years the actual increases were lower."[9] Representatives of the hospital industry would "still come in and say, 'You're cutting our rates,'" recalls Stuart Guterman. "But Congress never intended to have the hospitals receive payment rate increases at that level; it just created a phony baseline that was high in the federal budget's 'out-years,' so that members of Congress could then go back and claim budget savings when they 'fixed' it with lower payment rate increases."[10]

This fiscal technique became known as the "golden goose," because Congress used it to come up with annual "golden eggs" of Medicare savings for both deficit reduction and spending on other government programs, particularly Medicaid.[11] Medicare's baseline may have been "phony" in that policy makers did not have, in any individual year, a clear long-term intent about Medicare spending rates. And it may also have been phony in that policy makers never intended to have Medicare's rate of spending increase as much as the "market basket" of medical inflation would have allowed. But Medicare's baseline was not phony in other ways; it allowed policy makers—by adjusting downward from it—to both restrain the program's rate of spending growth and save an extraordinary amount of budgetary revenue that was put toward reducing annual deficits and increasing spending in other areas of the federal budget.[12]

During this period, then, budget imperatives essentially drove Medicare policy making.[13] "When people were looking for ways to lower the deficit," notes Representative Henry Waxman (D-CA), "Medicare became a particularly appealing program to reduce in terms of its spending because that's where the real money was!"[14] Policy makers' primary goal was to extract as much savings from Medicare as they could without significantly harming the hospital industry financially or compromising access for Medicare beneficiaries. "ProPAC and members of Congress would get the [market basket] number each year and they'd go through these shenanigans about hospital productivity and case mix, yada yada yada," recalls Allen Dobson. "But at the end of the day what they really looked at were hospitals' overall margins; if they were too high they would lower the rate of PPS increase, and if they were too low they'd increase the PPS payment rates."[15] What complicated this annual exercise was that the Medicare cost reports—which policy makers used to determine hospitals' financial margins—were typically eighteen to twenty-four months old.[16] And the difference between making decisions in "real time" versus "lag time" is significant. Adjusting Medicare payment rates was akin to trying to hit a moving target, because hospitals' financial situations had already changed (sometimes dramatically).

When the federal government's annual budget deficits continued to grow in the late 1980s, members of Congress sought even bigger Medicare savings.[17] "Medicare was the place to go," explains Rob Leonard, chief of staff for the House Ways and Means Committee from 1987 to 1993. "The Budget Committee would set global budget numbers or 'targets' in a fairly bipartisan manner and in consultation with the leaders of other congressional committees. But this frequently imposed a big part of the deficit reduction responsibility on Ways and Means, which invariably turned to Medicare Part A because it was more politically tolerable than taking from other entitlements."[18] The Budget Committee was not able to impose budget numbers or "targets" unilaterally. Usually the House Ways and Means and Senate Finance Committees established the targets for their own parts of the budget bills and negotiated with the Budget Committee. Nevertheless, Medicare was perceived as a huge "cash cow," to be milked for various purposes, according to the American Hospital Association's Rick Pollack and Robert Reischauer.[19] It was not solely a matter of cynicism. Medicare's spending was growing fast, making it a target for restraint for many leading budget analysts and policy makers.[20]

The other part of the pattern, notes Joseph White, was that Republicans would first go after beneficiaries, threatening to charge them more in order to balance the budget—thereby setting a budgetary "savings" target—which Democrats would then achieve by limiting payment increases to medical providers (first to hospitals and then later to physicians and other health care providers).[21] In order to pass the many deficit-reduction bills, however, congressional leaders needed a majority of senators and representatives. Yet conservative Republicans steadfastly refused to vote for bills that included tax increases, so every deficit-reduction package needed substantial support from at least some liberal Democrats (e.g., Henry Waxman). [22] The many Medicaid expansions between 1984 and 1990 were partly payoffs to Representative Waxman and other liberal Democrats—who were not overly concerned about medical providers receiving smaller payment increases—for going along with the Medicare savings. Thus, Medicaid expansions were part of the coalitional politics.[23] They were always much smaller than the Medicare savings, which were significant compared to what Medicare spending would have become without annual adjustments in the form of more modest payment increases.[24]

A casualty of Medicare policy's subordination to broader budget politics was the cordial relationship between Congress and the hospital industry, which deteriorated

TABLE 4.1

Hospitals' Inpatient (PPS) Medicare Margin* and Percentage of Hospitals with Overall Medicare Losses, 1984–92

	1984	1985	1986	1987	1988	1989	1990	1991	1992
Medicare's PPS margin*	14.5	14.0	9.5	6.6	3.9	1.4	−0.5	−1.4	−1.0
Percentage of hospitals losing money on their Medicare population	16.8	18.8	32.3	39.8	46.1	51.8	56.7	60.8	60.0

SOURCE: Prospective Payment Assessment Commission, *Medicare and the American Health Care System* (1994, 1996), 58, 68.

*Medicare's inpatient (PPS) margin = (hospitals' inpatient Medicare revenues − hospitals' inpatient Medicare costs) / hospitals' inpatient Medicare revenues

rapidly. Angry accusations of lying, fraud, and deceit arose on both sides.[25] Most of the spats occurred during public hearings on Medicare payment policy held by the Ways and Means Health Subcommittee.[26] The relationship between Congress and the hospital industry hit its nadir in 1989, when then AHA president Carol McCarthy and leading members of the Health Subcommittee argued vehemently over the issue of hospital closure rates.[27]

McCarthy and other hospital representatives may have "cried wolf" too frequently and too loudly, but over time the cumulative effect of Congress's repeated manipulation of Medicare payment policy for larger fiscal purposes did begin to affect hospitals financially (table 4.1 and figure 4.1). With the benefit of hindsight, acknowledges chairman of the Prospective Payment Assessment Commission Stuart Altman, "the hospitals had a legitimate case in the early 1990s that Congress had taken the industry's initial financial windfalls back and then some. We were heading into negative margins."[28] But because the data lagged almost two years behind, Altman was not persuaded at the time by the hospital industry's pleas.[29] Nor was Gail Wilensky, administrator of the Health Care Financing Administration in 1990, who maintained that there was "still some 'fat' in the hospital industry, which has hardly been starved for payments by Medicare."[30]

After years of Congress's ratcheting down the increases in Medicare's hospital payment rates, more and more hospitals began to lose money on their Medicare patients (particularly those with complicated diagnoses). They did so largely because the industry as a whole did not restrain its cost growth.[31] One major factor for hospitals' profligacy was the industry's general inclination for expansion of expensive medical services and hospital infrastructure regardless of demonstrated need.[32] "An awful lot of it has to do with C.E.O. ego," notes William McGuire, the chief executive of Kaleida Health, which owns several hospitals in New York. "We're kingdom builders as a group: 'I've got to have more beds than you do. I've got to have more hospitals than

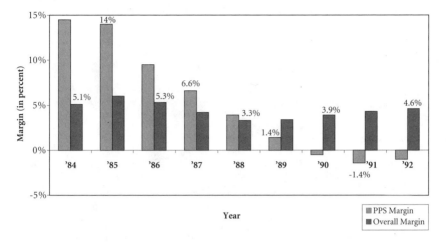

Figure 4.1. Hospitals' Inpatient (PPS) Medicare Profit Margin and Overall Profit Margin, 1984–92

Source: Prospective Payment Assessment Commission, *Medicare and the American Health Care System* (1996), 68.

you do. I've got to have the biggest empire.'"[33] Some members of Congress and HCFA wanted to incorporate reimbursement of hospitals' capital expenses into Medicare's PPS when the legislation passed in 1983, but the industry lobbied successfully to have capital expenses excluded from the PPS and reimbursed on the traditional cost basis until 1992.[34] The industry also succeeded in making the incorporation of hospitals' capital costs into the PPS a phased-in ten-year transition (until 2002).[35] As a result, the manner in which Medicare reimbursed capital expenses was a significant contributing factor to hospitals' rapid cost growth. According to Tom Scully:

We used to pay for capital in Medicare; it was a DRG add-on for capital expenditures. Well, if you're getting 40 percent of your revenues from Medicare and you want to build a new building, Medicare will pay for 40 percent of it, right? Then why not? So what you were getting all through the 1980s was a massive building spree up into the early 1990s and even through most of the '90s, because it was a ten-year phase out.

If you wanted to build a new hospital wing in 1990—even if you didn't have any patients for it—if you budgeted $100 million, Medicare would write you a check for $40 million. So what do you get? You got a hell of a lot of big new hospital wings, need them or not! This is one of the reasons we had such massive overcapacity in the hospital industry in the 1980s and for most of the '90s . . . You'd have to be an idiot *not* to put up a new building every couple of years, because Medicare paid for such a big part of it.[36]

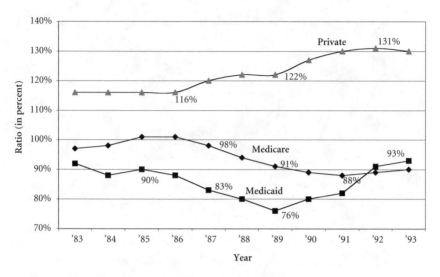

Figure 4.2. Hospital Payment-to-Cost Ratio by Payer, 1983–93

Source: Prospective Payment Assessment Commission, *Medicare and the American Health Care System* (1994), 29.
  Note: Medicare's payment-to-cost ratio in this table contrasts with the PPS margins in figure 5.1 and table 5.1. This is attributable to the broader scope of the payment-to-cost ratio, which reflects payments and costs for *all* Medicare services (inpatient and outpatient acute care, medical education programs, and hospital-based postacute care). See Guterman, Ashby, and Greene, "Hospital Cost Growth Down," 139, n. 14.

Hospitals' costs per case increased at an average annual rate of 8.6 percent between 1986 and 1992, more than 4 percent above the economy's overall rate of inflation.[37] As a result, by the end of the 1980s, hospitals' inpatient Medicare margins turned negative.[38] In 1991, the hospital industry's Medicare PPS margin and overall Medicare payment-to-cost ratio bottomed out at 1.4 percent and 88 percent, respectively (figure 4.2, and see table 4.1 and figure 4.1). These figures, however, did not show up in ProPAC's data analyses until two years later.[39]

The more policy makers used Medicare for larger fiscal imperatives, the more they sought to maintain the PPS's fairness by "targeting" a greater proportion of payment rate increases to specific segments of the hospital industry.[40] Rural hospitals and inner-city community hospitals that served a disproportionate share of indigent patients received badly needed increases beginning in 1990,[41] which helped stabilize Medicare and Medicaid's payment levels thereafter (figure 4.2).[42] With these targeted adjustments and many hospitals' ability to extract increased revenue from their private patients, select segments of the hospital industry were able to absorb Medicare's declining generosity.[43] According to Chip Kahn, former minority counsel (1986–93) for the Ways and Means Health Subcommittee, the hospital industry managed to find creative ways to compensate for less generous Medicare reimbursement of inpatient acute care.[44]

Hospitals Increase Their Cost Shifting
(or Price Discrimination or Differential Pricing)

When the 1990s began, the majority of hospitals were losing money on their Medicare patients.[45] According to ProPAC's chairman, Stuart Altman, they responded largely by turning to privately insured patients to make up for these losses, as well as for an increasing share of their Medicaid losses and unreimbursed charity care (figure 4.2).[46] Uwe Reinhardt has referred to this behavior as a form of "indirect taxation," whereby the public sector spreads "its constrained budgets over more people by paying prices below fully allocated costs for the health it finances—a practice commonly known as 'cost shifting.'"[47] Profits from private payers helped offset hospitals' losses on their inpatient Medicare population.[48]

In effect, cost shifting occurs when a hospital must increase prices charged to all payers to make up for shortfalls in reimbursement from some payers.[49] Hospitals have long received higher payments relative to costs from some payers than from others.[50] And surplus funds from at least some private payers have always been the primary method of financing hospitals' bad debts and charity care.[51] But cost shifting, explains Guterman, "refers to the relationship between changes in the prices paid by different groups; that is, an increase in losses (or a decrease in gains) from one source creates pressure to generate an offsetting increase in revenue from another source."[52] "Price discrimination" or "differential pricing" might be more accurate terms for this kind of hospital billing,[53] but ProPAC and health care analysts settled on "cost shifting" in the late 1980s, and it has remained the default nomenclature ever since.[54]

Economists argue that true cost shifting can only occur if two conditions are met. First, a hospital must have sufficient market power to raise prices. Second, the hospital not only has to have market power, but it must not have been fully utilizing it; if it had been fully utilizing its market power, it would have no ability to raise its prices still more.[55] Perhaps because the term *cost shifting* is open to competing definitions and conceptualizations, analysts often reach different empirical conclusions when researching the phenomenon. Some researchers reviewing data from the late 1980s and early 1990s could not find evidence of public- to private-payer cost shifting.[56] Conversely, a different set of researchers reviewing data from the 1980s and early 1990s found that lower Medicare prices were universally associated with statistically significant increases in hospital payments from private payers.[57]

Either way, most health economists agree that cost shifting exists. "It belongs to that group of actions, like predatory pricing," explains health economist Michael Morrisey, "that can exist but for which the underlying costs and benefits make most economists skeptical that an organization could successfully make it work."[58] What supports this economic theory is that hospitals essentially have to accept all Medicare patients, which constrains the options available to them.[59] As Kahn notes, "Hospitals can sword-rattle, but basically they can't walk away. Some specialties on the physician side can really marginalize their Medicare business, but that is rare thing for a hospital to be able to do regardless of where it's located."[60] Because hospitals take all Medicare patients, they may have no choice but to try to increase revenue from other payers. Thus, the economic debate turns semantic over whether differential pricing is framed in terms of "cost shifting," "cross-subsidization," or "price discrimination," because of the assumption that hospitals are "revenue maximizers," according to Donald Young, former executive director of the Medicare Payment Advisory Commission:

> And under a theory of revenue maximization, there is no such thing as cost shifting. Hospitals will get as much money as they can from as many places as they can. On the other hand, hospitals are still human service organizations; they operate in a community, many of them with a community board of trustees. And there are definitely limits to what these boards want their hospitals to do in order to maximize revenue. So most community hospitals would not go out and foreclose on somebody's home and put them out onto the street, because of the bad publicity it would generate. But a for-profit business would be more likely to do that, particularly a for-profit business that's three thousand miles away. Invariably, what hospitals will and won't do and how far they will go depends on how they are doing financially. But there have been cross-subsidies within our health care system from day one.[61]

Hospitals can and do exercise differential pricing in part because, like other service industries, they have high fixed costs and low variable costs.[62] In other words, the majority of a hospital's costs are consumed by its infrastructure and staff salaries (particularly nurses'), which do not change much depending on the amount of care the hospital provides. This kind of cost structure invites internal cross-subsidization, because it is very hard to disentangle precisely how much each and every individual medical service actually costs a hospital.[63] Other fixed costs include buildings, maintenance, utilities, equipment, capital, and some salaried labor costs. Variable costs are those that change with output.[64] Examples include medication, food, medical tests, and disposable supplies. On average, a hospital's fixed costs account for 75 to 85 percent of its total costs, whereas its variable costs account for 15 to 25 percent, depending on the type of hospital (teaching hospitals have the highest fixed costs because many of their physicians are salaried professors).[65]

Most hospitals' cost structures encourage creative billing practices, because hospital administrators essentially have two options for managing financial risk and maintaining their operations. The first is to reduce the cost per unit of each individual medical service. The second option is to increase reimbursements.[66] Because the majority of hospitals' costs are fixed and difficult to reduce other than by shrinking the number of salaried staff or closing whole departments, most hospital administrators have traditionally chosen to first pursue the latter option—increasing reimbursements from whichever payers they can—when faced with growing financial constraints.[67] According to James Mongan, CEO of Partners HealthCare in Boston, hospitals faced with serious cost pressures "are either going to go under or they're going to get it from their private payers."[68]

The hospital industry's Medicare PPS margins turned negative from 1990 to 1992 (see table 4.1 and figure 4.1), but it managed to maintain an overall profit margin of between 3 and 5 percent, primarily through cost shifting.[69] Evidence of hospitals' use of cost shifting even came in the form of public confession. In a written reply to a series of questions posed by the Senate Labor and Human Resources Committee, the AHA admitted that hospitals routinely shifted some of their costs to privately insured patients who then paid inflated bills.[70] Michael Bromberg, President of the Federation of American Hospitals—which represents the nation's investor-owned, for-profit hospitals—also admitted that hospitals regularly increased charges to private patients to compensate for reduced reimbursement for public patients.[71] The only surprising thing is how long it took for employers to pay attention to the resulting rise in their health insurance costs.[72]

Employers' Delayed but Dramatic Response

Both businesses and commercial insurers had long recognized the practice of cost shifting prior to the PPS's implementation,[73] but this form of cross-subsidization had traditionally remained at a modest enough level to avoid open conflict.[74] From 1984 to 1993, though, the average annual increase in per capita cost to privately insured patients was 22.7 percent more than the rate of increase in per capita cost to Medicare beneficiaries for the *same* hospital services.[75] Hospitals' payment-to-cost ratio for private payers peaked in 1992 at 131 percent (see figure 4.2). In more competitive markets without a large government presence, cost shifting of this magnitude would not and could not occur.[76] But medical providers are second only to defense contractors in their dependence on government payments, which provide approximately 45 percent of their total revenues.[77] So as Medicare and Medicaid tightened their reimbursement policies in the late 1980s and early 1990s, "they paid hospitals less than the hospitals believed was a fair share of total hospital expenses," notes health economist Rashi Fein. "Hospitals reacted by increasing charges to other payers, especially to commercial insurance carriers, in order to cover the shortfall in total receipts. In turn, private insurers raised their premiums in order to, as they would put it, 'subsidize' patient care only partly paid for by government."[78]

Employers recognized that, although cost shifting might be socially beneficial, the benefits did not accrue to their own individual firms,[79] especially when their health care costs skyrocketed in the late 1980s.[80] The cost of private health insurance premiums increased 90 percent between 1987 and 1993, which exceeded the 28 percent rise in workers' wages and salaries during this same period.[81] The subsequent drop in employer-provided health insurance coverage was pronounced.[82] From 1988 to 1993, the rate of employer coverage for the working poor fell 7 percentage points—from 51 percent to 44 percent.[83]

With the growth of hospital cost shifting and the related increase in the cost of private health insurance premiums (figure 4.3),[84] businesses concluded that their involvement in subsidizing the U.S. medical system had fundamentally changed.[85] A survey of 1,500 corporate chief executives in 1990 showed that of the health care issues with which executives were very concerned, "rising health insurance premium costs" ranked first.[86] The problem of escalating private insurance premiums was not new, but cost shifting exacerbated it and contributed significantly to unprecedented annual premium increases—often in excess of 20 percent—in the late 1980s.[87] Hewitt Associates, a benefits consulting firm, identified cost shifting as the single leading source of health plan premium increases in 1987 and 1988.[88] And "it will continue as long as the public sector payers know that the business community is a bunch of patsies and is accepting the cost-shift," said Walter Maher, director of federal relations for the Chrysler Corporation, in 1992.[89]

What is arguably most important about the concept of cost shifting is the extent to which employers believed it largely explained their rapidly increasing health care costs and then made health insurance decisions based on those beliefs.[90] Made prominent by ProPAC's reports on Medicare in the late 1980s and early 1990s (which repeatedly maintained that the phenomenon was large and growing), cost shifting emerged as the dominant explanation among employers for the rapid increase in private sector health insurance premiums.[91] "It became *the* mantra among employers," according to former vice president of the National Association of Manufacturers Sharon Canner.[92] Her colleague at the time, Christopher Bowlin (NAM's director of human resources policy), concurs: "Cost shifting was in every third sentence of employers' discussions about what to do with rising health care costs in the early '90s. It was considered *the* problem that we needed to address."[93] Representative John Dingell even initiated congressional hearings in 1991 to investigate Humana's and other hospitals' "controversial practice of cost shifting."[94] David McFadden argued that the

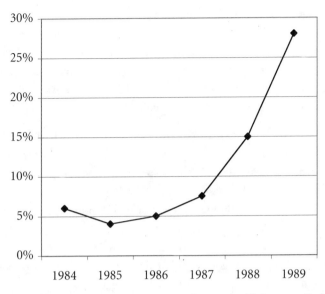

Figure 4.3. Average Annual Percentage Increase in Indemnity Health Insurance Premiums, 1984–89

Source: KPMG and A. Foster Higgins and Co., Inc., *National Survey of Employer-Sponsored Health Plans, 1981–1991.* http://mercerhr.com/ushealthplansurvey.

notorious "$7 aspirin" (a hospital's charge of $7 for a single aspirin tablet) had become an infamous legacy and a potent symbol of cost shifting.[95] And Malcolm Gladwell maintained in the *Washington Post* in March 1992 that cost shifting was one of the biggest reasons for the rapid increase in private health insurance costs.[96]

Employers' concerns over cost shifting peaked following the publication of an influential report to the Healthcare Financial Management Association in summer 1992 by Lewin/ICF. The report claimed that rising health care costs "were being allocated unevenly because some stakeholders are better than others at insulating themselves from paying their fair share of the costs," according to Allen Dobson and HFMA president Richard Clarke. "Stakeholders with significant purchasing power and those who purchase coordinated care are moving to protect themselves from what they believe is an untenable situation, leaving others, particularly small business and non-group purchasers, to fend for themselves. An important aspect of this interplay of stakeholders is the cost-shifting phenomenon."[97] As Dobson and Clarke argued, businesses and employers were essentially paying a "sick tax" to cover the additional costs that providers were shifting to them.[98]

As chairman of the Prudential Insurance Company and head of the Business Roundtable's Health Care Task Force between 1988 and 1994, Robert Winters had a unique vantage point from which to observe cost shifting. The Business Roundtable is an association of chief executive officers of the country's biggest companies, with a combined workforce of more than ten million employees.[99] Thus, the extent to which its members believed that cost shifting was primarily to blame for the nation's rapidly increasing private health care costs reflects how widespread the explanation had become throughout the entire business community. According to Winters:

> What happened in the late 1980s and in the early 1990s was that health care costs became such a significant part of corporate budgets that they attracted the very significant scrutiny of CEOs . . . More and more CEOs [were] saying, "G— d— it, this has to stop!" What was attracting CEOs' attention was costs, and they very quickly got animated by their recognition of cost shifting. So CEOs started to say: "Hey, providers are shifting costs to us to pick up the expenses that they had incurred for uninsured and underinsured patients. That's not fair. That's the government's job. The government should pay it and they'll tax people for it, tax us some, tax citizens some, tax property some, I don't care. But it's *not* fair to make my corporation and my shareholders pay for the care of people outside of our company . . . So, as I said before, CEOs finally began saying, "G— d— it, this has to stop!"[100]

Ultimately, the U.S. health care system stumbled when double-digit increases in health insurance premiums coincided with the recession of the early 1990s. As Uwe Reinhardt notes, "Eventually, the increasingly desperate American employers began to reevaluate the open-ended social contract they had written and supported for so long, and they looked around for an alternative deal. That deal was known as 'managed care.'"[101]

The Managed Care Revolution Takes Off

Managed care as a term hardly existed until the early 1990s. Yet the origins of managed care, prepaid group practice, stretched back more than fifty years and were rooted in a West Coast sense of progressive idealism. The direct forerunners of the HMOs that arose in the 1980s were founded in the late 1930s by physicians who were disgruntled with traditional practice. Some, especially those in rural areas, were organized as consumer cooperatives.[102] The core concept of prepaid group practice involved a group of physicians who would emphasize preventative medicine among their patients. For a single payment per month, each member was entitled to all necessary medical care without extra charges as long as the member sought care from physicians working in the medical group. Rooted as they were in populism, these health plans were strictly nonprofit.[103] By the 1950s, prepaid group practices, such as Kaiser Permanente and Health Insurance Plan in New York, had established particular niches in a few, mostly urban, communities.

The American Medical Association and local medical societies, however, despised prepaid group practices and exerted enormous amounts of political, legal, and social pressure against them whenever possible. This pressure succeeded in keeping prepaid group practices marginalized at the outer fringes of American medicine. Consequently, they could only appeal to a limited number of individuals who preferred the group practice style, the comprehensive benefits, and the protection from out-of-pocket expenses that conventional insurers charged.[104]

Prepaid group practice probably would have remained a marginalized outpost within the U.S. health care system were it not for an ironic twist of fate. Looking for ways to control runaway health care costs in 1970, Nixon Administration health officials came upon the work of an iconoclastic pediatric neurologist from Minnesota by the name of Paul Ellwood, who coined the term *health maintenance organization (HMO)*. According to Ellwood, the federal government could begin prepaying for services under Medicare and Medicaid and use its resources to stimulate development of prepaid plans, notes Paul Starr.[105] Largely because HMOs relied on private-sector initiative rather than a new government bureaucracy, many Republican administration officials embraced the HMO concept. In early 1971, President Nixon announced a new national health strategy based on the expansion of HMOs. The centerpiece of his strategy was the HMO Act of 1973, which provided start-up grants and loans for HMOs.[106] The act required that businesses that had more than twenty-five employees and that already offered health insurance make HMOs available to their employees. The Nixon administration hoped more than 1,300 HMOs would be caring for roughly sixty-five million people by the early 1980s. These projections proved overly optimistic. By 1981, only about three hundred HMO plans were serving ten million members.[107] Despite concerted government support, managed care could not overcome formidable economic barriers to entering local markets or organized medicine's opposition.[108] Nevertheless, the Nixon administration's optimistic projections did not prove wrong, just off by about ten years.

Eventually, cost control in the public sector with the success of Medicare's PPS contributed significantly to inflation in insurance premiums in the private sector, which triggered the private sector's response: a massive switch to managed care (figure 4.4).[109] Once employers learned of the cost-saving potential of managed care, they quickly began abandoning their traditional indemnity plans.[110] The shift by big employers began with Allied Signal Corporation, which in 1988 moved all its employees from indemnity insurance into a Cigna HMO.[111] By 1991, Allied Signal had demon-

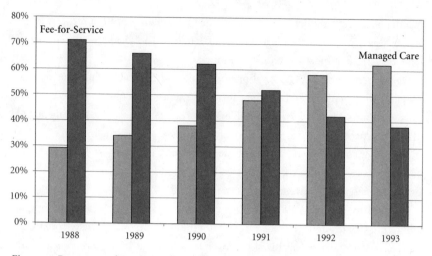

Figure 4.4. Percentage of Employees in Managed Care and Fee-for-Service Plans, 1988–93
Source: Kaiser Family Foundation and Health Research and Educational Trust, Employer Health Benefits Survey, 1999.

strated the cost-saving potential of managed care, reporting a 23 percent cut in health insurance expenditures.[112]

Employers' shifting of their workers away from fee-for-service health insurance was facilitated by the managed care industry's ability to quickly construct networks of participating providers.[113] Between 1988 and 1993, managed care organizations responded to employers' demands for more cost control by consolidating and applying extensive utilization review to their more traditional fee-for-service insurance offerings.[114] ("Utilization review" refers to the insurance company practice that decides if care recommended or provided to a patient is necessary.) The traditional managed care organizations, such as staff- or group-model HMOs (e.g., Kaiser Permanente), required significant expenditures in "bricks and mortar" when entering new markets, because they were vertically integrated organizations that operated their own physical facilities in different geographic locations, and whose physicians worked solely for the managed care organization.[115]

Beginning in the late 1980s, however, many new for-profit HMOs experienced rapid growth because they were "virtual organizations" or "organizations without walls," built largely on contractual (paper) relationships with community provid-·ers.[116] These new HMOs began competing with the traditional prepaid group practices by contracting with networks of private physicians called independent practice associations (IPAs). In this newer type of HMO, physicians would provide care for HMO patients in their own offices, not a shared clinic. This model kept health plans from having to invest in "bricks and mortar" or hire their own personnel. The IPA approach also enabled HMOs to enter new markets more quickly and with much lower capital expenses than the traditional prepaid group practices.

The initial shift to managed care had a self-reinforcing quality that fed back into the momentum away from fee-for-service insurance. Managed care organizations initially attracted and enrolled low-risk individuals who were least likely to object to restrictions on utilization of services and physician choice.[117] These low-risk individuals also tended to be healthier than the general population, so they did not increase spending on medical care; on the contrary, they increased the profitability of managed care organizations. So although the rates of change in premiums among the various forms of health insurance generally moved in tandem, premiums for fee-for-service indemnity insurance grew substantially more than managed care premiums between 1986 and 1991.[118] Moreover, the private health insurance market in the post–World War II era up to the mid-1980s essentially had been a "pooling equilibrium," according to health economists Mark Pauly and Sean Nicholson, "in which the risk of covering an individual patient's medical costs was spread out over a large pool of individuals who all paid generally the same, community-rated insurance premiums. Over 90 percent of employees had indemnity insurance, mostly with Blue Cross and Blue Shield, which experience rated only reluctantly," add Pauly and Nicholson. "This pooling equilibrium unraveled between 1984 and the early 1990s when [managed care] quadrupled its share of the large employer market."[119]

By expanding their provider base and involving in their systems more physicians whose predominant practice was fee-for-service, managed care organizations developed to the point that employers took them more seriously and found them significantly more attractive.[120] Why? Because by increasing their number of affiliated medical providers, managed care organizations essentially became more effective "managed *cost*" plans, which could negotiate lower prices on behalf of larger numbers of patients and then pass the savings on to employers.[121] Prior to this balance of power shifting temporarily to payers in the early 1990s, providers had set prices and determined fees in most markets.[122] In short, Medicare's success in controlling hospital prices encouraged the private sector to try to follow suit.

Policy makers' growing use of the PPS to both control Medicare's spending and reduce federal budget deficits led to a "paradox of liberal intervention." In seeking to control costs, notes sociologist Mary Ruggie, the government became "more involved in regulating the activities of both hospitals and physicians," not less.[123] Through a step-by-step expansion of government regulations in a political atmosphere that endorsed private enterprise and marketplace rate setting, she adds, Medicare's PPS enhanced the government's capacity to govern a sprawling health care system possessed of an endless appetite for additional spending.[124]

Much of the success in containing Medicare's costs, however, came at the expense of hospitals increasing their revenue from privately insured patients. Exactly how much hospital cost shifting was specifically caused by Medicare's PPS is difficult, if not impossible, to determine. Nevertheless, employers bought into the cost shifting argument made by ProPAC, health policy journalists, and others, regardless of how much empirical support there was for it. This confounds the causation question, because if employers *believed* that cost shifting was driving the inflation in their health care costs (and then acted on this belief), that is a powerful influence in its own right.

Moreover, causality comes in different forms.[125] To understand prospective payment, explains David Smith, the image of a river and flooding rains is helpful. The rain that comes down is the cost drivers—general inflation in nurses' salaries, overhead costs, bad debt—that continually raise the cost of medicine, and there are many tributaries—new medical technology, rising prices, more elderly patients—filling the river. The PPS functioned, in part, as a diverting dam that helped to keep the flood away from Medicare. Yet the water was simply diverted back into the river, to spill out elsewhere. In other words, only Medicare was (temporarily) sheltered from ever increasing medical inflation. After the PPS went into effect, a huge part of the medical establishment, Medicare, was no longer doing its part to absorb a significant portion of the river of ever-increasing medical inflation, flooding employers in the private sector who were left to make up the difference.[126]

This cost-shifting phenomenon became a major motivation for businesses to begin moving their workers into various forms of cheaper managed care. The responsibility for either paying more for medical care or accepting increased rationing, which the government chose not to accept, now fell squarely on employers and other purchasers in charge of health care spending.[127] They quickly moved many of their employees out of traditional indemnity insurance and into various forms of managed care. Yet HMOs sowed the seeds for future trouble by not fundamentally altering or improving the delivery of health care (as staff- and group-model HMOs had done for years in some areas of the country). Instead, insurers simply employed the term HMO and focused on using contracting leverage to both negotiate discounts from medical providers and impose distant controls on them. The health care that resulted from these new arrangements was hardly more "managed" than it had been under traditional indemnity insurance. For these reasons and others, the next chapter in the cost-controlling rationalization of U.S. health care would prove enormously unpopular and acrimonious.

CHAPTER FIVE

The Resource-Based Relative-Value Scale Reforms for Physician Payment

Although the "usual, customary and reasonable" concept may have been reasonable and workable as a basis for [physicians] billing individual patients, it has been a failure as a basis for reimbursement from insurance funds. Because it contains none of the limits or standards that are applied to other services covered by insurance, the charges for medical services have escalated, with little or no restraint, to the point at which current fee levels in several medical and surgical specialties are simply indefensible and deserving of public censure. In effect, usual, customary, and reasonable (UCR) has become a boondoggle.

—*Benson B. Roe, M.D.*, New England Journal of Medicine, *July 2, 1981*

Aside from being inequitable, confusing, and mysterious, however, the current system is alleged to have two major problems, which the RBRVS—it is hoped—will solve. First, expenditures for physicians' services are growing too fast, growing faster than spending for other medical care . . . The second major problem is that fees in the current system are distorted.

—*Jack Hadley,* Health Economist, *1991*

   With Medicare spending on hospitals under control, policy makers soon turned their focus to the nation's doctors.[1] Part of the political deal with the American Medical Association that helped create Medicare was to pay physicians based on physicians' own charges, rather than on the basis of fixed indemnity payments—a fee schedule—in which insurers maintained control of the prices of the services for which they were paying. A few local Blue Shield plans, whose boards of directors tra-

ditionally were dominated by physicians, had adopted what in private insurance par-
lance was called "usual, customary, and reasonable" (UCR) reimbursement.[2] Under
this approach, insurance payments made to physicians for services rendered were
based on the regular, "usual" charge of the physician, assuming the charge to be within
the range of "customary" fees in that geographic area for the same service, or if prece-
dent is lacking, to be "reasonable."[3] Because patients no longer had to pay most of the
charge out of pocket, but rather relied on their Blue Shield plan to pay physicians directly, the UCR payment system was a boon for physicians who continually raised
their usual charges. Because all physicians had incentives to raise their own charges,
(thereby raising the customary fees in an area), the UCR payment approach assured
that prices would rise continuously, seemingly without restraint.

Physician reimbursement based on UCR methods was actually rare until Medicare
adopted this approach.[4] It then spread rapidly through private insurance plans, beyond its initial limited use in Blue Shield plans. Medicare's adoption of UCR produced
some variations, both in terminology and in calculations. In its "customary, prevailing, and reasonable" (CPR) version, Medicare's payment for a service was an amount
equal to the least of three charges: (1) the actual, submitted charge, (2) the physician's
customary charge (that is, the median of the charges submitted by the physician for
that same service in the preceding year), and (3) the prevailing charge, which was the
seventy-fifth percentile of the distribution of the customary charges of all physicians
in the area for the same service.[5] The amount Medicare actually paid for the service
was called the "reasonable charge." It is not hard to see why analysts would regard this
system as "inequitable, confusing, and mysterious."[6] From the point of view of policy
makers, the bigger problem with the CPR system was that it rewarded physicians for
continually jacking up their charges.

Congress in 1972 had attempted to limit the incentive for physicians to keep raising their charges by placing onto the CPR payment method a limitation on annual
growth in prevailing charges known as the Medicare Economic Index (MEI). The MEI
reflected the annual increase in physicians' costs of doing business. The limit on permitted increases in prevailing rates did restrain increases in allowed charges and, in
effect, created an extremely complicated fee schedule, with some services constrained
by prevailing charge limits and others not so constrained.[7] Congress attempted to reinforce the effect of the MEI limitation, first in 1984 by freezing charges and then, later
in the decade, by making selective payment reductions in particular "overpriced" surgical procedures, such as cataract removal.[8]

Attempts to moderate spending by limiting physician fees without addressing aggregate expenditures for physician services were unsuccessful, however, because increases in the number of services physicians provided per beneficiary (volume) and

the average complexity and costliness of those services (intensity) continued to increase total spending.[9] Under the CPR reimbursement method, the annual growth rate of Medicare's spending on physician care between 1978 and 1987 had risen to the unsustainable annual compound rate of 16 percent.[10] In the late 1980s, Medicare's physician expenditures were growing at more than double the rate of its hospital expenditures.[11] This divergence in expenditure rates was partly driven by the hospital PPS's new incentives, which pushed more and more medical services out of inpatient hospital settings and into ambulatory settings, including physician offices.[12] By 1989, Medicare's Part B spending—most of which was for physician services—had become the single largest domestic program financed from general federal revenues.[13] The same kind of financial pressures that led to paying hospitals based on diagnosis-related groups drove the political imperative for policy makers to design and implement a new payment system for physicians.[14]

Rationalizing Medicare's Financial Relationship with Physicians

But in looking at designing a new system to address costs, policy makers also focused on other defects in the system used by Medicare to reimburse physicians. Under the CPR system, some services were reimbursed much more generously relative to the underlying costs of providing services than others. William Hsiao, a Harvard University researcher, had been studying physician competition under a Health Care Financing Administration contract in the late 1970s, when his research took a detour that proved hugely consequential. "Most of the physicians I interviewed," Hsiao notes, "told me that the prices of physicians' services were unfair."[15] He judged that the value of surgical procedures was overstated by much as four- to five-fold when compared to the value of a routine office visit.[16] Procedures that had become routine or automated as a result of advances in technology were especially profitable, because the rates that had been previously established were never adjusted downward when the same procedures became less costly and easier to perform.[17] Economists refer to these as "downward-sticky" prices. In a scathing critique of the payment system published in 1981 in the *New England Journal of Medicine*, Benson Roe, chair of the cardiothoracic surgery department at the University of California, San Francisco, described the impact of these downward-sticky prices for coronary artery bypass grafting (CABG):

> Historically, of course, there was justification for extraordinary fees in cardiac surgery . . . The early cardiac surgeons participated in the diagnostic studies and preoperative preparation, planned and directed the technical details of the

cardiopulmonary bypass, conducted the entire long operation, and personally supervised every detail of postoperative care, often spending late nights at the bedside. The circumstances were comparable to the challenges of aviation during World War I. Three or four cases a week was an exhausting endeavor in those days, and if extraordinary fees were ever warranted, that would have been the time.

But times have changed. Today, cardiac surgery, like commercial aviation, is provided on a huge scale with automated routines; although it remains highly complicated and fraught with danger, experience and improved methods have replaced "blood, sweat, and tears" with safety and seeming simplicity. Two or three open-heart cases a day are now common for many cardiac surgeons, and some do even more.[18]

Analysts calculated that with fees set high to reflect the initial difficulty of performing CABG surgery, thoracic surgeons could receive about $538,000 annually by performing just three bypass operations per week, or twelve hours of work weekly, based on the payment amounts allowed by Medicare in 1984.[19]

Hsiao and colleagues identified other factors that produced physician charges that were not consistent with those that would exist in a competitive market. They argued that because consumers differed in their sensitivity to prices, some services were priced much higher than others relative to their cost or value.[20] For example, patients might place a higher value on the work physicians provide in performing a minor surgical procedure than on the time spent in discussing with the patient management of a medical problem.

Variations in insurance coverage created distortions as well. Physician Mark Blumberg reviewed the available literature and found that insurance plans of the day typically covered hospitalizations and surgical procedures much better than outpatient visits and preventive services. That could lead to systematic distortion in what physicians charged for. "Some physician services had been systematically underpriced at times when physicians had considerable slack and there was little third party coverage," writes Blumberg. "There was an attempt to encourage new patients through underpricing of initial office visits and complete physical examinations. In any event, the marginal cost to a physician for his time when he has slack is negligible and any marginal revenue is welcome."[21]

Policy makers identified other important problems that had arisen under the CPR system. Prices across different geographic areas did not accurately reflect objective geographic differences in the cost of inputs such as rent and labor. In addition, varying implementation of the CPR system by different carriers (intermediaries for Medicare

Part A and administrators for Part B that receive and pay physician claims) over time resulted in different payments. That is, for surgical procedures, carriers paid a global surgical fee and had different rules for the extent of services the fee covered.[22] Policy makers held that a national fee schedule was needed to standardize the determination of prices across the country.

In short, physician charges for services were distorted because of the unique characteristics of local markets for physician services. Over time, Medicare's CPR reimbursement method—with the MEI limits providing a de facto fee schedule—effectively ratified these distortions.[23] Hsiao's original research for HCFA did not lead to immediate changes in physician payment policy, yet it did have an effect on a number of organized medicine's senior leaders. As Hsiao points out, they were growing concerned that "the medical profession was being torn asunder by different training and professional interests, and especially by the growing differences in income between specialties."[24]

With income disparities among the specialties increasing, primary care physicians such as general internists began to recognize that the CPR system worked against their interests. In 1981, the American Society of Internal Medicine (ASIM) published a white paper calling for the reduction of payment disparities between what they called "cognitive services" (e.g., nonprocedural physician services such as office visits and consultations) and surgical and other procedural services.[25] Relying on Hsiao's developing concepts, the ASIM called for Medicare payments based on the relative differences in physician service resource costs to produce each of the thousands of services physicians provide.

The American Medical Association ultimately lobbied against a Medicare fee schedule for physicians,[26] but until then it supplied expert advice to Hsiao's research team.[27] Hsiao received funding from Massachusetts' Medicaid program in 1984 to continue his research, which stimulated stronger interest in the medical and health policy communities, and he received substantial funding from HCFA in 1986 to develop an alternative physician reimbursement system that would make payments commensurate with the amount of effort involved in performing a medical procedure or service.[28] Work, Hsiao decided, "was a function of time spent, mental effort and judgment, technical skill and physical effort, and stress," explains Harvard surgeon and author Atul Gawande:

> He put together a large team that interviewed and surveyed thousands of physicians from almost two dozen specialties. They analyzed what was involved in everything from forty-five minutes of psychotherapy for a patient with panic attacks to a hysterectomy for a woman with cervical cancer. They determined

that the hysterectomy takes about twice as much time as the session of psychotherapy, 3.8 times as much mental effort, 4.47 times as much technical skill and physical effort, and 4.24 times as much risk. The total calculation: 4.99 times as much work. Estimates and extrapolations were made in this way for thousands of services. Overhead and training costs were factored in. Eventually, Hsiao and his team arrived at a relative value for every single thing doctors do.[29]

In the meantime, Congress tried to limit Medicare's escalating physician spending by instituting a freeze in payment rates between 1984 and 1986.[30] It only had a modest effect, though, because physicians compensated largely by increasing their volume of Medicare cases.[31] Congress responded by creating the Physician Payment Review Commission (PPRC).[32] Its mission was to provide technical advice for Congress on transforming Hsiao's research into a new payment method that would be accepted by the medical profession—an undertaking comparable to the implementation of hospital DRGs[33]—and to do so independently of the presidential administration and office (at that time, the Reagan administration).[34] In this capacity, the PPRC went a step beyond the advisory model that ProPAC had successfully promulgated to crafting policy that Congress could pass and HCFA could implement.[35]

In addition to laying the groundwork for an entirely new system of physician reimbursement, Congress also made some immediate decisions to alter CPR-based payments before a new fee schedule could be implemented. First, in the Omnibus Budget Reconciliation Act of 1987, based on recommendations from the PPRC, the Congress identified a number of "overvalued procedures," and implemented modest reductions in prevailing charges for them. PPRC recommended specific, high-frequency procedures, for example, CABG and cataract extraction, for payment reductions to achieve immediate savings based upon its assessment of the likely impact that a resource-based fee schedule would have on the prices for these procedures once implemented.[36]

Second, Congress replaced the payment freeze in 1987 with a new series of limits on how much physicians could increase their charges.[37] Referred to as maximum allowable actual charges (MAACs), the new limits essentially prohibited physicians from charging Medicare beneficiaries personally (or "balance billing" them)[38] more than 15 percent (subsequently changed a few times) above the prevailing fee for any service or procedure.[39] The MAACs were only supposed to last until the end of 1990, but Congress extended them until 1992 for financial and political reasons.[40] The MAACs were widely viewed—perhaps more in hindsight than at the time—as the physician equivalent of what the Tax Equity and Fiscal Responsibility Act had been to the hospitals, notes David Smith, "a regulatory scheme that would 'drive the doctors crazy,' and that would 'make life so difficult' that they would ask for and accept a more reasonable compromise, for instance a fee schedule."[41]

PPRC Recommends a New Physician Fee Schedule

Building on Hsiao's work, the PPRC ultimately submitted three recommendations to Congress in 1989 for overhauling Medicare's physician payment system.[42] First, it called for a relative-value scale that would raise reimbursement rates to some physicians and lower them to others by basing physician payments on the resources—work, time, and costs—required to provide services. This became known as the Resource-Based Relative-Value Scale (RBRVS). In brief, "The RBRVS was trying to mimic the competitive market, in which the cost of a product should come very close to the cost for producing that product," explains Hsiao.[43] Although the values of the RBRVS system were meant to simulate competitive market prices, it nevertheless was being adopted in Medicare as a complex and detailed set of administrative prices. In effect, the RBRVS was designed to replace a de facto fee schedule based on historically distorted physician charges with a new one that, arguably, better reflected actual production costs. Just as with hospital DRGs, the rhetoric of the market was invoked to create an improved administrative pricing system in Medicare.

The second major goal of the PPRC's recommendations was to restrain the overall growth rate of Medicare's physician expenditures.[44] As a volume control to keep physicians from offsetting lower reimbursement rates by simply performing more Medicare services, the PPRC called for annual expenditure targets. If total Medicare spending on physician services exceeded this target in one year, payment rates would be adjusted downward the following year. Policy makers referred to this mechanism as the volume performance standard (VPS).[45] The PPRC thought that the VPS, modeled after similar devices used in Germany and other countries to restrain spending,[46] would not only constrain expenditures, but do so in a desirable way by providing "an opportunity for physicians to help the program achieve its cost containment objectives through actions to slow the increase in utilization of services. A collective incentive would be given to the medical community to reduce services of little or no benefit to patients . . . Such a policy would encourage the leadership of medicine to become more active in the support of activities to better inform physicians of the medical benefits and risks of procedures and to play a more active and constructive role in peer review activities."[47] Although initially recommending an expenditure target for all physicians' services nationally, the PPRC expected the policy to evolve to incorporate a broader range of services and to include separate targets for regions and categories of physicians' services.[48] As it turned out, the VPS did evolve, but not in the ways envisioned by the PPRC.

Finally, concerned that physicians might respond to the first two initiatives by try-ing to charge their Medicare beneficiaries more out of pocket, the PPRC called for limits on how much physicians could charge Medicare beneficiaries in excess of the standard Medicare fee that had been in place since 1984 (with the previously described MAAC limits).[49] Four PPRC members called for a policy of requiring physicians to take mandatory assignment, that is, to accept Medicare allowed charges as their own charges and forgo the opportunity to balance bill the patient beyond the 20 percent share of the bill many Medicare beneficiaries face.[50] Not ready to recommend a pol-icy of mandatory assignment at that time, the PPRC nevertheless recommended a policy of strictly limiting how much—on top of the allowed charge—physicians could bill Medicare patients, a policy recommendation that was adopted and tight-ened over time.

Taken as a whole, the PPRC's recommendations were a signal to the medical pro-fession (especially to specialists) that Medicare policy objectives would now deter-mine the structure of the physician payment system as well as payment rates. Several surgical specialties immediately opposed the PPRC's recommendation because sim-ulations of Hsiao's new payment scale revealed that the average ophthalmologist could lose as much as 40 percent of current revenues, whereas the average family prac-titioner could receive more than a 60 percent increase in revenue (with all other spe-cialties falling somewhere in between).[51] Congress accepted the PPRC's recommen-dations and incorporated them as part of its 1989 budget reconciliation bill.[52]

The PPRC recommendation that most outraged organized medicine was the an-nual expenditure targets.[53] The AMA likened them to "rationing."[54] Physicians were so opposed to the expenditure targets that their opposition threatened to derail the entire proposal,[55] largely because the AMA had the support of most Republicans (particularly on the powerful House Ways and Means Committee).[56] What almost tipped the balanced in organized medicine's favor was that a leading Democrat, Rep-resentative Henry Waxman, supported their opposition to expenditure targets.[57] His objections could not be easily disregarded for a number of reasons, not the least of which was that the original idea for the PPRC came from one of his chief aides.[58]

High-ranking Bush administration officials desperately wanted tighter expendi-ture targets to help constrain the government's ever-increasing annual budget defic-its.[59] So it fell to Leon Panetta and Dan Rostenkowski (chairmen of the House Bud-get and Ways and Means Committees, respectively) to devise a plan for passing the legislation.[60] What they pulled off, recalls Tom Scully, "was the most amazing legisla-tive moment in my life and I've been doing this a long time."[61] Panetta and Rostenkowski's chiefs of staff created a "diversionary bill" that distracted Waxman and his staffers by allowing them to mark it up the way they wanted to in the House Commerce Committee. The trick was that select leaders of the House agreed in advance that the Commerce Committee bill would then be discarded for the "real" bill marked up by the Budget Committee, in which tighter expenditure targets were traded by Rostenkowski for increased funding from the Bush administration for teaching hospitals.[62] It was not, as Waxman noted later, a "procedure to be proud of."[63] But it worked. Congress passed the new physician fee schedule—together with annual expenditure targets—as the Omnibus Reconciliation Act of 1989, which became effective on January 1, 1992.[64]

Under the Medicare fee schedule that was fully phased in over ten years, beginning in 1992, a single fee is paid for each of the more than seven thousand services—such as hospital and office visits, surgical procedures, x-rays, and tests—delivered by physicians and certain other health professionals, regardless of the medical specialty providing the service. The fee was based on a relative-value scale, with each service's value determined according to three different types of resources required to provide each service. The physician work component of the scale provides payment for the physician's time, skill, and effort. The work value component was estimated by physicians, originally as part of the Hsiao research that HCFA commissioned and subsequently by members of physician specialty societies under the aegis of the AMA / Specialty Society's Relative-Value Scale Update Committee (RUC).[65] The second component, practice expense, provides payment for the expenses incurred in operating a practice, such as staff salaries, space, and equipment. Third, the professional liability component provides payment for the expenses physicians incur purchasing professional liability insurance. The values given to these three types of resources are adjusted by variations in the input prices in different markets, and then the total relative value is multiplied by a standard dollar amount—called the fee schedule's conversion factor—to arrive at the final payment amount.[66]

Transforming Medicare's financial relationships with hundreds of thousands of physicians was unprecedented. The RBRVS and related expenditure targets were extremely difficult to implement, according to HCFA's administrator Gail Wilensky, requiring an enormous mobilization of HCFA staff.[67] But when the new system finally began operation in 1992,[68] it triggered another seismic shift in American medicine. Just as DRGs had done less than a decade before with hospitals, Medicare's new fee schedule and expenditure targets shifted the balance of power between providers and the government, power that physicians had assiduously developed and solidified over decades.[69]

With the implementation of the RBRVS-based Medicare fee schedule, for the first

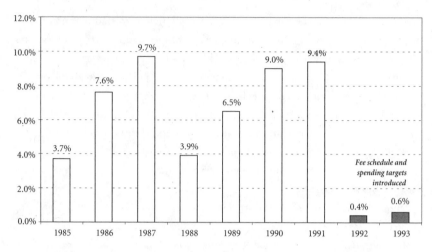

Figure 5.1. Growth in Volume and Intensity of Medicare Physician Services per Beneficiary, 1985–93

Source: GAO, "Medicare Physician Payments," (Washington, D.C.: Government Printing Office, 2002); 7, fig. 2. GAO-02-441T. www.gao.gov/cgi-bin/getrpt?GAO-02-441T (accessed May 10, 2006).

time ever, the government was able to regulate both the price and the volume of Medicare's spending on physician services.[70] The new expenditure targets went into effect immediately and had a noticeable impact (figure 5.1). In the five years after Medicare's fee schedule and expenditure targets went into effect, Part B spending rose at an average annual rate of just 4.4 percent (less than half the rate from the five-year period before the change).[71] Once the relative-value scale was fully in place, family and general practice physicians saw their Medicare fees increase by 36 percent, while ophthalmologists saw theirs decrease by 18 percent.[72]

Throughout most of the 1990s, Medicare's RBRVS-based fee schedule was viewed as a significant success by most observers. A sign of its acceptance is the fact that much more than with DRGs, the RBRVS system maintained by Medicare also became adopted by most private payers.[73] Before the RBRVS system, the private insurers that abandoned the inflationary UCR payment approach often used relative-value scales that had been based on historic charges, thereby perpetuating the alleged distortions among the various categories of services.[74] Private payers now typically rely on the RBRVS relativities, even if they often use different conversion factors to reflect local market factors that dictate their ability to negotiate fees with physicians.[75] Perhaps because organized medicine was given a major role in maintaining and updating the RBRVS system through the RUC,[76] physicians initially accepted the resultant shift in relativities of different services, even if they continued to strenuously object to expenditure limits.

An added benefit of the expenditure limitation mechanism was that it was formula-driven. Congress merely needed to tinker with some parts of the formula, based on recommendations from PPRC, and HCFA could make the necessary changes in the payment systems the contractors administered without any disruption in the flow of dollars to physicians for services rendered.[77] With control over budgetary expenditures for Medicare's Part B (physician services), Congress did not concern itself much with "winners and losers" among the medical profession. Congress and HCFA were more than happy to let the AMA preside over inevitable "food fights" within the profession after they cut the pie of physician expenditures. Having successfully limited physician expenditures, Congress did not need to include physician payment as a target of savings in the Balanced Budget Act of 1997 (see chapter 6), although, as we will see, the BBA made an important change in how the expenditure target was calculated.

That success obscured some of the inherent limitations of the RBRVS-based payment system. Many of these limitations had been observed before implementation of the new fee schedule but were mostly ignored in the near universal desire to do away with the difficult and fiscally unconstrained CPR payment system.[78]

A main difficulty with fee schedules is that they do not permit variation among physicians in absolute and relative fees. For example, it is hard to incorporate adjustments to the Medicare fee schedule to recognize higher quality and more efficiently produced services.[79] In the face of that limitation, policy makers and purchasers today have coined a new term, "pay for performance," for a potential approach to rewarding physicians and other providers for quality of care provided.[80]

More generally, paying on the basis of input costs ignores whether the services provide value for patients. Prior to the implementation of the RBRVS payment method, the assumption had been that what professionals decide to do with their professional time is the best determinant of value. Yet even in the mid-1980s some had argued that Medicare should set the relative values not just on how physicians combine inputs to produce services, but also on the value the fee schedule promotes in terms of benefit to beneficiaries and the program.[81] Relative values should reflect relative value, not merely resource costs. Today, with more than two decades of evidence that physician practice patterns and costs vary significantly without important differences in quality or patient satisfaction,[82] there is increasing recognition that purchasers, including Medicare, may not be getting their money's worth for their major investment in physician services.

Additionally, the initial redistribution of dollars away from procedures and toward evaluation and management services, a primary objective of the RBRVS system, has been frozen in place. Because of the continued introduction of new procedural services that are free to receive relative values unconstrained by the original values determined by the Harvard study, and because volume is increasing dramatically for radiology and other tests, the percentage of Medicare physician spending supporting evaluation and management services—for example, office and hospital visits and consultations—has essentially not changed over the first ten years of the fee schedule.[83]

The introduction of Medicare's physician payment reform also further complicated the doctor-hospital relationship. Many specialist surgeons petitioned their hospitals to help them make up their lost Medicare income,[84] while hospital administrators pursued joint ventures with physicians for outpatient services in order to increase their institutions' revenues, which they needed to offset the declining generosity of Medicare's hospital payments.[85]

Ultimately, though, the main problem with the Medicare physician fee schedule lies in the coupling of fixed budgets with fee-for-service reimbursements. The appropriate amount to be budgeted for physician services may be difficult to determine.[86] Using historic costs ignores the reality that technology changes, the population's burden of illness changes, and other factors may significantly alter how much should be allocated to any particular provider sector, such as physician services. The Balanced Budget Act altered the calculation of the volume performance standard by tying spending per beneficiary on physician services to the rate of growth in the national economy, as reflected in growth in the real gross domestic product, creating a new expenditure limitation called the sustainable growth rate.[87] Whatever the theoretical merits of tying Medicare beneficiary needs for physician services to how the national economy is doing, as we will examine in the Conclusion, the new SGR approach has proved unworkable and is currently subject to intense attention by Congress and its advisory bodies.

Second, in a fixed, national budget arrangement, all physicians have an incentive to overprovide, because gains from overprovision would typically exceed the losses from the pro rata reductions that the application of the expenditure limitation produces.[88] Under this system, prudent physicians are penalized financially, while profligate ones are rewarded. The PPRC had hoped that organized medicine would step up to the challenge of national expenditure limits by taking responsibility for rationalizing the volume of services through the establishment of clinical practice guidelines, enhanced peer review, and other professionally grounded approaches to reducing excessive volume and intensity of services.[89] This never happened.

The Calm before the Storm

Around the mid-1990s there was a respite of sorts . . . We weren't doing
the deficit reduction stuff every year. That probably led partially to the
BBA [Balanced Budget Act] in '97, which we've been trying to dig
ourselves out of ever since.

—*Rick Pollack, Vice President, American Hospital Association*

Medicare's inpatient hospital prospective payment system had these
various exclusions, particularly capital expenses and outpatient
services. And there's an awful lot of room within the rules to do some
creative cost allocation. And, so, as we learned while we spent roughly
ten years tearing our hair out trying to do outpatient PPS for Medicare,
part of the issue was that all sorts of Medicare costs had sort of slid into
the hospital outpatient side. And, obviously, that was something that
did not happen on day one [of Medicare's PPS], October 1, 1983. This
was a process that took place over a long period of time. But Medicare's
PPS really accelerated this movement of services [away from inpatient
acute settings] . . . There were enormous incentives throughout the
1980s and the first half of the '90s for hospital CFOs—again, clearly
within the realm of appropriate accounting—to slide costs over into
the less regulated areas of their institutions, whether into cost-based
outpatient settings or into capital reimbursement.

—*Bruce Vladeck, Administrator (1993–97),*
Health Care Financing Administration

In the mid-1990s, Republican and Democratic leaders found themselves unable to
forge a consensus on how to control Medicare's rate of spending growth. Consequently, the program became a relatively generous payer again, arguably too generous. In 1995, the program's trustees predicted that Medicare would run out of money

as early as 2002.[1] The subsequent political push to "save" Medicare coincided (conveniently) with a nasty partisan struggle between President Clinton and senior congressional Republicans over how best to achieve a balanced federal budget.[2] Republicans wanted substantial Medicare spending reductions to help balance the federal budget and pay for large tax cuts. President Clinton and congressional Democrats countered with smaller proposed spending reductions and charged Republicans with threatening both the financial integrity of Medicare and the welfare of the program's beneficiaries.[3] The impasse that ensued culminated in President Clinton vetoing the Republicans' Medicare legislation with the same pen that Lyndon Johnson had used to sign Medicare into law in 1965.[4] Clinton's veto triggered the infamous government shutdown in late 1995, from which he emerged victorious politically at the expense of congressional Republicans and House Speaker Newt Gingrich, who saw their public opinion ratings tumble.[5]

The legislative turmoil stemming from the debate over Medicare in 1995, together with an improving economy and President Clinton's landslide reelection in 1996, realigned political incentives for Republicans and Democrats. Rather than risk another government shutdown, leaders of both parties endeavored to reach a bipartisan compromise over Medicare and the federal budget.[6] The product of their pragmatic and conciliatory negotiations—the Balanced Budget Act of 1997—involved another major subordination of Medicare payment policy to larger fiscal policy goals.[7]

The BBA also created a new and convoluted politics for Medicare. It expanded on the success of Medicare's hospital and physician payment reforms by enacting new prospective payment systems for Medicare's remaining cost-based programs, including outpatient and postacute care.[8] The BBA also embraced the rigors of the free market—with an assumption or wishful thinking that more Medicare beneficiaries would move to private HMOs—just as the backlash against managed care was gaining significant momentum. Yet virtually all of the budgetary savings derived from the BBA's changes to Medicare were projected to come *not* from the free market and expanded competition associated with managed care but from increased government regulation and cuts in payments to medical providers.[9] "In 1997, as in 1983," notes political scientist Jonathan Oberlander, "policymakers talked right, but ultimately moved left."[10]

Managed Care Reduces Cost Inflation and Private Payments

The mid-1990s marked a transition for the U.S. health care system in which the balance of power temporarily shifted from the providers of medical care to its purchasers. This paradigm shift to various forms and styles of managed care did not "corporatize" U.S. health care; the majority of hospitals and physicians did not switch to "for-profit" status.[11] But medicine in the United States did take on a far more corporate orientation, due in large part to the increased competition and imposition of administrative controls associated with managed care.[12] Managed care appeared to solve the two main problems associated with traditional indemnity health insurance: the "moral hazard" problem, in which insured individuals tend to spend more of someone else's money than they would of their own,[13] and the "demand inducement" problem, in which physicians and hospitals tend to oversupply medical services and technology for the same reason.[14] And as health costs slowed dramatically, notes political scientist Lawrence Brown, "many analysts credited this managed care revolution with savings that flowed from the rebuff, perhaps repeal, of provider dominance."[15]

Only two years after the failure of President Clinton's ambitious effort at comprehensive health care reform, managed care—in all of its different forms and levels of restrictiveness—had taken over the bulk of the private health sector. It covered roughly 75 percent of employees or approximately one hundred million Americans (up from just fifteen million in the mid-1980s).[16] The limitations that managed care organizations placed on covered services—coupled with their use of selective contracting within which medical providers felt pressured to offer deep discounts—sent shock waves through the country's health care system. For the first time, the laws of supply and demand favored the purchasers of medical care rather than its providers. Employers' demands concerning cost growth for health insurance premiums became severe: "no or low growth."[17]

The term "managed care" only came into wide usage in the early 1990s and encompassed a variety of organizational designs and reimbursement methods.[18] As distinct from traditional indemnity health insurance, though, managed care essentially restricted patients' access to and choice of medical provider.[19] The original health maintenance organization, which was based on prepaid group practices, morphed into a cornucopia of acronyms and different management models built on contracts with individual medical providers: a preferred provider organization (PPO), a point of service plan (POS), or an individual practice association (IPA).[20] Managed care organizations essentially became effective "managed cost" plans. The lower prices they received from negotiating with a limited number of participating providers (on behalf of a larger number of patients) were passed on as savings to employers.[21]

Eager to attract market share and increase their revenues, for-profit managed care organizations promised to meet employers' demands for cost control.[22] Two major consequences emerged from this new arrangement: managed care became employ-

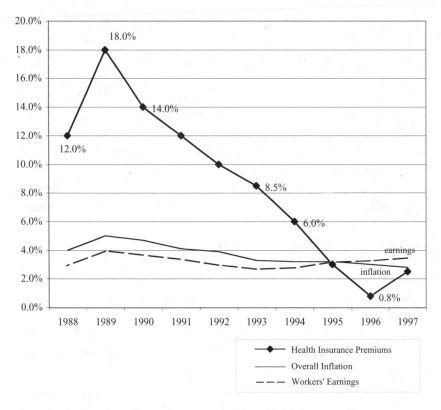

Figure 6.1. Average Annual Percentage Increase in Private Health Insurance Premiums, 1988–97

Sources: Adapted and modified from Mercer/Foster Higgins; Health Association of America/KPMG Peat Marwick Survey (1998), C3; U.S. Dept. of Labor, Bureau of Labor Statistics, "Annual Change in CPI." www.bls.gov/cpi.

ers' vehicle for cost control and, in the process, employers shifted a significant portion of financial risk to managed care organizations that could no longer simply pass along large annual premium increases to employers.[23] At the same time, the accumulation of enrollment in managed care organizations provided them with greater negotiating leverage with providers.

Businesses often encouraged their employees to enroll in more restrictive health plans by restructuring their financial incentives.[24] In other words, they either offered only one insurance option or made their employees pay more for a higher-cost policy.[25] By 1996, slightly more than half of all U.S. businesses offered only one health insurance option to their workers, usually a managed care plan.[26] The effects were dramatic (figure 6.1). In 1996, premium growth was almost nonexistent.[27]

Hospitals Slow Their Rate of Spending as Postacute Care Grows

With the rise of managed care, hospitals' ability to cost shift rapidly dwindled.[28] Instead of the average increase of 11 percent per year that hospitals had received from their private payers between 1986 and 1992, their payment per case *decreased* in real terms by an average of 0.7 percent per year between 1993 and 1997.[29] As a result, private payers' payment-to-cost ratio fell from a high of 131 percent in 1992 to 118 percent by 1997 (table 6.1). With excess bed capacity widespread, many hospitals entered into multi-year contracts with private payers in the early 1990s in order to maintain their patient volume.[30] Securing these contracts, however, required that hospitals agree to lower payments.[31] "A lot of hospital executives cut deals that they later came to regret," notes the AHA's Rick Pollack.[32] Areas of the country that experienced greater managed care penetration saw significantly lower rates of hospital cost growth, especially those areas with a high level of hospital competition.[33]

Out of financial necessity, therefore, most hospitals finally managed to achieve substantial cost control in the mid-1990s. The industry as a whole held its overall cost growth down to an average of just 1.6 percent per year between 1994 and 1997, which led to Medicare's payments rising faster than the costs of treating the program's beneficiaries (figure 6.2).[34] This phenomenon occurred during the mid-1990s, observes John Iglehart, when Medicare was left untouched by budget cuts because Congress and the Clinton administration could not agree on how to curb the program's rate of growth.[35]

Hospitals' success in reducing their cost growth stemmed primarily from two major strategies: restructuring their workforce and shifting a greater proportion of med-

TABLE 6.1
Hospitals' Overall Payment-to-Cost Ratio by Payer, 1988–97

Year	Total Medicare	Total Medicaid	Total Private Payer
1988	0.94	0.80	1.22
1989	0.91	0.76	1.22
1990	0.89	0.80	1.27
1991	0.88	0.82	1.30
1992	0.89	0.91	1.31
1993	0.90	0.93	1.30
1994	0.96	0.94	1.25
1995	0.99	0.94	1.24
1996	1.03	0.95	1.21
1997	1.04	0.96	1.18

SOURCE: Medicare Payment Advisory Commission, *Report to the Congress: Medicare Payment Policy* (2003).

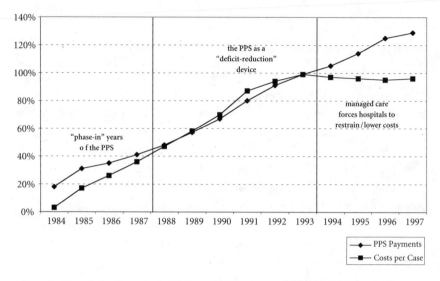

Figure 6.2. Cumulative Increases in Medicare PPS Payments and Hospitals' Costs per Case, 1984–97

Source: Medicare Payment Advisory Commission, *Report to the Congress* (1999): 52, fig. 3.1

ical care away from inpatient settings. First, beginning around 1993 and 1994, hospitals set about reducing the size and cost of their salaried workforce.[36] In particular, they replaced many of their registered nurses (RNs) and licensed practical nurses (LPNs) with less-educated, cheaper aides and clerks.[37] Annual employment growth for RNs had averaged almost 4 percent between 1983 and 1994, nearly double the rate of employment growth among all occupations over the same period.[38] But after 1994, employment growth for RNs slowed to less than 2 percent, and virtually all of it occurred in non-hospital settings (home health services, freestanding clinics, and nursing homes).[39] Moreover, the deceleration in the rate of employment growth for RNs coincided with a noticeable decline in their earnings. RNs had experienced solid wage growth during the 1980s, but it leveled off between 1990 and 1994, and then fell 1.5 percent annually over the next three years.[40]

The hospital industry's other leading cost-containment strategy was to shift the locus of patient care.[41] Until the implementation of Medicare's inpatient hospital PPS, postacute care accounted for only a small part of Medicare spending and was viewed generally as a cost-effective and less intensive alternative to extended inpatient hospital stays. However, the hospital PPS—with its fixed payments per stay—created strong incentives for hospitals to attempt to discharge patients as quickly as possible ("quicker and sicker"), thereby increasing the number of people needing postacute care services.[42] This incentive for early discharge was reinforced by the fact that postacute providers still operated on the basis of cost-based reimbursement.[43] Some hospitals even chose to acquire postacute care facilities to take advantage of these incentives.[44] For fiscal year 1996, on the eve of the BBA, 23 percent of Medicare beneficiaries discharged from an acute care hospital were discharged not to home, but to rehabilitation facilities, skilled nursing facilities (SNFs), or home health agencies (HHAs).[45] The increase in postacute care was not solely a function of payment incentives. Advances in technology that allowed more complex services to be delivered in less intensive settings contributed as well.

The growth in postacute care was further stimulated by several court rulings in the mid-1980s, which had the effect of liberalizing and expanding Medicare coverage for postacute care services.[46] In response to expenditure increases for skilled nursing services, the Health Care Financing Administration had increased the stringency with which Medicare fiscal intermediaries scrutinized claims.[47] The intermediaries, which are private insurance companies that serve as the federal government's agents in the administration of the Medicare program (including the payment of claims), developed "rules of thumb" that reduced the need for detailed claim review on an individual basis. In 1986, as a result of *Fox v. Bowen*, the fiscal intermediaries were expressly forbidden from using rules of thumb to deny coverage. Furthermore, they were not permitted to deny any physician-ordered SNF (or home health) care—even if such care was only for maintenance therapy—without providing specific clinical evidence about why a particular service should not be covered. The clinical evidence requirement made it much more difficult (as well as more costly) for intermediaries to deny claims. Predictably, claim denials decreased and SNF Medicare expenditures increased.

In *Duggan v. Brown*, a class action suit brought in 1988, a U.S. District Court held that HCFA's guidelines on who could receive home health services were contrary to the intent of the Medicare statute.[48] The effect of the ruling was to allow home health care that was part time or intermittent and to liberalize the definition of "homebound" patients—for whom the home benefit was designed—to include those who were able occasionally to leave the home.[49] On July 1, 1989, HCFA formally introduced the liberalized rules, and both the number of beneficiaries receiving home health services and the number of home health visits per user climbed significantly.[50]

During this period, the number of SNFs grew 6.8 percent annually, and the number of home health agencies grew 9.3 percent annually.[51] Between 1988 and 1995, home health care experienced an enormous employment increase (168 percent), which made it the single fastest growing segment of the U.S. health care system.[52] The number of home health agencies skyrocketed from 5,663 in 1990 to 9,838 by 1996.[53] "It seemed every person in the state of Louisiana in 1996 opened a home health agency," jokes Tom Scully. "You just had tons of hospitals and individuals coming in and chasing the carrot."[54]

The same phenomenon was taking place in the neighboring state of Texas. Visiting a small, rural hospital in East Texas in a town of a few thousand people, Robert Berenson asked the hospital administrator why this small town could barely support a twelve-bed hospital, yet had had six home agencies just a few years before. He replied, "For a while there, it seemed like every 'mom and pop' gas station that was having problems from gasoline shortages decided to become a home health agency in order to take advantage of easy Medicare payments. Now the hospital is the only home health provider, and we are doing fine."

With all of these factors contributing, Medicare spending for postacute providers—including SNFs, HHAs, rehabilitation facilities, and long-term care hospitals—grew rapidly. Payments to SNFs and HHAs increased at double-digit rates from the late 1980s on, averaging 35 percent a year for SNFs and 25 percent for home health care.[55] Between 1974 and 1983, hospital inpatient payments accounted for 64 percent of the growth in total Medicare payments, whereas SNF and home health services accounted for only 3.5 percent of the growth. Between 1990 and 1995, inpatient hospital services accounted for only a little more of the growth in Medicare payments than did SNF and HHA payments—38.6 percent compared to 30 percent.[56] Expressed a different way, the ratio of Medicare hospital expenditures to the combined expenditures for skilled nursing and home health care fell from twenty to one to just over three to one between 1986 and 1996.[57]

A similar explosion of services was happening in hospital outpatient services, also facilitated by technological innovations in medicine, including the development of many new, less invasive surgical techniques.[58] Between 1980 and 1994, expenditures for hospital outpatient services as a share of total Medicare spending nearly tripled, from 2.9 percent to 8.1 percent of total payments.[59] Outpatient expenditures, which represented only 6 percent of Medicare payments to hospitals in 1980, had increased to 20 percent by 1997.[60] Compounding the problem of spending increases, the hospital outpatient payment system had become a patchwork of payment approaches, making it difficult to administer for both Medicare contractors and hospitals.[61] In addition, the arcane method for calculating program payments and beneficiary coinsurance obligations resulted in beneficiaries having to pay a disproportionate share of total payments to hospitals, as much as 50 percent of the payment, compared with 20 percent for most services covered under Part B (as called for in the Medicare statute).[62]

The shift of care away from inpatient settings led to a 30 percent reduction in Medicare patients' average length-of-stay between the early and late 1990s, compared

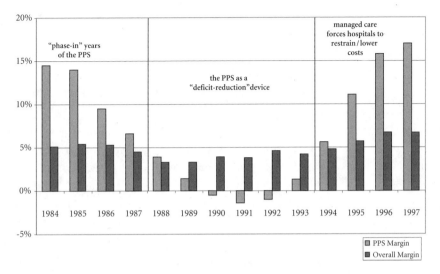

Figure 6.3. Hospitals' Inpatient (PPS) Medicare Margin and Overall Margin, 1984–97
Source: Medicare Payment Advisory Commission, *Report to the Congress* (1999): 53, fig. 3.2; 55, fig. 3.4.

to a less than 10 percent reduction in non-Medicare patients' average length-of-stay during this same period.[63] But the shift was not painless. Half of the total projected increase in Medicare spending between 1996 and 2002 was accounted for by hospital outpatient, skilled nursing, and home health services combined; this form of cost-shifting to other providers was Medicare's (and taxpayers') problem.[64]

Ultimately, the hospital industry reaped significant financial rewards from the changes it made. By 1996, hospitals were enjoying their highest Medicare and overall margins since the first two years of the PPS's operation (figure 6.3).[65] Between 1994 and 1997, while the industry's rate of cost growth increased only 1.6 percent per year, Medicare's average annual increase in spending per beneficiary was a comparatively generous 4.7 percent.[66] As a result, by 1997, "health care providers were all way over-paid by Medicare," argues Scully.[67] It was not surprising, therefore, to find articles in hospital trade industry journals with titles like "Changing Tunes: No More 'Whining for Dollars' by Healthcare Lobbyists in Washington."[68] By 1997, the hospital industry's profits were such that they didn't need to whine.

Medicare's Antifraud Campaign Triggers a "Big Chill"

Another reason why hospital executives did not pay especially close attention to Congress' deliberation over the BBA legislation in 1997, besides the fact that the majority of their institutions were doing well financially, was that for the first time fraud had become the talk of the industry.[69] After the 1996 Health Insurance Portability and Accountability Act (HIPAA) dramatically increased the federal government's funding of antifraud efforts, prosecution of Medicare fraud cases became the Justice Department's top priority, after violent crime.[70] FBI investigations of health care fraud jumped from 650 in 1992 to nearly 2,500 by 1997.[71]

Medicare's different reimbursement systems made it a target to aggressive entrepreneurs whose tactics had become attractive to a growing number of hospital executives worried about the effects of managed care on their institutions.[72] With corporate forces gaining influence, for-profit hospital chains found a niche and became a growth industry.[73] The chains focused much of their efforts on combining partial physician ownership with networks that vertically integrated inpatient care with outpatient surgical centers, home health care, and rehabilitation and diagnostic services.[74] Their goal was to consolidate a hospital's market share in order to present a more unified front in negotiations with insurance companies and large employers. But in a predominantly not-for-profit industry, the for-profit hospital chains made enemies.[75] They also raised the suspicions of government investigators who recognized that Medicare's mix of prospective and cost-based reimbursement systems made it particularly vulnerable to fraud and abuse.[76]

The government stepped up investigative efforts as part of its program "Operation Restore Trust," which began in 1995 and targeted fraud and abuse in three high-growth areas of the health care industry (home health agencies, nursing homes, and durable medical equipment suppliers).[77] Federal investigators aggressively pursued fraud within the home health industry.[78] They were spurred on by reports that organized crime had become heavily involved in setting up fraudulent medical clinics and home health agencies in states with large Medicare populations (particularly Florida).[79] According to numerous convicted criminals, the penalty-to-risk ratio for Medicare fraud—relative to narcotics and racketeering—was considered "extremely positive," with low penalties and "stratospheric rewards."[80] Medicare had always included a home health benefit, but Congress's expansion of eligibility and coverage rules in 1989 sparked a period of extraordinary growth for the industry. According to HCFA, the proportion of enrollees using the home health benefit more than doubled between 1988 and 1996, rising from 4.8 to 10.7 percent.[81] During this period, notes health economist Harriet Komisar, the number of visits received by home health users nearly tripled from an average of twenty-four to seventy-four visits. Medicare's home health spending grew from $83 per enrollee in 1988 to $528 in 1996 (in inflation-adjusted terms), which represented an average annual rate of increase of more than 25 percent.

TABLE 6.2

The Growth of Columbia/HCA, 1988–96

	1988	1989	1990	1991	1992	1993	1994	1995	1996
No. of hospitals	4	4	11	12	24	115	207	332	351
Gross revenue (in millions)	$45	$153	$290	$500	$819	$10,252	$14,543	$17,646	$19,900
Net profits (in millions)	$1.7	$6.3	$10	$15	$26	$507	$814	$988	$1,500

SOURCE: Adapted and modified from Kuttner, "Columbia/HCA and the Resurgence of the For-Profit Hospital Business," 364, table 1.

Consequently, home health increased from 2.4 percent of Medicare's total spending in 1988 to 10 percent by 1996.[82]

The Justice Department's most celebrated and high-profile investigations were within the hospital industry. No case more epitomized the conflict between Medicare's complicated array of reimbursement systems and the government's increasingly serious attitude about investigating fraud than Columbia/HCA.[83] The company began on the day of the stock market crash in October 1987, when Richard Scott and Richard Rainwater each invested $125,000 to create Columbia Hospital Corporation.[84] Through extremely aggressive acquisitions of individual hospitals and then a series of for-profit hospital chains, the company owned more than 350 hospitals and half of the for-profit hospital sector by 1996 (table 6.2).[85] The core of the company's enormous financial success was its hypercompetitive vision of medical care, noted the *New York Times,* "one that applies the practices of corporate America to an industry still dominated by not-for-profit institutions."[86] In 1997, however, the company ousted Scott as its CEO and become the subject of the biggest health care fraud investigation ever pursued by the federal government.[87]

The origins of Columbia/HCA's legal woes stemmed from its corporate philosophy, which was known as the "three As" (acquire, affiliate, or annihilate).[88] Based on this philosophy, the company's *modus operandi* was to aggressively exploit the gray areas and incentive structures of existing reimbursement systems that were prone to abuse, especially Medicare's payment methods for home health and outpatient rehabilitation care.[89] The industry's larger strategy of shifting care to outpatient and postacute settings led some Columbia/HCA hospitals to maximize their Medicare reimbursement in ways that bordered on the unethical. In a practice commonly referred to as "double-dipping" or "unbundling," a hospital could get the standard Medicare payment for an inpatient admission and then also receive an additional payment by substituting cheaper postacute care services for the last days of a standard inpatient stay.[90] In addition, by offering physicians equity positions within Columbia/HCA or simply buying their practices outright, the company aligned financial incentives between physicians and hospitals in such a way as to all but invite kickbacks to physicians for referring often excessive patient care to Columbia/HCA hospitals.[91] The alignments were not explicitly illegal but rather "a barely legal but ethically indefensible cousin of fee splitting."[92]

What specifically led to the government's investigation of Columbia/HCA was outright billing fraud.[93] The company would often instruct its member hospitals to shift acquisition costs and overhead expenses to its home health care operations, where Medicare still used less effective, cost-based reimbursement methods.[94] Other Columbia/HCA hospitals systematically over-billed Medicare by "upcoding" (overstating) the severity of their Medicare patients' illnesses.[95] And the most egregious behavior, which triggered a whistleblower's False Claims Act, involved the company's practice of encouraging a handful of its member hospitals to keep two sets of billing books—one in accordance with Medicare's rules on allowable costs and another with exaggerated cost claims to see if Medicare would accept them.[96]

The Justice Department's investigation of Columbia/HCA served as a warning to the rest of the nation's medical providers that the government was adopting a much higher level of scrutiny of Medicare reimbursements. Even prestigious teaching hospitals—such as the Hospital of the University of Pennsylvania and Dartmouth-Hitchcock Medical Center—were audited for Medicare billing fraud, due to allegations that they frequently claimed an attending physician had provided medical services that had actually been provided by a younger, less-trained hospital resident.[97] By the end of 1997, thousands of hospital executives across the country had received notification that their cost reports—which they had personally signed over several years—were going to be reviewed by criminal investigators and federal prosecutors.[98] It sent a chill through the hospital industry and signaled the beginning of tough financial times ahead.

The Balanced Budget Act and Medicare's Ultimate Subordination to Fiscal Policy

After winning reelection in 1996, President Clinton was ready and eager to leave a major legacy: the first balanced budget in thirty years.[99] What the president and Republican leaders in Congress already knew, based on previous legislative experience, was that the only means by which they could achieve this goal was to return to using Medicare as the ultimate budgetary "slush fund." Any significant budgetary savings would—as many times before—have to come from substantial reductions in future

Medicare spending. Unfortunately, the program did not have surplus funds to share. In 1995, the annual report of Medicare's trustees showed that the program's hospital trust fund would run out of money by 2002.[100]

Republicans in Congress seized upon the dire report as an opportunity to dramatically change Medicare while balancing the federal budget and providing tax cuts. Fresh from defeating Clinton's ambitious attempt at comprehensive health care reform and an enormous electoral victory in fall 1994—in which Republicans gained control of both the House of Representatives and the Senate for the first time since 1954—Republican congressional leaders proposed $270 billion in Medicare spending reductions over seven years as part of a "Save Medicare" campaign.[101] President Clinton countered with $128 billion in projected Medicare spending reductions. An impasse developed, notes Ted Marmor, with "Republican charges of demagoguery against the Democrats and Democratic charges of Republican heartlessness."[102]

Clinton's veto of the Republicans' Medicare and other budget legislation triggered the infamous government shutdown of late 1995. He emerged the political winner from his battle with House Speaker Newt Gingrich and Gingrich's colleagues after public opinion turned against the Republican party.[103] Polls showed that the public viewed Clinton and the Democratic party as the defenders of a beloved government program.[104] When President Clinton won reelection handily in late 1996, any desire for continued partisan conflict disappeared.[105] In its place emerged a broad bipartisan drive to both achieve a balanced federal budget and "save" Medicare.[106]

In August 1997, President Clinton and Congress enacted some of the most extensive Medicare reforms in the program's history through the passage of the BBA.[107] The BBA called for $115 billion in budgetary savings from reductions in future Medicare spending (between 1998 and 2002).[108] The figure was just slightly less than half of the BBA's total projected savings, despite the fact that Medicare only constituted 12 percent of federal spending.[109]

The BBA represented the height of Medicare politics' subordination to fiscal partisan politics. According to Representative Henry Waxman, "the Clinton administration and congressional Republicans used Medicare strictly as a piggy-bank."[110] Nancy-Ann DeParle, Clinton's associate director for health and personnel at the White House's Office of Management and Budget (before she became administrator of HCFA in 1997), elaborates:

> We looked at five or six different factors [with regard to changing Medicare] . . .
> The first one was *not* what was happening with health care spending or, particularly, what was happening with Medicare spending. The thing that drove us to the [bargaining] table was the overall level of the federal budget deficit. That

was the number one thing we thought about in looking at health care policy. I'm not sure I agree that that's what we should have been thinking about, but that was what precipitated the discussion.[111]

As long as leading Medicare analysts and members of Congress were persuaded that hospitals' overall margins were positive—they were the best they had been in a decade (see figure 6.3)—and because hospitals still represented a large proportion of Medicare spending, they generally felt comfortable manipulating Medicare's payment policy to suit larger budgetary purposes.

While the changes to Medicare were primarily budget-driven, this time they were also policy-driven to an extent.[112] "There was considerable evidence that spending in some sectors of the program had been increasing at annual rates that many of us thought were unsustainable for Medicare, 20 to 30 percent," explains DeParle. "So that was another big focus of our efforts to look at what we should be doing with Medicare as part of this Balanced Budget Act."[113] In addition to reducing future payment increases for important provider types, including hospitals, HHAs, and SNFs, the BBA substantially altered the framework of the Medicare program by mandating new payment systems that would nearly complete Medicare's shift from cost-and charge-based reimbursement to prospective payment systems. And these new systems were to take effect quickly.

The experience with Medicare's DRGs for hospitals and its fee schedule (with the RBRVS) for physicians had made the concept of prospective payment seem easy. "Prospective payment had become a magical phrase for 'cost control,'" recalls Stuart Guterman. "All you had to do was develop a prospective payment system and assume that you were going to be able to save a ton on Medicare payments. The problem was that we knew a lot more about hospital and physician services when we put them into prospective payment systems than we knew about most of Medicare's other services."[114]

According to the BBA, which was enacted on July 31, 1997, SNFs were to begin a transition to prospective payment on July 1, 1998; the new PPS for hospital outpatient services was to start on January 1, 1999; and payment systems for inpatient rehabilitation facilities and HHAs were scheduled to start on October 1, 1999, with an interim payment system to limit expenditures in effect in 1998.[115] Other PPSs were to follow in short order. Furthermore, the BBA addressed the issue of hospitals profiting from quick transfers of patients to other facilities with a major expansion of the hospital transfer policy. Under the expanded policy, acute care hospitals would no longer receive a full DRG payment for shorter-than-average inpatient stays in ten high-cost DRGs when these short-stay cases were transferred to postacute care facilities. Instead, the hospital would now receive per-diem payments that would be less than the full DRG amounts.[116]

It turned out that HCFA could not implement all of the new PPSs and myriad, complementary policies on the overly-ambitious BBA timetable. For HCFA to produce the required "notice and comment" rule-making and then implement changes to the various electronic systems required for correctly processing and paying claims would have been daunting under normal circumstances. And these were not normal circumstances. While the BBA was being debated and enacted, HCFA was undergoing a major reorganization that included both administrative reassignment and physical relocation for most key personnel. These changes left the agency poorly prepared to take on the task of putting all the pieces together to pay providers differently.[117] By 1998, HCFA also started confronting the potential threat of the Y2K problem. In many circumstances, Y2K readiness took precedence over demands of the new payment systems, and senior HCFA officials had to decide which payment systems to postpone. For example, a proposed rule for outpatient PPS was published on September 8, 1998, only five weeks after the rule for SNFs. But as it was publishing the details of the new payment approach, HCFA also announced it was delaying the implementation date by more than a year, citing the priority of Y2K-related preparedness.[118]

Nevertheless, over a period of a few years, HCFA did accomplish the transformation of the Medicare program through the adoption of fifteen payment systems in which payments were based on predetermined rates and were mostly unaffected by medical providers' costs or posted charges; that is, they were all prospective payment systems.[119] And they have largely been successful in changing incentives by placing providers at some financial risk for the services they provide.

The BBA's Medicare + Choice Program

Another prominent feature of the 1997 Medicare reforms was policymakers' creation of Medicare + Choice ("M + C"). Republicans' broad vision was to dramatically increase the number of Medicare beneficiaries in participating (private) managed care plans.[120] The concept of shifting financial risk away from the government by moving Medicare beneficiaries into managed care plans originated in the early 1970s, but the enrollment in such plans had been trivial. Moving Medicare beneficiaries into private managed care plans gained additional momentum with the 1982 Tax Equity and Financial Responsibility Act,[121] which mandated that HMOs would be paid 95 percent of the adjusted average per capita payments made for Medicare beneficiaries in each county, with plans being allowed to keep the difference between the cost of care and the amount of payment. HMOs were allowed the normal level of profit, or retained earnings, they customarily received in their private sector products. Under this payment methodology, the Medicare HMO program expanded greatly, especially in the early to mid-1990s.

By 1997, there were five million Medicare beneficiaries enrolled in various managed care plans (14 percent of the program's total population).[122] Republicans had ambitions to significantly increase that number and make progress on four separate goals: (1) expanding beneficiaries' health care choices, (2) providing additional benefits, such as prescription drug coverage, (3) restraining the growth of federal Medicare spending by encouraging competition among private health plans, and (4) reducing the need for direct government regulation of provider payment policies.[123]

The BBA provided a redesigned payment formula that was intended to address earlier methodology problems that had resulted in significant geographic disparities, with most enrollment in M + C clustered in counties where payment rates to HMOs were very high and plans could purchase care for their members at lower costs. The main thrust of the BBA formula was to increase payments to plans in areas of the country with low payment rates based on fee-for-service spending, while limiting increases in plan payments in relatively high-payment counties, thereby compressing the range of payments and reducing the linkage between M + C payments and county-level spending for the fee-for-service part of the Medicare program.[124]

The BBA's Cross-Cutting and Paradoxical Politics

The BBA represented a political deal between Democrats and Republicans. Both parties needed cost controls that would be scored by the Congressional Budget Office in such a way as to achieve a balanced budget. Along with spending reductions, the BBA gave private plans a supportive boost and a handful of free market demonstration projects (e.g., medical savings accounts).[125] Thus, the BBA was a historic milestone, because it significantly expanded private, managed-care elements within the Medicare program (M + C).[126] Yet it also continued the process of giving Medicare more authority to control costs by calling for the development of prospective payment systems for Medicare's remaining cost-based components.[127] As Jonathan Oberlander explains:

> These new regulatory reforms, as well as reducing payments to providers under already established regulations, generated the savings in program spending, not the procompetitive elements of the legislation. In this the BBA echoed a familiar theme from Medicare politics during the 1980s. In 1997, as in 1983, when the prospective payment system for hospitals was adopted, the rhetoric

was all about markets and competition. But the reality was that the savings were all from regulation. The secret of the BBA was that the move to competition was not projected to save Medicare any money. Given budgetary pressures for Medicare savings, Republicans and Democrats once again embraced more regulation and lower payments to providers as the best way to achieve short-term budgetary goals.[128]

In essence, the BBA allowed Republicans and Democrats to test two theories of cost control: the efficiency of regulation (pushed mostly by Democrats) versus competitive markets (championed largely by Republicans). As the following chapter demonstrates, the "public" regulatory approach proved infinitely more effective than the "private" free-market approach.

Using Medicare again for larger budgetary purposes meant another round of *increasing*, rather than decreasing, government regulation in the form of new prospective payment systems. Nevertheless, in terms of what the Congress set out to accomplish—balancing the budget largely by reducing the rate of increase in Medicare spending—the BBA's new payment policies were a remarkable success.[129] The further paradox is that the lowered payments to M + C plans that caused plans to pull out of the program and reduce their benefits occurred because of the success of the BBA in decreasing payments to providers in the traditional program. Congress had for a long time based its payments to private plans on what it was spending in the traditional program. By doing so well in decreasing these provider payments, Congress inadvertently reduced payments to private plans, just as these plans were losing control over spending.[130]

Following a decade in which Medicare operated as the leading "change agent" within the U.S. health care system, the private sector temporarily rose to the fore in the mid-1990s. The failure of President Clinton's attempt at comprehensive reform left managed care as the hoped-for solution for cost control. And for a period it worked, largely because while managed care organizations did not radically transform health delivery or organization, they were able to squeeze payments to medical providers and significantly reduce inpatient hospital stays.[131] There was a lot of "fat" in the nation's patchwork system of health care that could be eliminated through competitive negotiations between medical providers and insurers, employers, or managed care organizations. The success of managed care, however, turned out to be short-lived and partly due to what insurance experts call the "underwriting cycle," which typically results in several years of profitability followed by several years of losses.[132] In their ongoing efforts to control costs and remain profitable, the behavior of many managed care organizations (particularly for-profit HMOs) and for-profit hospital chains eventually triggered a populist backlash.[133]

Perhaps the best way to understand managed care, and the backlash it eventually spawned, is to view it as the private sector's response to the effects of Medicare's PPS. As Chapter 4 explained, the success of the PPS in controlling Medicare's rate of expenditure growth fueled inflation in the private health sector, in turn triggering employers' demand for cost control.[134] Managed care operated partly as a systematic suppression of cost shifting, as managed care organizations qua purchasing agents prevented hospitals from summarily raising prices to privately insured patients to meet their financial requirements. The key difference, however, is that Medicare's payment reforms rarely (if ever) triggered a backlash. Why? Partly because the budget deficit overwhelmed Medicare politics through about 1997, but mostly because the dramatic changes associated with Medicare's PPS remained hidden from the program's beneficiaries, who continued operating under the same fee-for-service model as they always had. Medical providers and administrators were the ones who changed their behavior in response to Medicare's new payment incentives. Managed care, on the other hand, did alter patients' traditional and customary medical arrangements. By its very nature, it undermined the basic principles that had made traditional indemnity health insurance acceptable.[135] Managed care created incentives for medical providers to withhold care instead of oversupplying it, and then it began restricting patients' choices and access—in ways that Medicare never did—while also threatening the decision-making autonomy of medical providers, which fostered a confrontational environment.[136]

In response to intense pressure from managed care, the hospital industry finally managed to achieve extraordinary cost control in the mid-1990s. Beginning in 1994, hospital cost inflation fell for four consecutive years, bottoming out in 1997 at less than 2 percent. Apart from 1973 (when Nixon's price controls were in effect), this represented the only year on record in which hospital cost inflation was lower than general economic inflation.[137] The industry's success at reducing the cost of its workforce and shifting an increasing proportion of care to less expensive outpatient and postacute settings led to sizeable financial gains. By 1997, hospitals' Medicare and total margins were even bigger than they had been in the first two years of the PPS' operation.

Thus, when the Clinton administration and Republican leaders in Congress sought to achieve a balanced federal budget, playing with Medicare's payment policy became the prime means again of generating enormous savings. Similar to the many budget reconciliation acts that preceded it, the BBA's significant deficit reduction came largely from cuts in future Medicare payments to medical providers. Most policy makers were not overly concerned about the effects of these reductions because, by 1997, market forces appeared to have tamed medical inflation and made medical providers more efficient. Hospitals and other medical providers seemed to be in a position to withstand a modest financial "hit." With the BBA's call for new Medicare prospective payment systems and its creation of Medicare + Choice, everyone could emerge a winner from the BBA. The government could balance its budget and provide tax cuts; Medicare's solvency could be solidified as the program was modernized; and medical providers—if they were not under federal investigation—could continue to receive fair prices for the services and care they provided. What could go wrong?

CHAPTER SEVEN

The Reckoning and Reversal

Hospital lobbyists typically get paid every year to come in and—it's like Pavlov's bell—yell and scream, "We need more money!" But if you do that and then get overpaid, Congress will come back—as it did in 1997—and whack you! That was part of the problem in '97, when I was lobbying for the hospitals. I knew those [Medicare] cuts were too big and everyone else involved knew it as well. But nobody in Congress would listen to us, because hospitals had always come in and whined the same things whether they were underpaid or overpaid. After a while, it was like crying wolf.

Besides, my member hospitals were so fat, dumb, and happy at the time that they didn't even really notice. They were doing so well financially that they didn't really understand what was coming. They hadn't had a Medicare cut since '93 and a real big one since '90. They'd been doing great! So getting them all stoked up to come in and lobby and scream and moan for anything more than just the general stuff was hard. But then in '98, when those cuts started kicking in, oh my . . . they just could not believe it.

—Tom Scully, President and CEO (1995–2001),
Federation of American Hospitals

The U.S. health care system experienced something of a structural and economic reckoning in the late 1990s. Health care reform based on private competing plans offered only a temporary solution to the nation's ongoing struggle with medical inflation.[1] Eventually, renewed cost pressures, the Balanced Budget Act's significant Medicare cuts, and years of minimal (or nonexistent) payment increases from private payers left the hospital industry with its lowest overall margins in a decade; most physicians with increased workloads, less autonomy and often reduced incomes; and a slew of bankruptcies and near-bankruptcies among a wide variety of health care management and delivery organizations.[2] Yet medical providers were not alone. Even as managed care organizations experienced their own severe "profitability crisis," the consumer and physician backlash against them led to an aggressive legislative and legal assault on the industry. The general public came to view commercial managed care as responsible for turning doctors "into entrepreneurs who maximize profits by minimizing care."[3] The result is that the managed care "revolution"—which, despite the rhetoric about improving the quality and efficiency of health care delivery, was principally about forcing medical providers (primarily hospitals and physicians) to provide discounts to health plans, essentially stalled.

Medical providers hastened the demise of managed care by consolidating into larger networks and practice groups, which vastly improved their bargaining leverage. A roaring economy in the late 1990s aided their efforts, because it led employers to request more generous and less restrictive health plans. By the early 2000s, most hospitals and physicians were receiving sizeable payment increases. Private health plans followed suit and pursued their own consolidation strategy. Many managed care organizations and traditional health insurance companies either merged or exited the market altogether. The surviving plans, facing less competition and more employer willingness to pay higher costs, quickly restored their profitability by dropping money-losing patient populations and increasing premiums. Insurers also dropped some of their most objectionable approaches to containing costs. Employers shifted more and more of their employees out of low-cost health maintenance organizations into less restrictive preferred provider organizations, increasing their employees' level of cost sharing as an alternative approach to limiting employer's financial liability.[4]

The resurgence in medical inflation that resulted from these changes, together with a recession in 2001 and a period of sluggish economic growth thereafter, triggered the rise of another health care crisis in the United States.[5] As the cost of private health insurance soared, growing numbers of employers either shifted more of the costs to their workers or ceased to provide coverage altogether. Enrollment in public health insurance programs—such as Medicaid and the State Children's Health Insurance Program (SCHIP)—increased substantially; and the programs became huge financial burdens for state governments already struggling under reduced tax revenue. Even worse, despite these public program expansions, millions of individuals fell through the cracks completely. Between 2001 and 2003, the number of uninsured increased by 5.2 million individuals.[6] One in every three non-elderly Americans (81.8 million people) experienced a lapse in health insurance coverage for all or part of 2002 and 2003.[7] And health-related problems became a leading cause of the increasing rate of personal bankruptcy in the United States.

In the midst of these deteriorating health care trends and growing federal budget deficits, President George W. Bush and a Republican-controlled Congress narrowly passed the biggest expansion of Medicare since the program's creation in 1965. The 2003 Medicare Prescription Drug, Improvement, and Modernization Act added a more than $700 billion prescription drug benefit to the program. It also expanded the role of private health plans in Medicare, renaming the struggling Medicare + Choice program "Medicare Advantage" and substantially increasing payments to participating plans. The MMA, however, departed from the dominant pattern of Medicare policy making that had existed for two decades. It was born out of the political impasse that developed within the National Bipartisan Commission on the Future of Medicare (1998–99). With Medicare fully "prospectivized," the MMA made no pretense to either save money or prolong Medicare's solvency. Instead, President Bush and a slim majority of mostly Republicans and a handful of Democrats in Congress filled a widely acknowledged gap in the program's coverage with a controversial catastrophic prescription drug benefit and moved Medicare in the direction of increased privatization.[8] Ironically, many conservatives disliked the MMA as much as (if not more than) liberals,[9] because it provided a huge new Medicare benefit without significant programmatic restructuring or fiscal discipline.

Medical Providers' "Perfect Storm"

The late 1990s marked one of the more difficult financial periods in recent memory for many of the nation's medical providers. After years of reluctantly giving discounts to health plans and making a myriad of often painful cost-cutting reforms, growing numbers of medical providers found themselves at a crossroads. Their revenues were flat or even declining, but their costs were increasing.[10] Some hospitals and physicians began to try to "push back" against (or receive higher reimbursement rates from) managed care at this time.[11] But the managed care industry was still a force—despite the growing backlash against it—in part because of its continued, albeit slowed, rate of enrollment growth.[12] If anything, managed care organizations were more desperate than ever in the late 1990s to pay medical providers less, or only marginally more, than they had before, because the majority of managed care organizations were losing money.[13]

Hospitals, in particular, faced a confluence of financial pressures. In 1998, private and public payments to hospitals decreased at the same time (a first), while health care costs jumped after more than four years of very low and even negative growth.[14] These two phenomena—decreasing revenue and increasing costs—continued the following year. As a result, the hospital industry's average overall margin fell from 6 percent

TABLE 7.1

Changes in Medicare Spending and Hospitals' Financial Conditions, 1996–2000

	1996	1997	1998	1999	2000
Real Medicare spending (in billions of 2000 dollars)	$214.2	$224.0	$221.0	$217.3	$221.8
Percentage increase or decrease in real Medicare spending (deflated)	6.7%	4.6%	−1.3%	−1.7%	−2.1%
Hospitals' average total medicare margin	9.9	10.4	6.0	5.6	5.1
Hospitals' average overall margin	6.1	6.0	4.3	3.0	3.4
Percentage of hospitals with negative overall margins	22%	26%	34%	37%	35%

SOURCES: Newhouse, "Medicare," table 10; Medicare Payment Advisory Commission, *Report to the Congress: Medicare Payment Policy* (2001), 60–71; Medicare Payment Advisory Commission, *Report to the Congress* (2003), 6–39.

in 1997 to 3 percent in 1999, its lowest level in more than a decade.[15] That same year, 37 percent of the nation's hospitals reported a financial operating loss, which represented an 80 percent increase from 1996 (table 7.1).

The BBA succeeded in dramatically slowing Medicare's rate of expenditure growth, especially in the postacute areas of home health care and skilled nursing.[16] Prior to the BBA's implementation, Medicare spending on both home health care services and skilled nursing facilities was growing annually at the unsustainable rates of more than 30 percent.[17] From 1998 to 1999, after the BBA went into effect, Medicare payments to skilled nursing facilities fell by 17 percent, as the average SNF rehabilitation charge per hospital stay dropped by 45 percent.[18] And Medicare spending on home health care decreased by roughly 50 percent.[19] The number of home health care visits in 1999 was less than half of the number in 1997,[20] as a third of all home health agencies went out of business in 1998 and 1999.[21] Although there was a great hue and cry from the home health care industry that the BBA's changes were disastrous, most of the carnage was concentrated in the four states (Texas, California, Oklahoma, and Louisiana) where there was an excessive number of home health agencies.[22]

Even the annual growth in Medicare spending on inpatient hospital care—which represents the bulk of the program's Part A expenditures—virtually ground to a halt, increasing only 0.1 percent between 1998 and 2000.[23] The nationwide effects of this radical spending slowdown were striking.[24] Real, inflation-adjusted Medicare spending did not return to its 1997 levels until 2001 (see table 7.1).[25] The BBA's impact did vary depending on the type of hospital. All hospitals received lower payments, but the reduction in Medicare spending came disproportionately at the expense of teaching hospitals and hospitals that treat large numbers of poor patients, which are often the same hospitals.[26] Consequently, many policy makers who led the charge in passing the BBA were the first to change their minds afterwards and push for "fixing" the BBA.[27]

The BBA was not solely responsible, however, for Medicare's significant spending reductions between 1998 and 2000. The federal government's aggressive efforts to deter Medicare fraud and abuse, vividly illustrated by its high-profile investigation of Columbia/HCA, led many hospitals to submit more conservative claims to avoid the risk of large retroactive payment settlements to Medicare. For the first time since the PPS began in 1984, Medicare's Case Mix Index for inpatient admissions (which measures the severity of a hospital's medical cases) fell, decreasing 0.5 percent in 1998 and again in 1999.[28] HCFA found that this decline was "primarily attributable to changes in the coding of certain hospital admissions, particularly shifts in coding from 'respiratory infection' to 'simple pneumonia,' and from cases 'with complications' to those 'without complications.' Not coincidentally, these coding categories were the focus of an investigation by the U.S. Department of Justice."[29] Medicare fraud and abuse did not cease to exist,[30] but its frequency and scope did decrease, which contributed to the slowdown in Medicare spending.[31] Policy makers had estimated that the BBA would reduce Medicare expenditures by $115 billion; that figure rose to $217 billion by the summer of 1999.[32]

Squeezed financially by both their public and private payers (as well as their own increasingly conservative billing practices), hospitals lobbied Congress intensively for two successive BBA relief bills. They argued that their "Medicare margins were approaching zero; their total margins including Medicare and private payers were in the 2–3 percent range (regarded as unsafe by the AHA); their bond ratings were plunging; and that their industry's average obscured an alarming proportion of hospitals with negative overall margins."[33] Their efforts paid off. The hospital industry managed to get two relief or "give-back" bills—one in 1999, the Balanced Budget Refinement Act, and another in 2000, the Budget Improvement and Protection Act—which increased payment rates for almost all hospitals, SNFs, and home health agencies.[34] Tom Scully, president and CEO of the Federation of American Hospitals at the time, maintains that while the "relief" bills were financially necessary, the purpose of Medicare payment policy should not be to make *every* hospital profitable:

> The hospitals deserved to get some money back. They went from having a picnic in '96 and '97 to having the worst years they'd had in thirty years in '98 and '99 . . . Yet 33 percent [of hospitals losing money] is the historical average going back to 1965 . . . That's a fact. So when 25 percent of the hospitals are losing

money, like they were in '96 and '97, you know they're being paid too much. But when almost 40 percent are losing money, like they were in '98 and '99, you know you've got a problem . . .

The majority of hospitals are wonderful, but there are always those ratty little hospitals that aren't very good that are probably losing money and are close to closing. That's not necessarily bad. Not *every* hospital should *always* be making money. If it's a well-run hospital, if it's well managed, it should be making a reasonable return.[35]

The two give-back bills were still modest on the scale of the entire program, notes Joseph Newhouse, former vice chair of the Medicare Payment Advisory Commission. They only raised Medicare spending above what it otherwise would have been by about 3 percent.[36]

Many medical providers found themselves struggling financially in the late 1990s. Physicians' average net income dropped 5 percent in real (inflation-adjusted) terms during the latter half of the 1990s.[37] This trend represented a dramatic shift from 1991 to 1995, when other professional occupations lagged behind the growth in physicians' income.[38] Executives at teaching hospitals spoke of having to make "difficult choices" about their services and programs.[39] Thousands of home health agencies went out of business. As the late John Eisenberg, former administrator of the Agency for Healthcare Research and Quality, lamented, "It's survival of the fittest, and when the fittest are trying to survive, their generosity and charity care are diminished."[40] Medical providers were not alone, however, as they underwent tumultuous change. The managed care industry also found itself at a crisis point.[41]

Managed Care's "Perfect Storm"

The origins of the managed care backlash were principally financial. In the early years, managed care organizations found it relatively easy to lower patients' hospital use and obtain significant discounts from medical providers worried about their loss of patient volume if they were not included on managed care plans' lists of "participating providers."[42] The discounts were necessary for managed care plans to make a profit. But the ability of managed care organizations to continue lowering hospital use and obtaining discounts from medical providers proved harder as time went along. There were fewer "one-time" cost savings to be had.[43] Nearly 90 percent of all HMOs were profitable in 1994, but slightly less than half were by 1997, notes health economist Marsha Gold, and the average profit margin by then was only 1.2 percent.[44] When the price of health care services invariably went up, many managed care organizations turned to unpopular strategies in order to remain profitable and keep their contracts with employers. They limited or eliminated coverage for many medical services and increased employee cost sharing (in the form of higher deductibles and co-payments).[45]

Consequently, the mid-1990s marked a sea change in the public's perception of managed care.[46] Even though only a few patients reported a "threatening and dramatic" event with managed care, frustrations became commonplace.[47] "Drive-through deliveries," in which new mothers were limited to twenty-four-hour maternity stays in the hospital, became a leading symbol of managed care's "reprehensible focus" on the financial bottom line.[48] Nitpicking utilization management (such as requiring health plan approval for routine outpatient referrals) and outpatient mastectomies added additional fuel to the public relations fire.[49] Managed care achieved what everyone considered necessary cost control, but in the process it demonstrated that cost control was inherently unpopular with both medical providers and the general public.

Rightly or wrongly, then, managed care executives essentially became the new health care villains. Opponents of Clinton's health care reform proposal in 1993–94 protested vehemently at the time that his model would lead to government rationing of medical care.[50] Instead, private health plans, less able to achieve price concessions from medical providers, imposed restrictions that generated the backlash. How ironic it was, as Uwe Reinhardt explains, that so soon after embracing the free market idea of managed care, the "rugged individualists" of the United States began "to show their more tender side, as self-pitifully and pitiably they plead with the White House, with the Congress, with their state governments and with the courts to jump right back onto their backs, to protect them from the forces of the private markets that, in their more rugged moments, they had professed to adore."[51]

By the late 1990s, managed care organizations were struggling under intensifying pressures on multiple fronts: political, economic, purchaser (employers), and consumer (patients). First, just as older regulations were beginning to take effect, state legislators passed new ones requiring that health plans provide additional benefits and an expanding array of consumer protection measures.[52] The timing could hardly have been worse. A resurgence in cost growth and continued internecine price competition within the industry forced managed care organizations to abandon their leading strategy of increasing market share and enrollment. Instead, they had to shift their focus to restoring profitability.[53] Meanwhile, a tight labor market and a roaring economy led employers to demand less restrictive health plans as part of their efforts to attract and retain valuable workers.[54] And, finally, the growing ranks of angry consumers and physicians made managed care organizations more unpopular than ever, which resulted in many individual and class-action lawsuits against the industry.[55] Examining in depth these pressures—and how they interacted with each other—helps explain why the managed care revolution stalled and then retreated so quickly.[56]

State legislators added new and extensive HMO regulations with broad bipartisan enthusiasm in the late 1990s.[57] In fact, many of the states leading the nation in implementing new managed care laws (New York, New Jersey, and Connecticut) had Republican governors and Democratic legislatures, note Richard Sorian and Judith Feder.[58] Elected officials were responding to the general public's hatred of managed care.[59] As the media made managed care the leading "pariah" industry—and before that honor passed to pharmaceutical companies a few years later—state legislators passed hundreds of new laws requiring that health plans: (1) offer richer benefits packages, (2) explicitly outline the physician-patient relationship with full disclosure of all treatment options and physicians' financial incentives, and (3) provide for independent patient appeals for coverage denials.[60] Close to one thousand managed care regulations were passed between 1995 and 1999, with four states (Texas, Missouri, California, and Georgia) allowing patients to sue for damages caused by denials or delays in coverage of necessary medical care.[61]

Managed care organizations found it harder and harder in the late 1990s to achieve profitability.[62] For years, their primary business strategy had been to both increase the number of people enrolled in their plans (in order to wield greater bargaining power in their negotiations with medical providers) and achieve economies of scale. In other words, managed care organizations wanted to get as big as possible, and then use their size to become more efficient and negotiate better contracts.[63] Yet market expansion proved to be a costly endeavor.[64] When new health plans entered local and national markets in the early and mid-1990s, they routinely offered their products at prices significantly below those of their competitors. This "below-margin" pricing strategy works when medical inflation remains minimal, which it did for a few years. But the period of low cost growth ended in 1997.[65] The following year, health care inflation rose at twice the rate of consumer price inflation.[66] As a result, the strategy of gaining market share by keeping premiums artificially low proved unsustainable.[67] In 1998, almost two-thirds of managed care organizations lost money, including major losses by some of the biggest plans: United Healthcare ($900 million), Oxford Health Plan ($508 million), and Kaiser Permanente ($266 million).[68] Humana, which had converted from a hospital chain to one of the nation's largest health insurers, lost more than half of its stock market value in 1998.[69] By the late 1990s, growing numbers of managed care plans were teetering on the verge of bankruptcy.[70]

On the demand side, employers were once again driving change. This time, though, they were pushing in the opposite direction of the restrictive forms of managed care that they had clamored for and received in the early to mid-1990s. Price competition among health plans was largely a response to employers' willingness to switch plans for even slightly lower premiums.[71] By the time this strategy proved unsustainable in the late 1990s, the country's economic recovery had turned into a boom and dramatically altered employers' attitudes about health insurance. When unemployment reached thirty-year lows in 1999 and 2000, businesses became desperate to attract and keep good workers.[72] Offering their employees health plans with broader networks of medical providers and fewer restrictions to health care services was more expensive.[73] But with strong corporate earnings, employers were once again able and willing to absorb large premium increases.[74]

Finally, the main force behind managed care's retreat was the growing consumer backlash, which was backed by state legislators and employers. Once the consumer backlash merged with the physician backlash, notes James Robinson "it quickly turned into an unstoppable political tornado."[75] The industry found itself on the receiving end of a famous tirade of profanity in the popular 1997 film, "As Good As It Gets," starring Jack Nicholson and Helen Hunt. (Hunt's character rants, "Those f—ing HMO bastard pieces of s—! It's okay. Actually, I think that's their technical name.") *Newsweek*'s November 8, 1999 edition included an angry patient on its cover with a lead story entitled "HMO Hell: The Backlash."[76] The medical directors of many managed care organizations—whose job involved determining what services would be covered and which medical providers patients could see—became targets of malpractice suits for "intentional infliction of emotional distress, breach of contract, fraud, and unfair claims practices."[77] For years health insurance companies and managed care organizations had considered themselves immune from medical liability lawsuits due to a federal law passed in 1974, the Employee Retirement Income Security Act (ERISA).[78] ERISA's original purpose was to keep individual states from meddling with the benefits packages of multistate employers.[79] As long as fee-for-service insurance dominated the industry, employees never had medical care denied.

After employers shifted most of their workers into managed care, increasing numbers of consumers accused their health plans of "practicing medicine" negligently by making medical decisions that should have been left solely to physicians.[80] The backlash arguably reached its zenith in October 1999, when a team of lawyers led by prominent attorney David Boies filed a class-action suit against Humana, "demanding that the company pay billions of dollars to health plan members for failing to honor its promises to pay for medically necessary care."[81] The suit was ultimately thrown out two years later, but by that time the managed care industry had moved away from most of the business and administrative practices that had initially triggered the lawsuit.[82] When a Florida district court certified a class-action suit on behalf of the nation's physicians against eight of the largest health plans in the United States in September 2002, the two largest—Aetna and Cigna—became the first health plans to settle and agree to "injunctive stipulations and hundreds of millions of dollars in payments."[83]

One final development emerged in the late 1990s, provider consolidation, which forced health plans to expedite the changes they were already beginning to make.[84] Large numbers of medical providers formed networks, physician-hospital organizations (PHOs), independent practice associations (IPAs), and system affiliations.[85] Their goal was to increase their bargaining position with managed care organizations, many of which were already eager to mend their damaged and frayed relationships with physicians and hospitals.

Medical Providers and Managed Care Organizations Respond

Pushed to the financial edge by a convergence of economic forces, hospitals led the way among medical providers in seeking to shift the balance of power from the purchasers of medical care to those who provide it. Building on a busy period of mergers in the mid-1990s,[86] many hospitals in the late 1990s formed concentrated systems by affiliating themselves with other local hospitals.[87] The amount of consolidation that subsequently occurred was substantial.[88] The proportion of the nation's hospitals in some form of local multihospital system increased from approximately 30 percent in 1995 to 65 percent by 2001.[89] The extent of this consolidation varied across the country; hospitals in areas where managed care controlled a larger share of the market were more likely to be part of a local system than those in areas of lower managed care penetration.[90] Yet, by 2001, hospitals in the majority of the nation's largest markets were concentrated in just two to four hospital systems.[91] And they were not shy about their use of cost shifting. Hospital executives frequently justified asking for large payment rate increases as necessary for "offsetting the impact of reduced state and federal reimbursements."[92] Their efforts paid off. The hospital industry's financial health improved dramatically beginning in 2000.[93]

In addition to pursuing consolidation, a sense of financial desperation emboldened many hospital executives to take their negotiations with private health plans to a level of brinkmanship.[94] The late 1990s had been the hospital industry's worst period in decades. While Congress did increase Medicare's payment rates in two "giveback" bills in 1999 and 2000, the adjustments were not large enough to do much more than stabilize Medicare's otherwise declining payment level (figure 7.1). Moreover, hospitals' labor costs were growing again.[95] Consequently, increasing numbers of hospital executives returned to the bargaining table in 2000 and 2001, threatening to

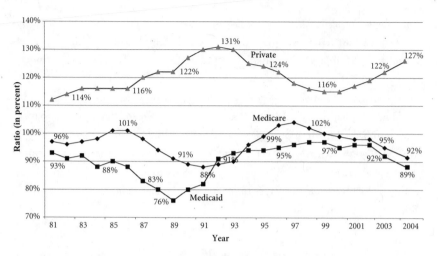

Figure 7.1. Hospital Payment-to-Cost Ratio by Payer, 1981–2004

Source: Data from Mayes and Lee, "Medicare Payment Policy," 157.

Note: Because Medicare is a "first mover" in the annual payment game and reimburses a prospectively set administered price that medical providers cannot negotiate, arguably the best measure of any relationship between a change in public payment and an aggregate change in private payment would be to compare Medicare and Medicaid's payment-to-cost ratios from 1984–96 and 1981–2003 with private payment-to-cost ratios from 1985–97 and 1981–2004, respectively:

Correlations:
1984–97: Medicare and Private ratios: $r = -.86$
1981–2004: Medicare and Private ratios: $r = -.73$
1984–97: Medicaid and Private ratios: $r = -.39$
1981–2004: Medicaid and Private ratios: $r = -.56$

walk away if their demands for increased payments were not met.[96] Acrimonious contract negotiations between hospitals and health plans were common across the country at this time.[97] By winning most of these showdowns, hospitals became "contract breakers," rather than the "takers" they had been in the mid-1990s.[98]

The major improvement in hospitals' bargaining position coincided with extensive changes within the managed care industry. Bowing to ever increasing pressures from consumers, politicians, lawyers, and physicians, managed care plans essentially surrendered. They either dropped most of their older, restrictive HMO plans or changed them to more closely resemble the increasingly popular PPO plans, which provided access to a much wider array of physicians.[99] Managed care plans also pulled back on the control mechanisms that limited patients' access to medical services. They relaxed or eliminated their pre-authorization requirements, which forced patients to obtain approval from a health-plan nurse or benefits manager before being admitted to a hospital, having a test or procedure done, or seeing a specialist.[100] They also loosened their grip on physicians' autonomy and financial remuneration.[101] With employers demanding less restrictive health plans and demonstrating a willingness (however unhappily) to pay more for them, managed care plans were only too willing to ditch many of the rules and practices that were causing them so much grief.[102] And when they capitulated, they gave up any claim to be transforming the U.S. health care delivery system.

Another key change that managed care organizations made at this time was to follow the hospital industry's example and pursue consolidation within the larger health insurance industry. As previously mentioned, when new managed care plans flooded the market in the early and mid-1990s, they increased price competition considerably and, in so doing, lowered insurance premiums. But there were limits to how long this competition could continue. Eventually, all health plans had to restore or achieve some measure of profitability. "Continuing losses on top of the declining interest in HMOs associated with the backlash against managed care drove a number of plans from the market, which, in combination with the large-scale mergers of national plans, led to a more concentrated industry," note Joy Grossman and Paul Ginsburg of the Center for Studying Health System Change.[103] By the early 2000s, virtually every state in the country was dominated by three large health plans.[104] With fewer competitors, the surviving plans—now much larger—raised premiums and dropped unprofitable lines of business.[105]

For many of the surviving health plans, the first unprofitable line of business to go was their participation in Medicare + Choice. The number of plans participating in the government's managed care program for Medicare beneficiaries fell from a high of 346 in 1998 to 155 by 2003.[106] The number of senior citizens in Medicare + Choice peaked at 17 percent of the program's beneficiaries in 1999, falling to less than 13 percent by 2003.[107] In 1999 and 2000, more than a million Medicare beneficiaries were abruptly dropped by health plans leaving the program.[108] The private health plans that remained increased premiums and beneficiary cost sharing, which left many Medicare beneficiaries with much higher out-of-pocket expenses. The plans also dramatically limited or dropped benefits such as prescription drugs.[109]

It quickly became clear that Medicare + Choice had failed as a vehicle for policy makers to expand market reforms of Medicare.[110] Medicare payments to participating managed care plans were linked to spending in the traditional fee-for-service part of the program, which after the BBA grew much more slowly than Congress and the Congressional Budget Office anticipated. Moreover, Medicare payments were not risk adjusted, which gave extra money to many M + C plans that actually had less sick and costly beneficiaries than beneficiaries in fee-for-service Medicare.[111] In the end, Republicans and Democrats disagreed over why Medicare + Choice failed—either the plans were over-regulated and underpaid by the government or the Medicare population is simply unsuited for profit-oriented managed care plans that are less able than traditional Medicare to manage costs.

In addition, the timing of Medicare + Choice was inauspicious. During the period in which federal policy makers tried to inject greater market forces into Medicare, restrictive managed care went into retreat, medical inflation returned, and health plans abandoned their pursuit of enrollment growth.[112] In other words, just as managed care organizations were giving up their tools and their will to restrain costs, the federal government actively encouraged millions of Medicare beneficiaries to enroll in private health plans—and spent a lot of money to do so. There was plenty of blame and fault to go around, according to Leonard Schaeffer, former HCFA administrator and founding chairman of WellPoint (the nation's largest private health insurer): "When Medicare + Choice came along, the plans all rolled out the red carpets. Those companies had been making enormous windfall profits. The government screws around, wakes up one day, figures out that it's overpaying everybody—which it's been doing for years—and says, "Look, we're not going to overpay you anymore." Then the companies all run for cover, and seniors get left high and dry. That is, I think, a failure of enormous proportions: bad social policy, bad business, bad for people."[113] Schaeffer's argument obscures the fact that reducing payments to private health plans was not policy makers' intent under the 1997 BBA. Instead, it was an unintended consequence of the success of cost control in the traditional Medicare program in the late 1990s. The BBA's success in controlling the cost increases in Medicare's fee-for-service program inadvertently reduced payment increases to participating M + C private health plans.[114]

Ultimately, the changing strategies of hospitals and managed care organizations in the late 1990s and early 2000s restored both industries to profitability. Spending on hospital services surged beginning in 2000 (figure 7.2). By 2002, hospital operating margins were the highest they had been in five years.[115] Similarly, after consolidating, raising premiums, and dropping unprofitable patient populations, the surviving health plans saw their profits soar from $4 billion in 2001 to slightly more than $10 billion in 2003.[116] Renewed profitability helped managed care plans and medical providers repair their acrimonious relationship. Major disputes between health plans and medical providers, particularly hospitals, became rare after 2001. Health plans largely acquiesced to medical providers' demands for higher payments and more than passed on the increased costs to employers in the form of double-digit increases to their health insurance premiums (figure 7.2).[117] Market forces were no longer strong enough to deliver cost control.[118]

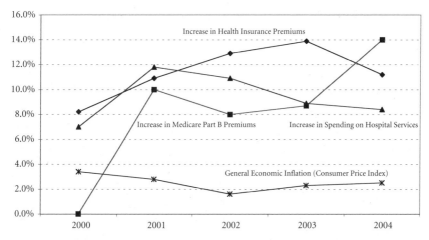

Figure 7.2. Resurgence of Medical Inflation in the United States, 2000–2004
Sources: Data from Census Bureau; Bureau of Labor Statistics; CMS.

A Resurgence of Medical Inflation and Its Consequences

Reopening the floodgates of private health care spending after a decade of cost control and rationalization had extraordinary consequences. The same problems that drove health care reform to the top of the nation's political agenda in the early 1990s returned—only worse—and new ones appeared.[119] First, employers' health insurance premiums skyrocketed. Between 2000 and 2004, the cost of employer-provided health insurance increased by more than 50 percent, five times the rate of inflation and growth in workers' earnings (figure 7.2).[120] Employers absorbed most of the initial increases, but eventually they shifted a larger proportion of them to their workers in the form of increased co-payments, deductibles, and monthly salary deductions.[121] More and more employers across the country also ceased to provide health insurance coverage to their retired workers. By 2003, fewer than 35 percent of U.S. companies provided health benefits to their retirees.[122]

Second, as health insurance became significantly more expensive, fewer businesses and workers could afford it.[123] Whereas 68 percent of U.S. businesses with fewer than two hundred employees offered health coverage to their workers in 2000, only 63 percent did so in 2003.[124] As a result, the total number of jobs in the United States that provided health insurance fell by five million.[125] This downward trend in coverage—together with the effects of a recession in 2001 and a sluggish recovery thereafter—increased the number of uninsured individuals from forty-one million in 2001 to forty-five million in 2003.[126] The growth in the number of uninsured people would have been far greater were it not for a major expansion of public coverage (Medicaid and SCHIP).

A third problem that stemmed from both rising medical inflation and declining private health insurance coverage was that Medicaid costs increased substantially.[127] Many individuals and families who lost their private coverage between 2000 and 2004 became eligible for Medicaid. Consequently, the program's enrollment grew by more than eight million people during this period, and its spending increased by more than 50 percent from $206 billion in 2000 to $311 billion in 2004.[128] State leaders became alarmed by their soaring Medicaid costs, because the program is jointly funded by the federal and state governments. "Medicaid is a cancer on our budget," noted Mississippi governor Haley Barbour.[129] Facing their worst fiscal shortfalls in decades, some states reduced benefits, increased patients' co-payments, and restricted eligibility or removed people from their programs.[130] The tragedy of these efforts is that they have come at the very time when the public's need for Medicaid has grown.

Last, the number of Americans with debilitating medical debt, as well as the number filing for bankruptcy due to health care expenses, increased sharply beginning in the early 2000s. Between 2001 and 2003, the proportion of low-income, chronically ill people with private insurance who spent more than 5 percent of their income on out-of-pocket health care costs grew by 50 percent to 2.2 million people.[131] In 1999, more than half a million families cited either substantial medical bills, a lapse in health insurance, or insufficient coverage as reasons for their insolvency.[132] Surprisingly, three-quarters of families who cited medical reasons for their bankruptcy had health insurance coverage.[133] Researchers found that medical debtors were mostly middle-class individuals who were injured or became ill. But they differed from others filing for bankruptcy in one important respect: "They were more likely to have experienced a lapse in health coverage," the researchers observed. "Many had coverage at the onset of their illness but lost it. In other cases, even continuous coverage left families with ruinous medical bills" due to large and uncovered out-of-pocket expenses (deductibles, co-payments, uncovered services).[134]

Bipartisan Commission on the Future of Medicare and the Push for "Premium Support"

The 1997 BBA included a provision calling for the creation of a National Bipartisan Commission on the Future of Medicare. The commission's mandate was to study the long-term financial condition of Medicare and provide recommendations on how best to prepare the program for the aging of the American population.[135] Co-chaired by House Ways and Means chair Bill Thomas (R-CA) and Senator John Breaux (D-LA), the commission first met in April 1998 and was made up of seventeen members appointed by the leaders of both parties in Congress. Breaux and Thomas led a subgroup of eight commission members who were strongly committed to switching Medicare to a defined contribution approach (or "premium support").[136] In other words, instead of providing Medicare as a defined benefit, the program would provide its beneficiaries with a defined contribution—something akin to a voucher—that they could use to purchase a private health insurance policy.[137] The premium support model was intended to make Medicare more closely resemble the Federal Employees Health Benefits Program (FEHBP), in which government employees purchase their health insurance coverage from a number of private plans that compete for their enrollment; and the federal government provides them with a financial contribution that covers most of the premium for a standard health plan.[138]

Under a premium support plan, argue health economists Henry Aaron and Robert Reischauer, "Medicare would pay a defined sum toward the purchase of an insurance policy that provided a defined set of benefits . . . All Medicare beneficiaries ultimately would receive a predetermined amount to be applied to the purchase of a health plan providing defined services."[139] To some, the result of the premium support proposal would be a fundamental transformation of Medicare's social insurance model.[140] Instead of offering the same entitlement to a uniform national benefit to entire demographic groups (senior citizens and people with disabilities), Medicare would provide the financing for beneficiaries to join hundreds of different private health plans across the country. The universality and collective philosophy of the program would have been replaced by a new paradigm that championed individualism and privatization.[141] Theoretically, competition among the nation's private health plans and managed care organizations for Medicare beneficiaries would serve to limit federal outlays, transfer financial risk from the government to the private sector, and allow medical providers to escape the heavy regulatory hand of HCFA (now the Centers for Medicare and Medicaid Services).[142]

What gave the push for moving to premium support a boost was that enthusiasm for market-oriented strategies went beyond just Republicans.[143] Commission members Senator Bob Kerrey of Nebraska and Senator Breaux of Louisiana, represented a number of conservative Democrats in Congress eager for a major restructuring of Medicare. In short, "premium support reaffirmed the 'technological wish' embodied by the prospective payment system for hospitals in the 1980s," notes Jonathan Oberlander, "the aspiration to adopt a policy system that would operate rationally and according to an automatic logic (of the market, in this case) that was self-regulating, without political interference, resulting in efficient and desirable outcomes."[144]

To secure the required "supermajority" of the commission's members (eleven of seventeen votes) for premium support, Breaux and Thomas were forced to consider including a provision calling for the adoption of a prescription drug benefit by Medicare.[145] They also had to recommend that 15 percent of the federal government's projected budget surplus be set aside to buttress Medicare's long-term solvency.[146] Including these two items may have procured the support of the commission's two swing voters: former chair of the Prospective Payment Assessment Commission Stuart Altman, and Laura Tyson, who was a senior economic advisor to President Clinton.[147] Unable to reach a compromise agreement, however, the commission ultimately deadlocked at ten in favor of premium support and seven against (one vote short), and then disbanded in spring 1999 without issuing a final report.[148] "Now begins the hard part," said Breaux.[149]

Later that same year, the commission's co-chairs proposed their premium support plan to Congress first as the Breaux-Thomas initiative and then officially as the Breaux-Frist Medicare Preservation and Improvement Act (with Senator Bill Frist, R-TN).[150] The bill was never debated in Congress, but it essentially became Republican policy and was adopted, in general terms, by George W. Bush in his campaign for the presidency in 2000.[151] The bill was revived early the following year as Breaux-Frist II and made considerable political progress in the Senate until the terrorist attacks of September 11, 2001. After this, major Medicare policy making was put on hold for more than a year, as domestic issues receded amidst the rise of intense foreign policy and national security concerns.[152]

The Medicare Prescription Drug, Improvement, and Modernization Act

The original impetus for the Bipartisan Commission on the Future of Medicare and for the first Breaux-Thomas initiative was to restructure Medicare, but the political focus shifted to providing prescription drug coverage. The shift was largely due to President George W. Bush and congressional Republicans' desire to garner the electoral support of senior citizens, particularly in Florida. In December 2003, President Bush and a Republican-controlled Congress enacted the largest expansion of Medicare in the program's history: the Medicare Prescription Drug, Improvement, and Modernization Act.[153] Beginning in 2006, Medicare provides the opportunity for prescription drug coverage to the program's 42 million beneficiaries. At a time of large and growing annual budget deficits, the MMA's cost[154] struck many observers as both fiscally irresponsible and politically paradoxical.[155] The neoconservative editorial board of the *Wall Street Journal* denounced the legislation as anathema and warned

Republicans who supported the bill that "they were fooling themselves . . . Republicans can never win an entitlement bidding war."[156] On the other end of the political spectrum, many liberal Democratic leaders in Congress found themselves in the awkward position of vehemently opposing a benefit expansion that they had pursued for more than a decade. They considered the drug benefit to be too meager and balked at the stipulation that the federal government would not be allowed to directly negotiate with pharmaceutical companies for lower prices.

In hindsight, the MMA seemed as much imposed as it was enacted. Senior citizens were facing larger and larger out-of-pocket costs for prescription drugs,[157] which contributed to the political momentum for adding a prescription drug benefit to Medicare. Yet, as John Iglehart observes, "Never before had Congress enacted major Medicare legislation about which the divisions between the political parties ran so deep."[158] Only two Democrats among the seven who had been appointed to the seventeen-member conference committee were actually allowed to participate in the final and most sensitive deliberations.[159] The House of Representatives passed the bill by a razor-thin 220 to 215 margin, with the Senate following suit by a narrow 54 to 44 margin.[160] One of country's leading congressional analysts, Norman Ornstein, described the tactics used to pass the bill in the House as "the ugliest and most outrageous breach of standards in the modern history of the House."[161] The House of Representatives was kept open for an additional three hours—for the longest roll call in House history—so that President Bush and the House Republican leadership could "resort to some extraordinary last-minute tactics to persuade some of the party's more conservative members to vote for it."[162] In a public poll taken the week that President Bush signed the legislation into law, almost 50 percent of senior citizens said they opposed the plan, with only 23 percent in support of it.[163]

Unlike the period following the passage of the BBA in 1997 or the Social Security reform bill in 1983, there was no sense of bipartisan gratification following the passage of the MMA.[164] "We have only just begun to fight," said Senator Edward Kennedy (D-MA) on the day that President Bush signed the MMA into law. "If Republicans think this fight is over, they are wrong." He and other Democratic congressional leaders pledged to attack specific parts of the law until they were repealed.[165] The MMA's opposition gained growing numbers of Republicans in February 2005, when the Bush administration released new estimates projecting the cost of Medicare's prescription drug benefit to be approximately $724 billion between 2006 and 2015 (a different time period than the previous $534 and $395 billion estimates, which were for 2004 to 2013).[166]

Critical to understanding the paradoxical politics of the MMA is recognizing that for many Republicans, and conservatives in general, Medicare is viewed as a huge, outdated, and inefficient government program.[167] Ever since taking control of Congress in 1994, leading Republicans have wanted to fundamentally change Medicare from a universal government benefit to a program that provides its beneficiaries with a defined contribution toward the purchase of a private health plan.[168] Private health plans competing for Medicare beneficiaries, Republicans argue, will help constrain the program's costs while also providing beneficiaries with new benefits such as prescription drug coverage.[169] The centerpiece of the BBA's 1997 Medicare reforms, Medicare + Choice, was the vehicle that they hoped would greatly accelerate this market-oriented transformation. It ultimately failed. But Republicans remained undeterred, as evidenced by the behavior of the leaders of the Bipartisan Commission on the Future of Medicare.

In early 2003, as the drive to add prescription drug coverage to Medicare was gaining political momentum, the Bush administration proposed that only beneficiaries enrolled in a private plan should receive any new drug benefit.[170] The proposal met with a definite lack of enthusiasm from members of both parties and was eventually abandoned.[171] But it revealed the administration's underlying motivation, which was to undermine the traditional Medicare program by continuing to freeze in place an outmoded benefit structure that lacked both prescription drug coverage and coverage for catastrophic illness, while assuring that private plans did provide these enhanced benefits. It tried to move more Medicare beneficiaries into private health plans, shifting a greater proportion of the program's financial risk to the private plans and even to beneficiaries themselves.

For years there had been widespread agreement among policy makers that some type of drug benefit needed to be added to Medicare. Yet two-thirds of the program's beneficiaries already had some form of prescription drug coverage (through plans they continued to receive from their previous employers, private Medigap policies, Medicaid, or a Medicare + Choice plan).[172] Policy makers were nervous that too generous a benefit would encourage other sources of drug coverage to recede or vanish altogether. Thus, Republican leaders in Congress did not craft a universal, seamless, and comprehensive prescription drug benefit. Instead, they made participation in Medicare's new prescription drug program voluntary (similar to Part B); they gave the responsibility for providing the drug benefit to private companies (not to the federal government); and they limited the plan's coverage.[173]

The enormity of the new drug benefit (Title I of the MMA) overshadowed and diverted attention from two other components of the law that represented a dramatic change in Medicare's traditional design and philosophy. First, the MMA broke with more than thirty years of social insurance tradition by providing a means-testing measure to charge wealthier beneficiaries more for their Part B benefits (physician and outpatient services). Medicare had always charged every beneficiary—regardless of their income—the same monthly premium for participation in Part B of the program. The entire Medicare population, therefore, shared equally in paying for 25 percent of Part B's annual costs. The MMA changed this. As of 2007, individual Medicare beneficiaries with adjusted gross incomes over $80,000 (or $160,000 for married couples) pay higher premiums for the same Part B benefit that less affluent beneficiaries will receive with lower premiums.[174] Moreover, low-income beneficiaries—those whose incomes are below 135 percent of the poverty level—will pay lower premiums than other Medicare beneficiaries for an even more generous prescription drug benefit.[175] "Proposals to means-test Medicare benefits are as old as the program itself," notes health economist Marilyn Moon.[176] But the MMA heralded the first time that Medicare's premiums and insurance benefits would vary depending on beneficiaries' income.

The MMA's other dramatic change is that it significantly expanded the law's bias toward the role of private health plans in Medicare. It did so by renaming the Medicare + Choice program "Medicare Advantage," adding billions of dollars in higher payments to participating managed care plans, and promoting the expansion of PPOs in private fee-for-service plans.[177] At first glance, recommitting to the same principles embodied in the failed Medicare + Choice program seems contradictory if Republicans' goal is to control Medicare's costs.[178] Private health plans in M + C did not save Medicare money; rather, they proved to be more expensive.[179] In 2003, Medicare paid private health plans participating in M + C an average of 4 percent more than if those Medicare beneficiaries had remained in the traditional program.[180] In 2004, the program renamed as Medicare Advantage paid private health plans 8.4 percent more on average than if the beneficiaries had remained in Medicare's traditional program (the figure rises to 15 percent if one takes into account the fact that many private plans enroll Medicare beneficiaries who are healthier than average).[181] And in 2005, Medicare is estimated to have spent 6.6 percent more—or an average of $546—for each of the almost five million Medicare beneficiaries enrolled in participating private health care plans than it did for the average beneficiary in its traditional fee-for-service arrangements (for a total of $2.72 billion in extra Medicare spending).[182]

The major recommitment that the MMA made to private managed care plans stems from the belief of several prominent leaders (mostly Republicans) in Congress, including former House Ways and Means chair Bill Thomas (R-CA) that "private plans and competition will help drive down the explosive growth of Medicare spending."[183] Given the numerous empirical analyses that find that health plans participating in the

Medicare Advantage program consistently cost more to taxpayers than the traditional fee-for-service program,[184] one is tempted to categorize Medicare Advantage as something of a "faith-based" initiative.

A unique convergence of severe political and financial pressures in the late 1990s ended the nation's brief experiment with restrictive managed care; it also ended its longest sustained period of below-average growth in per capita national health spending.[185] Steep Medicare cuts in spending on hospitals and postacute providers, imposed by the 1997 BBA, made it impossible for many medical providers to compensate for years of declining payment generosity from private payers. Prior to the BBA, the annual growth in Medicare spending had managed to outpace general medical inflation. After the BBA, both public and private health care payments decreased simultaneously for the first time. In desperation, large segments of the medical provider community turned to consolidation in order to survive financially. In the face of BBA cuts, they returned to their habit of tried-and-true cost shifting to increase revenues from private payers. They were aided in their efforts by an onslaught of regulatory and legal restrictions on private health plans by state governments responding to the public backlash against managed care. When private health plans surrendered the drive for cost control, health care spending returned to its long-term pattern of rapid acceleration.

The resulting surge in medical inflation triggered another in the nation's series of health care crises.[186] Beginning in 2001, public health insurance programs experienced rapid enrollment growth and the number of uninsured Americans increased significantly. More and more employers shifted a larger proportion of their growing health insurance costs to their workers and many ceased to provide coverage altogether. Medical debt and the number of health-related bankruptcies in the United States soared. "I know what you're thinking. Hillary Clinton and health care? Been there. Didn't do that!" wrote Senator Hillary Clinton. "No, it's not 1994; it's 2004. And believe it or not, we have more problems today than we had back then."[187]

Finally, the future of Medicare, both in financial and programmatic terms, was complicated by a Republican exercise of political muscle to narrowly pass the MMA in late 2003. The MMA made Medicare a more complete health insurance program for the elderly by adding prescription drug coverage. But it did so at a high price—more than $700 billion over ten years—with large subsidies for employers that continue to provide drug coverage to their retired workers, low-income subsidies for poor beneficiaries, and major payoffs for private health plans that participate in Medicare Advantage. Thus, the "MMA was a significant achievement, and in many ways an improvement," notes Eric Cohen. "But one can also understand why so many people—

Left, Right, and Center—see the bill as irresponsible or inadequate, and why no one really believes it is what Medicare needs over the long-term."[188] The same financial necessity, which became the mother of Medicare's payment innovation in the late 1970s, is bound to return in the near future. Fiscal exigencies will virtually require it.

As the history of Medicare policy making suggests, Congress will likely want to (and have to) reduce Medicare payments in the future as part of larger efforts to reduce federal budget deficits. The difficulty with this time-honored tradition, however, is that the country's baby-boom generation begins retiring in 2010. Each year thereafter, until 2030, the number of Medicare beneficiaries will increase significantly (from 46 to 77 million individuals by 2030).[189] As a result, Medicare's costs will increase significantly as well, and the immense budgetary "cushion" that the program has provided national policy makers for two decades will cease to exist. Even worse, the program's solvency beyond 2020 has become a matter of serious concern.[190]

How Medicare Does and Should Shape U.S. Health Care

So what we are trying to do, first of all, is say, "Okay, here is a government monopoly plan. We're designing a free-market plan ... " Now we didn't get rid of it [the "government monopoly plan," Medicare] in round one because we don't think that's politically smart and we don't think that's the right way to go through a transition ... But we think it's going to wither on the vine, because we think people are going to voluntarily leave it.

—*Newt Gingrich, Speaker of the House of Representatives (1994–98), in a speech to a Blue Cross Conference, October 24, 1995*

The pricing practices of the medical industry depart sharply from the competitive norm ... It is clear from everyday observation that the behavior expected of sellers of medical care is different from that of business men in general. These expectations are relevant because medical care belongs to the category of commodities for which the product and the activity of production are identical. In all such cases, the customer cannot test the product before consuming it, and there is an element of trust in the relation. But the ethically understood restrictions on the activities of a physician are much more severe than on those of, say, a barber. His behavior is supposed to be governed by a concern for the customer's welfare, which would not be expected of a salesman.

—*Kenneth Arrow, recipient of the 1972 Nobel Prize in Economics*

Prospective payment approaches in Medicare represent an important story of success. Although often derided by free market advocates—such as the editors of the *Wall Street Journal*[1]—as imposing an ineffectual "Soviet-style bureaucracy" by applying arbitrary and rigid price controls on the health care system, in fact, Medicare has successfully helped shape U.S. health care by converting inflationary cost- and charge-based payments into prospective payments based on predetermined rates. In most cases, these new payment systems have provided important incentives for economizing on care, while at the same time permitting Medicare beneficiaries access to virtually all the clinicians and institutional providers in the market.

Medicare's administrative prices may not be the prices that would be set by a well-functioning market. But as Kenneth Arrow has persuasively argued, we do not want to try to subject health care to the invisible hand of the market.[2] We want physicians and other clinicians to act not as marketplace sellers of services to wary consumers, but as trusted professionals with a duty to serve patients' best interests.

Victor Fuchs, the dean of American health economists, made the same point in arguing not only that the conditions for market competition do not exist in health care, but also that—even if the necessary market conditions were present—there is something fundamentally different about health care: "The production function for health is a peculiar one; it usually requires patients and health professionals to work cooperatively rather than as adversarial buyers and sellers. Mutual trust and confidence contribute to the efficiency of production. Thus the model of atomistic competition usually set as the ideal in economics textbooks often is not the right goal for health."[3]

Although Internet access permits some individuals the opportunity to learn about illnesses and the performance of providers at their leisure, persistent information asymmetries between providers and patients continue to make the idea of a well-functioning market in health care unlikely. That is, the patient cannot really be a wise and prudent shopper for services because she is dependent on the vendor—in this case, the physician—for specialized information on which to base decisions that the physician has acquired through many years of training and clinical practice. Moreover, a lot of health care does not take place at anyone's leisure. Rather, health problems may arise at times and under circumstances when individuals must question but ultimately trust the judgments of the professionals they have selected—acting as patients, not consumers.

Surely, health care needs to deemphasize reliance on often paternalistic physicians oblivious to the particular preferences and needs of the individuals they are caring for. However, this reorientation should promote patients' sharing decision making with professionals, not taking it over altogether.[4] The vision promoted by some market advocates—especially those promoting so-called consumer-directed health care (CDHC), in which patients are empowered to become wary consumers carefully navigating a retail marketplace of health care providers who need to promote their own services through aggressive marketing—is not one we endorse.

Due to the potential high costs associated with a sudden illness and the cumulative high costs of chronic conditions, our society wants the protection that third party insurance provides. Admittedly, broad insurance protection against health care costs creates what economists call "moral hazard," the natural tendency of individuals to spend more of someone else's money than their own. Some would seek to address this by decreasing the essential role of health insurance. New insurance products, built on tax-advantaged medical savings accounts (MSAs), impose large deductibles and significant co-payments at the point of service to encourage patients to "take more responsibility for their choices."[5] Yet patients, especially older and disabled persons with serious chronic health conditions, are naturally reluctant to give up the economic and psychological security of good health insurance coverage in exchange for more control over how their money is spent. Rather, they want the payers—in this case the Medicare program—and the providers to determine how best to moderate health care cost increases.

Not only, in our judgment, is the public not interested, willing, or able to become the same kind of prudent shoppers for health care services that they are when purchasing cell phones and airline tickets, but the CDHC model will not actually restrain costs very much, because of the uneven distribution of health care spending among the population. Certainly, higher cost sharing might lead a weekend sports enthusiast to defer obtaining a physician-recommended MRI for recurring knee pain, a prototypical example of supposed wasteful health care spending that might be reduced if the person faced the MRI costs directly without health insurance. And health care costs might be reduced somewhat (but so might be the person's physical and emotional well-being.) Yet, in health insurance programs both public and private, the most costly 20 percent of patients account for 80 percent of health care spending.[6] Many of the patients who generate high spending have one or more persistent, advancing chronic conditions and, therefore, have annual costs far in excess of what any insurance plan would impose in out-of-pocket expenses.

Thus, turning patients into price-wary consumers will not save the system much. Studies continue to document the excessive, and probably wasteful, spending associated with the care of patients with multiple chronic conditions and those in their last year of life.[7] Yet insurance products that reasonably provide financial protection—with limits on deductible and annual out-of-pocket spending limits—serve the purpose insurance was designed for, leaving patients cost-unconscious once they reach the deductible or the out-of-pocket spending limit.[8] Although full insurance coverage surely does produce some excessive spending, as noted, for those who most depend on it, insurance protection provides needed comfort. If anything, Medicare's basic benefits should be expanded, not only to fill in the donut hole in the new prescription drug benefit, but also to provide better catastrophic coverage, which nonpoor beneficiaries now obtain only if they are fortunate enough to have retiree supplemental coverage or can afford to purchase a supplemental Medigap policy.[9]

Should Medicare Be Allowed to Wither on the Vine?

In contrast to the consumer-directed health care approach—which would minimize the role of insurance and create more traditional retail markets like those that exist in most other sectors of the economy—Alain Enthoven, a Stanford health economist, has long proposed a markedly different, market-based model of health system reform, one that he has called "managed competition." The approach relies heavily on group purchasing, competition among an array of private health plans, and restructuring of the health delivery system into organized, integrated delivery systems,[10] which involve the incorporation of large physician group practices with hospitals and other providers into single organizations with the size, scope, and mission to better manage care across a continuum of services that patients need. Kaiser Permanente exemplifies the kind of system that Enthoven wants to see promoted nationally.[11] This prescription specifically rejects relying on retail consumer markets where individuals choose among competing professionals and other providers at the point of service.[12]

In the context of the future of Medicare, one can plausibly argue that managed competition makes good policy sense because private health plans are better positioned than a national Medicare program to respond to both the geographic diversity in the preferences of patients and providers and to the particular circumstances that characterize the local markets where health care is delivered.[13] We are sympathetic with managed competition's particular vision for reorganizing health care around integrated health care delivery systems. And although some social insurance advocates would disagree, we think that strictly regulated competition among private plans can be made compatible with the basic principles of social insurance.[14]

In fact, in some ways, the Medicare environment may be better suited to Enthoven-style managed competition than are private insurance markets. For example, in contrast to employers that typically do not offer a choice of all eligible health plans and do not make equal, fixed-dollar contributions to the employee's chosen plan, Medicare Advantage provides a choice of all eligible plans and makes a fixed government contribution to plans who submit bids in relation to that contribution. It also adjusts the payments to health plans based on the underlying health status of enrollees. These and other elements of Medicare's approach to private plan contracting is closer to Enthoven's approach to competition than currently is present in commercial markets.[15]

Unfortunately, although managed health plan competition in Medicare, where there is a competent buyer of services able to shape the competition among the private health plans, might work in theory, as we detailed in Chapter 7, it would very likely fail in practice. And if it can't work in Medicare, it surely won't work for the entire health care system. As Victor Fuchs—who was clearly sympathetic to Enthoven's call for health system restructuring based around health plan competition—documented, the basic conditions for desirable competition do not exist in health care.[16]

In many ways, the competitive situation is even worse today than when Fuchs was writing in the 1980s. As providers have learned that contract negotiations with plans over prices are crucial to their financial well-being, they have engaged in various activities to buttress their negotiating strength that, among other things, permits them often to cost shift to private payers when Medicare reduces its prices. Hospitals have consolidated through mergers and acquisitions, and physician specialists have consolidated into larger medical groups, providing hospitals and many physicians the opportunity to exert market power over health plans to push prices up.[17] Contributing to the imbalance in negotiating leverage, hospitals have less excess capacity of hospital beds and fewer physicians have openings on their appointment schedules.[18] At the same time, health insurers have consolidated extensively and are currently enjoying the extraordinary profitability associated with the near-monopoly status they have achieved in many regions throughout most of the country.[19] These and other worsening barriers to efficient market outcomes have led to increased doubts that even well-structured and appropriately regulated market competition among fewer and fewer (but also larger and more profitable) health plans would be able to accomplish the ambitious and laudable goals that market competition advocates have proposed.

The reality is that the admittedly cumbersome Medicare program uses its governmental authority to get better prices than private health plans are able to obtain in most, but certainly not all, local health care markets.[20] And although private plans theoretically can do a better job than the traditional Medicare program in restraining the use of services (which, when multiplied by applicable prices, determines program expenditures), in fact, these plans have not done a better job in limiting cost increases than the traditional Medicare program. Over the long term, the rates of growth in per capita spending for Medicare and private insurance have been remarkably similar.

When comparing spending for benefits that private insurance and Medicare have in common—notably excluding prescription drugs—Medicare's per enrollee spending grew at a rate that was about one percentage point lower than that for private insurance over the 1970–2002 period.[21] This should not be surprising since both private insurance and Medicare have been essentially passive payers of what providers determine is needed for patients.

Medicare has done a good job holding down cost increases through prospective payment, but for the most part has not been allowed to proactively address the ever-increasing volume and intensity of services. Having mostly abandoned their managed care tools in the face of the public backlash,[22] private plans have even less ability to actually manage costs than does traditional Medicare, which at least has market power as the health care system's largest payer. With the recent migration of insured individuals from HMOs to PPO products whose predominant function is to obtain price discounts from providers but who are not as successful at doing so as Medicare is, even the theoretical advantages of private plans over the traditional Medicare program are disappearing.[23]

Except for group- and staff-model HMOs such as Kaiser Permanente, commercial health insurance plans now function much as Medicare, but with no ability to mandate reasonable payment rates. Private plans also have much higher administrative costs and need to make profits to satisfy stockholders and provide often outrageously exorbitant executive salaries.[24] As we showed in Chapter 7, private plans need to spend more than the traditional Medicare program does in order to make serving Medicare beneficiaries a profitable business proposition. The evidence of private health plan failure has not deterred the Republican Party, which for more than a decade has been attempting to dismantle the traditional Medicare program. Newt Gingrich explained a decade ago that the goal was to have Medicare "wither on the vine,"[25] by which he surely meant the traditional Medicare program, with its "Soviet-style bureaucracy" that relies on price controls.

Medicare has long paid a little more to private plans than it would pay in traditional fee-for-service Medicare, but the Medicare Modernization Act now has it paying private plans much more.[26] The MMA's architects apparently hope that over time these overpayments will lead beneficiaries to seek out the additional benefits that private plans will be able to offer. For example, private plans are able to use the extra funds they receive to decrease enrollee's out-of-pocket expenses, provide additional benefits for prevention services, provide good catastrophic coverage, and enhance the rather meager prescription drug benefits that are available to beneficiaries who remain in the regular Medicare program. With the higher payments plans should be able to offer providers, they might also hope providers will steer their patients into the private plans, because the providers will receive higher reimbursements from the private plans than from traditional Medicare. Consistent with Gingrich's strategy, such an approach would lead to traditional Medicare's demise, not through an explicit political decision that—given Medicare's enormous popularity—would be very difficult, but rather through the decentralized and diffused decisions of beneficiaries and providers making choices on an unlevel playing field decisively tilted in favor of private plans.

Medicare Shapes Health Care Markets

Conservative rhetoric notwithstanding, Medicare's payment levels are not arbitrarily set by a large government bureaucracy impervious to the needs of patients and providers. Instead, Medicare's prices attempt to reflect the underlying costs providers bear for caring for Medicare beneficiaries. Congress, counseled by its Medicare Payment Advisory Commission, attempts to have Medicare pay "the approved costs in full that are incurred by efficient providers when they offer necessary and appropriate care to Medicare beneficiaries," according to Robert Reischauer, vice-chair of Med-PAC. "What this means, in short, is that Medicare should not consider the level of payments relative to costs that other purchasers are paying providers. It should set rates as if it were in a sense the only payer."[27] This discipline generally leads to fair, if sometimes inflated, payment levels. As part of the goal of assuring fair payments, MedPAC and others continually conduct beneficiary surveys and collect other data to assess whether payment levels continue to support adequate beneficiary access to care.

The only major exception to the general proposition that Medicare should pay the costs for its own beneficiaries are the explicit subsidies Congress provides for two hospital sectors whose missions often overlap—teaching hospitals and hospitals that constitute the nation's safety net for the uninsured—through financial support of the education of thousands of hospital residents-in-training and special financial supplements to so-called disproportionate share hospitals serving the poor.[28] And although a less explicit consideration, when budgetary conditions permit, Congress may sometimes pay extra to assure the solvency of important community health care resources.[29]

Even the United States Supreme Court recently weighed in on whether Medicare payments are designed solely to pay the costs of care for Medicare beneficiaries or to be a primary financial support for providers. In 2000, in a criminal fraud case, *Fisher v. United States,* the Court considered whether participating hospitals should receive actual "benefits" from the Medicare program and not merely compensation for services rendered.[30] The Court concluded, in a 7–2 decision, "We do not accept the view that the Medicare payments in question are for the limited purposes of compensating providers or reimbursing them for ordinary expenditures . . . The payments are made not simply to reimburse for treatment for qualifying patients but to assist the hospital in making available and maintaining a certain level and quality of medical care, all in the interest of both the hospital and the greater community."[31]

So far the Court's dictum, which was provided on a case unrelated to the generosity of Medicare's actual payment rates, has not been invoked to challenge payment policies that pay providers only for their "ordinary expenditures," perhaps because Congress has been relatively generous with Medicare provider payments. Because it must assure acceptable quality care for beneficiaries, Medicare needs to take into account the financial well-being of providers, a consideration to which the invisible hand of a marketplace would be completely indifferent.[32]

For example, current payment policy favors the preservation of small, rural hospitals that are viewed as important community resources in rural communities, both as major employers and as part of the basic health care delivery systems in these areas.[33] Thus, Medicare's payment approach has been highly successful not only in paying for the costs of care provided to Medicare beneficiaries, but also for providing important financial support for the nation's health care infrastructure.

In addition, the 1997 Balanced Budget Act demonstrated that imposing relatively modest limits on provider payment increases can generate a substantial reduction in expenditures (at least for a few years). The so-called giveback bills that returned some of the unanticipated savings to hospitals and certain other providers may suggest to some that the cuts were excessive, but no one has shown that Medicare beneficiaries experienced lack of access to needed care or received reduced-quality care. In short, administratively determined, prospective payment can be an effective tool for controlling costs. What is at issue is whether Congress has the political will to apply the tools to control costs for the long term.

The United States spends much more on health care than other developed country, not primarily because more health care services are provided but because we have a more expensive health care enterprise, with more personnel who receive higher wages relative to their counterparts in other industrialized nations.[34] Consequently, high prices are driving spending, and Medicare's success in converting payment to prospectively set rates is an important strategy in controlling health care spending. Again, in most local health care markets, Medicare's prices are lower than those of private purchasers and health insurance plans.

Medicare's ability to impose prices on providers derives from the fact that it is a dominant payer, but that dominant position also tempers Medicare's use of its market power. Because relatively few clinicians and institutional providers can afford not to care for the program's beneficiaries as patients, Medicare could probably get away with driving rates down below what a well-functioning marketplace would produce. After all, hospitals, home health agencies, inpatient rehabilitation hospitals, the part of the nursing home industry that provides skilled nursing, and other providers and suppliers would be out of business without Medicare revenues. But Medicare has an interest in assuring access to needed services for the beneficiaries it serves; correspondingly, it has no interest in abusing its position of market power to the detriment of its beneficiaries and the delivery system.

Even now, when Medicare tempers its market power by tying its payment rates fairly explicitly to estimated provider costs, some medical providers try to cost shift to other payers and, as we demonstrated earlier, often succeed. Indeed, because of the possibility of cost shifting in what can euphemistically be labeled our "pluralistic" health care system, Medicare's discipline in restraining payment increases does not necessarily guarantee that the health care system as a whole restrains overall cost increases. But the reality of cost shifting, due in part to noncompetitive private health care markets, is not Medicare's fault.

Some are concerned that aggressive price cutting by Medicare would lead providers to view Medicare beneficiaries as second-class patients, a concern that motivated the failed efforts by the Carter administration to impose all-payer hospital cost limits. Although there have been suggestive anecdotes, so far there is no evidence that providers are turning away Medicare patients or subjecting them to second-rate care. MedPAC has looked closely at surveys of Medicare beneficiaries' ability to access physician services and of physicians' willingness to serve Medicare patients; it concluded that beneficiary access to physicians remains good overall.[35]

Medicare's Problematic Relationship with Physicians

The current problems faced by Medicare's prospective payment system for physicians illustrate a number of challenges for Medicare payment policies. As emphasized in Chapter 5, Medicare spending for physician services is supposed to be restrained by an expenditure limit, initially called a "volume performance standard" and replaced in the 1997 BBA by the "sustainable growth rate." The SGR formula ties physician payment rate updates to a number of factors, including growth in input prices for goods and services used in physician practices, the effects of laws and regulations on the kinds of services physicians provide, the growth in enrollment in the traditional Medicare program, and the growth of physician services in relation to growth in the national economy as measured by the gross domestic product. Remarkably, the GDP linkage was an attempt to determine how much volume growth in physician services society can afford.[36] It is the only part of Medicare that attempts to formally limit spending by linking it to the contemporary state of the economy rather than to more relevant measures of inflation that medical providers face.[37]

The basic SGR mechanism compares actual Medicare Part B spending to a spending target calculated through the SGR formula and then adjusts the annual payment update accordingly.[38] If Medicare spending for physician services remains on target, the annual increase in physician fees is set equal to the estimated change in physicians' cost of providing care—that is, the change in the Medicare Economic Index, which measures input prices for the resources physician practices use to provide services. However, if the growth in the volume and intensity of services is high enough that Medicare Part B spending exceeds the SGR target, future physician fee increases will be lower than the MEI. And if the gap is wide enough, Medicare's fee update may even be negative, producing fee reductions (as occurred in 2002, when physician fees *decreased* by 5.4 percent).[39] Conversely, physicians receive fee increases exceeding the MEI if actual spending is less than that set by the SGR target.

Although the growth in physician volume slowed significantly during the 1990s, following the initial imposition of the VPS,[40] the situation changed dramatically thereafter. Since 2000, spending has remained above the target in large part because the growth in the volume of services has been greater than the growth allowed by the SGR. From 1999 to 2003, growth in volume of physician services per beneficiary averaged about 5 percent per year. By contrast, the allowance in the target for volume growth—driven mostly by the trend in growth in real GDP per capita—was only about 2 percent.[41] That volume growth, however, pales in comparison to what happened in 1994. In a 2005 letter to the chairman of MedPAC, the Centers for Medicare and Medicaid Services described unprecedented volume increases in physician services. CMS found that expenditures for physician services had increased 15 percent in 2004 due to increases in the volume and intensity of services.[42]

The services that displayed rapid growth were discretionary ones that do not involve significant potential risk to patients, and therefore can be ordered and provided with relative impunity. The costs from unnecessary use of services are the only major problem for beneficiaries and taxpayers, and do not affect the physicians, who actually benefit from increased revenues. The main sources of these spending increases were payment claims for longer office visits and increased provision of laboratory, radiology, and other tests. For example, the number of claims submitted from the service category labeled "advanced imaging" (CT, MRI, and PET scans) increased 25 percent in just one year.[43]

Based on Medicare's SGR formula, physicians would have received an estimated 4.3 percent reduction in 2006. However, as it did for 2004 and 2005, Congress in the Deficit Reduction Act of 2006 prevented the formula-driven reduction, freezing 2006 payments at 2005 levels but not raising the spending targets.[44] The reduction would have been even larger based on the 15 percent physician spending increase, but there is a limit on how much the physician spending update rate can be cut in any one year.[45] Nevertheless, the deficits from SGR-allowed spending are cumulative, affecting future years' spending. In other words, excess spending that is not offset in one year accumulates in succeeding years until it is recouped. With Congressional temporizing to fix the SGR mechanism, the CMS Office of the Actuary has projected physician updates of about −5 percent per year for at least nine consecutive years, from 2007 through 2015.[46]

Yet it is unlikely that physicians will actually be asked to absorb a 40 percent decrease in their Medicare fee schedule payments over the next nine years, because just the specter of this level of cutting has raised concerns that many physicians would view Medicare patients as second class, avoid caring for them in non-emergency situations, and replace them with better paying, "easier," younger patients. This scenario needs to be avoided and will be, because Medicare payment levels are responsive to the marketplace—not through an invisible hand but rather through a political process. We are confident that Medicare beneficiaries will not lack access to physician care as payment procedures and payment levels are reconsidered.

Congress and its advisory committees, including MedPAC and the Government Accountability Office (GAO), are studying how to change the SGR mechanism to correct its apparent flaws and are rethinking the assumption that there should be a relationship between Medicare beneficiaries' needs for services and the vagaries of the U.S. economy. If, as most expect, physicians are protected from most of the formula-driven payment cuts, a result will be even more Part B spending and even higher Part B premiums for Medicare beneficiaries. CMS recently reported that the monthly premium for 2007 will rise from the current $89.50 to $98.20.[47] But that assumes the SGR mechanism is in place and working. Relief to physicians will increase the Part B premium substantially. In short, Medicare beneficiaries will bear part of the cost for protecting physician fees.

Ironically, an expenditure limit on physician services was designed, among other things, to protect Medicare beneficiaries from the full effect of volume and cost increases in physician services. By law, the federal government pays 75 percent of the cost of Medicare's Part B benefits—for physician services and outpatient medical care—with beneficiaries' Part B premiums, paid out of pocket or by supplemental insurance, covering the remaining 25 percent. In 2004, a few months before the presidential election, the Bush administration announced that the Part B premium for 2005 would increase from $66.60 to $78.20 (a record 17 percent increase that received considerable attention during the presidential campaign).[48] And now the premiums have risen substantially twice more, to $88.50 in 2006 and $98.20 for 2007. Without an expenditure limit in place, the increase in the Part B premium would surely have been even greater.

In sum, after years of cost stability in the aftermath of the BBA, Medicare again has begun to experience the consequences of health care inflation that far exceeds general inflation, putting pressure on the monthly Part B premiums paid by the program's beneficiaries. Due to the rapid rate of growth in the program's spending on physician and other outpatient services in the early 2000s, a growing proportion of Medicare beneficiaries' Social Security income has become consumed by medical inflation.[49] The cost of their monthly Part B premiums, which are automatically deducted from their monthly Social Security checks, increased by more than 50 percent during this period (see figure 7.2). Congress may be able to assure that the SGR expenditure control mechanism does not affect beneficiaries' access to physician services, but that assurance comes at a high cost.

It's the Expenditures, Not the Prices, That Finally Matter

The current issues faced in physician payment reform provide timely examples of the broad challenges faced by Medicare's prospective payment systems. In some ways the physician payment system presents these challenges most starkly because it is the payment system that most closely resembles the traditional cost- or charge-based reimbursement that preceded prospective payment. Medicare's payments to physicians, based on the resource-based relative-value scale, are prospective in that payment amounts are predetermined for the class of providers—in this case, physicians and related clinical professionals—and, accordingly, are not related to the actual costs or charges of those submitting claims.

However, physician payment remains fee-for-service in that payments are made for discrete individual transactions, each of which is described using one of thousands of standardized codes. In contrast, as detailed earlier, the more successful prospective payment systems have bundled services or pay for aggregated services over a period of time—whether for a hospital discharge, which covers the costs of care for the duration of a hospitalization, or for sixty days of home health care. The providers under these more advanced prospective payment approaches have incentives to conserve resources, because they receive a lump sum no matter how many services are provided.

Nevertheless, the current problem created by Medicare SGR limits on expenditures for physician services strongly suggests that, at least for some kinds of services, it is not enough to just control prices. Prospective payment has been a very effective tool, first for hospital payment and subsequently for most other providers. Over time, however, the volume and intensity of services may increase total Medicare expenditures despite (or even as a result of) the savings generated through pricing controls.

In all prospective payment systems, providers receive greater revenues by increasing the number of reimbursable units of service, whether those units are individual services (such as physician services), packages of individual services (such as outpatient hospital services), per diems (skilled nursing and inpatient rehabilitation services), or episodes of care (hospitals and home health services). Health professionals, be they clinicians or administrative staff, believe highly in the value of the services they provide to Medicare patients. And if unconstrained, they will want to offer more services, especially if by doing so they also help their own financial bottom lines.

There are natural limits to providers' opportunity to induce patient demand to meet revenue expectations. We trust that professionals do not knowingly jeopardize patient well-being to support their own incomes. A commitment to such professionalism is one plausible explanation for the fact that the double-digit rise in physician expenditures in 2004 resulted from major increases in the duration of office visits and major increases in provision of diagnostic tests and imaging services, not in invasive surgical procedures, which could place patients in danger.

At the same time, because a great deal of health care is discretionary in nature, the decision whether to provide a medical service often is not clear-cut. Three decades of research by John Wennberg and colleagues at Dartmouth showing major variations in the rates of medical interventions—ranging from simple surgical procedures such as tonsillectomies to days spent in intensive care units for patients in their last months of life—strongly suggests that the practice of medicine currently is as much art as science[50] and is often practiced without the elegance associated with fine art.

Different practitioners and providers do not make the same decisions when confronted with seemingly identical clinical problems.[51] Patient preferences might explain some of the variation, but Wennberg has found that physician practice styles and the supply of physicians and hospital beds often explain these significant practice variations. Although professionalism surely does provide some constraint on provider generation of services to increase revenues for the practice or institution, the discretionary nature of much medical care suggests that the financial incentives inherent in fee-for-service payments (including prospective payment systems to varying degrees) lead to increased volume and intensity of services and, consequently, to increased expenditures.

Medicare does police the behavior of medical providers, monitoring for activity that is solely intended to generate increased reimbursable services. The success of Operation Restore Trust and other initiatives to crack down on fraud and abuse demonstrates that Medicare can protect spending when provider behavior blatantly crosses the line. At the same time, though, most overspending does not constitute fraud. And Medicare is allowed to use only gentle, generally unobtrusive approaches to prevent excessive use of services. For example, CMS tries to monitor hospital coding practices to detect systematic "DRG creep" and relies on financially disinterested physicians to certify the need for episodes of home health services. Yet straightforward surveillance can only accomplish so much, especially as providers, with some justification, argue that more ambitious regulatory interventions could become too intrusive or exert a chilling effect on innovation.

Creating incentives for providers to restrain their interest in generating extra services remains a challenge for prospective payment systems that reward provision of additional reimbursable units of care. Julian Pettengill, formerly Research Director for MedPAC, argues that "the eleventh commandment states, 'Thou shalt not tempt' . . . Don't put a pot of money on the table in front of people who could just reach out and take from it. If you don't want providers to behave badly, then don't give them the chance."[52] Relatively crude approaches, such as a sector-specific expenditure limit or budget, worked for a decade for physician payment but seem to be unraveling now.

Administered Prices Can Lead to Market Distortions

Another problem prospective payment systems face derives from the fact that they are not set by a well functioning market but rather are administered prices set to some extent through a political process. It is difficult to get administered prices "right," especially in industries such as health care in which technology changes rapidly.[53] Payment rates may become "ossified," set in stone, even when technological change, professional experience, economies of scale and scope, and other factors are interacting to make the established rates of some services no longer accurate. But once set, the generosity of some payments—relative to their changing underlying costs—may distort the behavior of some medical providers, who take advantage of this generosity by steering patients toward more profitable services.[54]

Distorted Medicare payments had a lot to do with the recent proliferation of physician-owned specialty hospitals, which have been built in several communities.[55] Partially owned by physicians, who are in a position to selectively refer their own patients, these cardiac, orthopedic, and general surgical hospitals are described by advocates as "focused factories."[56] By offering a limited range of services and allowing physicians to have more control than they have in a general community hospital, such hospitals can arguably care for patients more efficiently and with better outcomes.[57] However, critics contend that such hospitals skim off the most profitable patients, undermining a community hospital's ability to subsidize the less-profitable services their communities need, such as emergency services, burn units, inpatient psychiatric facilities, and care for the underinsured and uninsured.[58]

The point here is not to take sides in this ongoing debate, but rather to show that distortions in Medicare DRG payments for inpatient services were a catalyst not only for stimulating a major expansion in specialty hospitals but also for orienting community general hospitals toward overprovision of surgical services in general and cardiac surgical services in particular.[59] Mandated by Congress to study the specialty hospital issue, MedPAC found that the average relative profitability of these institutions varies considerably by DRG and masks even larger differences in relative profitability by the level of severity of illness for patients within each group. Calculating relative profitability ratios—by comparing DRG payments to underlying costs for providing various services—MedPAC found that surgical cardiovascular DRGs were highly profitable, whereas medical DRGs—DRGs for hospital stays without surgical procedures performed—were relative losers.[60] Thus, hospitals receive much greater profits for performing cardiac bypass graft operations than for treating patients with uncomplicated heart attacks or congestive heart failure. Indeed, some believe that these distorted payments have been a major contributor to the current "medical arms race," whereby hospitals try to outdo each other with provision of the same high-tech, high-profit service lines.[61]

Serious price distortions also persist in Medicare's physician RBRVS-based fee schedule, for the most part because adjusting the relative values is largely a political process under the auspices of the American Medical Association, rather than an objective, technical process. Although the elaborate RBRVS process undertaken by Hsiao and colleagues to estimate resource costs for individual physician services corrected some of the worst distortions of the historic, charge-based fee schedules, the process for monitoring and revising relative values established under the new approach does not adequately address the issue of "downward- sticky" prices. In other words, once relative values have been set for new procedures, it remains nearly impossible to revalue them downward even after the procedures become easier, cheaper, and routine.[62] This is one main reason why the shift away from technologically oriented services toward evaluation and management has been frozen in place for the past decade.[63]

The health care system relies on professionals to do the right thing for their patients. But there is little question that the tendency for hospitals to invest more heavily in and compete for cardiac surgical services resulted, at least partly, from the distorted profitability signals sent by the Medicare hospital payment system. MedPAC has identified similar problems in the physician fee schedules. Now that particular price distortions have been found and defined, we will see whether the desire to get administered prices "right" will be able to overcome resistance from those who profit from the current distortions.

Prospective Payment May Reinforce Provider Silos

Medicare payment approaches initially were designed to reflect the organization of health care delivery, with clearly differentiated provider types. Until relatively recently, the functions and clinical jurisdiction of hospitals were decidedly separate from that of the physician office or the nursing home. The lines between different entities providing health care services have become blurred over time, however, as technological and organizational developments permit similar care to be provided in any number of settings. Yet Medicare's prospective payment systems still assume and, in fact, reinforce existing "silos" of care. Medicare's payment policies have even generated altogether new provider types (e.g., long-term care hospitals), for which Medicare has created still more prospective payment systems.[64]

Because of provider-specific prospective payment, patients with similar needs are currently served by different types of providers paid on different bases; the amount Medicare pays on behalf of similar patients varies simply by where they receive their care. This is particularly true for postacute care. Patients with similar rehabilitation needs might be cared for at home with outpatient therapy, in a skilled nursing facility, in a rehabilitation hospital, or in a long-term care hospital. Medicare payment, eligibility, coverage, and certification policies for each type of postacute care provider continue to differ even though the variation among the types of providers in services offered, service intensity, and conditions of patients served are becoming less distinct. Completely distinct payment systems derive from the unique perspectives each provider group brought to the table when prospective payment options were researched and developed.[65]

Medicare faces the same situation when paying for acute care services. For example, a patient might undergo a routine colonoscopy in an outpatient department of a hospital, in an ambulatory surgery center, or in a physician's office. In some ways, given the diversity of health delivery systems across the country, the flexibility to pay on behalf of patients served in different types of facilities makes sense. However, Medicare's payment methods produce payment levels that are based more on the underlying costs of different provider types than on the costs needed to care for patients with particular health problems.[66]

Further, if changes in technology allow resources to be shifted, for example, out of the hospital and into the community, it will be difficult for the government payer to redistribute the funds from the hospital sector to support the increased financial burden of ambulatory care.[67] The result is that patients may be cared for in ways that suit the purposes of the providers, rather than the needs of patients, with financial incentives rather than clinical considerations driving decisions about the setting in which care is delivered.

For example, when Robert Berenson was a senior official at CMS, he met with a group of gastroenterologists who came to complain that Medicare was paying too much for performing colonoscopies in physicians' offices. They argued that the much too generous payment was enticing them to perform the procedures in their offices— exposing their patients to risk—rather than in the safety of ambulatory surgery centers (ASCs). In effect, the physicians were asking CMS to "protect them from themselves" by cutting their payments, which was a fairly unusual request, to say the least.

Only later did the rationale for this not entirely selfless plea become apparent. Some gastroenterologists own ASCs, which were losing the business of gastroenterologists now able to perform the procedure in their own offices rather than provide a facility fee for the ASCs. It took a full investigation and report by the GAO to confirm the safety of the office-based colonoscopy in most clinical situations, and to expose the fact that the clinicians' concerns were about the payment differentials (and not really about patients' interests).[68]

Furthermore, siloed payments with incentives to move patients contribute to the growing problem of uncoordinated care, with patients falling through the cracks during transitions across practice settings.[69] Patients are often transferred without the proper discharge arrangements made to assure a seamless and safe transition to a different facility, again in response to the provider-specific payment incentives that reward earlier hospital discharges.

One of the new challenges Medicare faces is the growing number of beneficiaries with one or more chronic conditions. Twenty percent of Medicare patients have five or more chronic conditions and are responsible for about 66 percent of Medicare spending.[70] These beneficiaries have, on average, thirty-seven physician visits in a year and see almost fourteen different physicians.[71] One important implication of these findings is that care needs to be carefully coordinated across different provider domains to reduce medical error and improve efficiency. Unfortunately, provider-specific payment policies frustrate new efforts to improve safe transitions across settings and to make sure that patients' needs, rather than providers' needs, are met.

Another implication is that the current payment orientation that tilts in favor of technically oriented, acute-care services provided by medical specialists in acute-care settings—such as hospitals and ambulatory surgery centers—needs to be reoriented to care provided by generalist physicians in non-acute-care settings, including the physician's office and the patient's residence, whether it be her own home or a long-term care facility. In short, for many beneficiaries, Medicare needs to be altered from a classic acute illness insurance program to one that also provides high-quality palliative services for persons in their last months of life.[72]

The potential to shift funds across existing payment silos provides one of the theoretical rationales for private plans being allowed to attempt what Medicare has difficulty accomplishing because of political constraints.[73] However, with their broad abandonment of global capitation as a dominant payment method and with their dependence on contractual relationships with providers, such as hospitals, that have substantial market power to assure that the flow of funds continues to support current operations, private health insurance plans have not been more successful than Medicare in shifting health care priorities. Again, although health plan competition makes sense in theory, it fails in fact.

Barriers to Value-Based Purchasing

Rather than using its market power to drive prices below competitive market rates, as some critics feared, it appears that Congress is focused more on satisfying the financial needs of the various provider group interests than on what is good for the program or the taxpayers who support it. Former CMS administrator Bruce Vladeck argued that restrictions on how Medicare pays (and even the payment levels that are written into law) frustrate efforts to permit the program to behave like a "prudent purchaser" or "value-based purchaser," obtaining greater value for the dollars spent.[74] Medicare pays providers and other suppliers more than the prices a purchaser of its size could obtain in the marketplace. And now, in administering the Medicare Modernization Act's new prescription drug benefit, CMS has been precluded by Congress not only from setting prescription drug rates but also from even negotiating with pharmaceutical manufacturers over prices.[75]

Vladeck remains a strong advocate for maintaining the traditional Medicare program's prominent role in any future redesign of Medicare. Nevertheless, he is concerned that the program is turning "from one that provides a legal entitlement to beneficiaries to one that provides a de facto political entitlement to providers."[76] This reality contributes to the difficulty of designing modified payment approaches that better address the needs of beneficiaries and the program overall.

The major challenges Medicare faces going forward are not primarily technical. For example, it is surely technically possible to thoroughly address the distorted payments that contribute to the medical arms race involving hospitals and physician entrepreneurs. The main problem lies in the politics of making changes that could detrimentally affect the financial interests of device manufacturers, pharmaceutical companies, specialty-hospital investors, physicians who perform well-remunerated procedures, and others who directly benefit from the technological orientation of current payment policies.

Moreover, Medicare is now at a stage of evolution where even "smarter" payment policies would not suffice to assure that it produced higher value (e.g., higher quality at lower cost) for its substantial and growing investment. We have tried to show that, overall, Medicare does a fairly good job at getting prices right in its various prospective payment systems. Yet the program makes payments to all providers at equivalent rates regardless of the quality or efficiency of their performance.

Standard payment approaches using uniform, national formulas will not address the geographic variations in health care spending that result in as much as 30 percent of Medicare spending serving no useful purpose (other than providing decent incomes for health care professionals and other health workers.)[77] Clearly, a single national payer permitted to use uniform payment formulas would not be well positioned to address local area practice variations or to apply policies on a discretionary basis to accomplish particular policy objectives, as a value-based purchaser would.

Instead of privatizing Medicare, as the MMA would do, we believe the wiser policy course would be to allow Medicare to use some of the tools that in some cases have been pioneered by private purchasers and health plans, introducing them carefully and selectively into the much more publicly accountable Medicare program.[78] The various political and legal constraints that apply to Medicare—such as the Administrative Procedure Act's requirements that limit agency discretion and create a lengthy decision-making process with assured public input—would temper the kinds of activities that got many HMOs into so much trouble with the public and produced the managed care backlash.[79] For example, Medicare could selectively apply prior authorization of expensive, discretionary services, but in a transparent process and based on professionally considered, evidence-based guidelines that would also take into account cultural values, individual patient preferences, and administrative feasibility.[80]

We believe there are a variety of tools available that would permit Medicare to become a purchaser that uses its dominant position to shape the market by forcing suppliers to adjust to its needs and that could pass statutory and constitutional legal challenge.[81] The MMA has sanctioned a few demonstrations of innovative approaches to modernizing the program, with particular emphasis on new payment approaches such as "pay-for-performance," which rewards providers for achieving specified performance targets with small percentage bonuses, in addition to the uniform payment that comes from application of a national formula.[82]

Although these demonstrations represent an important departure for Medicare by moving beyond its traditional focus on payment formulas, CMS needs much greater authority (and far more resources) to become a value purchaser than is implied by existing demonstrations. A series of administrative, resource, and political barriers stand in the way of Medicare achieving its potential as a value purchaser.

For example, a major barrier lies in the division of the Medicare budget between "mandatory" dollars to pay for services and "discretionary" dollars to pay for program administration.[83] Currently, Medicare spends less than two percent of program outlays on administration, compared to the over ten percent spent by private insurers.[84] In fact, two percent for administration is too low for a program as complex as Medicare. Adopting important cost-saving administrative tools would involve increased spending on program administration, but the savings would accrue to the trust funds. Currently Medicare cannot spend $1 million beyond the appropriated administrative budget, even to save $5 million in decreased health care spending.

A value purchaser would also use tools to influence care that go well beyond the current focus on payment and prospective payment systems. The companion of payment policy is coverage policy, that is, the benefit package of specific items and services to which beneficiaries are entitled. For more than twenty-five years, Medicare has tried to promulgate administrative rules to implement the Medicare statutory directive to cover those items and services that are "reasonable and necessary," for the treatment of illness and injury. The rules are needed in a public program to clarify CMS's legal authority and to describe specific criteria for determining which new technologies would be covered and paid for.

CMS administrators in both Republican and Democratic presidential administrations have attempted to develop criteria that emphasize coverage decisions based on scientific evidence of effectiveness. They have proposed introducing considerations of costs and cost-effectiveness to such decision making. Yet when CMS attempted in various ways to issue rules defining the statutory "reasonable and necessary" language, it was defeated by coalitions headed by the medical device industry, which have an interest in the approval of new technology, regardless of the relative worth of the technology under consideration.[85]

As a value purchaser, Medicare should be allowed to prioritize which services it makes available to its beneficiaries, given the growing recognition of a need for budgetary restraints to program spending. Furthermore, such a purchaser would require convincing, scientific evidence to justify that a particular technological innovation would provide greater benefit than harm, much less that it would represent a good use of program funds. Yet, most of the time CMS determines that a new service is reasonable and necessary based on evidence from scientific studies that the agency itself thinks is only fair or even poor.[86]

Furthermore, the coverage determination process is very much subject to political pressures, usually subtle but sometimes unabashedly overt, such as on the various occasions when the chairman of the Senate Appropriations Committee, Republican senator Ted Stevens of Alaska, essentially mandated that CMS approve expanded coverage for PET scans, regardless of what the relevant evidence from medical research studies showed.[87] More generally, Congress's seemingly unassailable requirements that Medicare assure greater procedural transparency to promote consistency, predictability, and accountability in coverage decision making often serves stakeholder interests more than the public interest.

In many areas of public policy, parties with a strongly concentrated interest in a particular issue are much more likely to take action to influence legislation and administrative decisions than are either the public at large or the Medicare beneficiary population, which has a more diffuse interest in any particular action. Coverage of new technology is an example where the general interest in promoting cost-effective, evidence-based decisions is much weaker than the dedicated interest of the owner or promoter of a new technology.[88] Although the public agency, in this case CMS, attempts to evaluate new technologies primarily based on their scientific merits, arguably transparency only strengthens the hand of the proponents of the technology, who are consistently monitoring and using all available procedural avenues to influence the process. Indeed, some argue that the device industry's push for more formal processes and transparency, which has been resisted at times by CMS, has actually represented a battle for control of the decision-making process, with the manufacturers winning as a result of Congress-imposed procedural requirements.[89]

PET scans are another example of how influential Medicare policies are in shaping the behavior of the health delivery system. Medicare's decision to cover PET scans for use in a variety of clinical conditions, without restrictions—and to reimburse their use generously—has had an important impact on health care delivery. Given Medicare's coverage decision, private insurers have little choice but to also cover PET scans under similar clinical circumstances. Again, although one can plausibly argue that private insurers might be better able to resist what Victor Fuchs labeled the "technological imperative"[90] to adopt and use the newest and best of new technology regardless of the value it provides, health plan executives acknowledge that the adoption of medical innovation is mostly driven by factors outside of their control.[91] As a result of decisions by Medicare and private insurers to cover the scans, hospitals and, increasingly, medical specialty groups (such as oncologists) have made business decisions to acquire PET scanners and refer their own patients for scans.[92]

Medicare's coverage and payment policies, in this case, directly increase the health care system's PET scanner capacity and have made patient access to obtaining a PET scan easier, but at a major cost not only to Medicare but to private payers as well. Although in this book we have emphasized that Medicare payment policies may lead to cost shifting from public to private payers, often Medicare and private payers actually share a common interest in resisting unfettered access to new technology—much as they share a common interest in reinforcing each others' payment methods, sharing data on provider performance, and collaborating on a myriad of other activities.

Though its attempt to rate and rank every nation's health system on multiple dimensions of performance in the *World Health Report 2000* (in which the United States ranked thirty-seventh in the world) was controversial and probably overly ambitious, the World Health Organization (WHO) nevertheless identified an attribute that needs to be addressed in all health systems.[93] The WHO asserted that governments should be the "stewards of their national resources, maintaining and improving them for the benefits of their populations. In health, this means being ultimately responsible for the careful management of their citizens' well-being."[94] Even in systems that rely extensively on private sector financing and delivery of services, the WHO argued, government's health policy and strategies help assure that health systems are oriented to the public interest.[95]

The lack of government stewardship over health care is becoming increasingly evident in the United States. Even private-sector market leaders in organization, delivery, and financing of health care are growing pessimistic about the future of local health care systems left to unfettered market forces. Although usually not supportive of moving to a government-run, single-payer system, these market participants nevertheless see a role for more government intervention to try to bring greater order to the health care systems in the core areas of insurance coverage, cost, and quality.[96]

In short, government needs to assume much greater responsibility as steward of the health care system, not necessarily to take over a larger share of financing and delivery, but rather to oversee the deployment of existing resources in the public interest. Unfortunately, the public overall does not support major expansions of government responsibilities, even in areas such as health care where market failures are manifest.

We think the Medicare program is well positioned to take on many of the most important stewardship responsibilities for the government, while continuing to serve as a crucial social insurance program for the more than forty-two million seniors and people with disabilities who depend on the program. Medicare's prospective payment systems have created a stable funding base for the nation's providers. They have led to important changes in how providers deliver care, producing improved quality and efficiency that have spilled over to better the care provided to Americans. Medicare can shape health care in other ways as well—such as improving access to care, expanding individuals' protection against the cost of illness, and lowering administrative costs—if allowed to do so.

Interviews

All interviews were conducted over the telephone by Rick Mayes.

David Abernethy, formerly of the staff of the House Ways and Means Committee, June 19, 2002

Stuart Altman, formerly chair of Medicare's Prospective Payment Assessment Commission, (ProPAC), July 22, 2002

Jack Ashby, formerly of the staff of the Health Care Financing Administration and currently of the staff of the Medicare Payment Advisory Commission (MedPAC), September 6, 2002

Larry Atkins, formerly of the staff of the Senate Special Committee on Aging, January 3, 2003

Richard Averill, formerly of the faculty of the Yale School of Management, March 19, 2003

Brian Biles, formerly staff director of the Subcommittee on Health of the House Ways and Means Committee, July 2, 2002

Robert Boorstin, formerly of the Clinton administration's communications team, September 20, 2002

Kenneth Bowler, formerly of the staff of the House Ways and Means Committee, June 28, 2002

Christopher Bowlin, formerly of the staff of the National Association of Manufacturers, the staff of the House Committee on Education, and the staff of the Department of Labor, September 3, 2002

Michael Bromberg, formerly the president of the Federation of American Hospitals, July 23, 2002

Sheila Burke, formerly of the staff of the Senate Finance Committee and chief of staff to Senate majority leader Bob Dole, October 2, 2002

Sharon Canner, formerly vice president of entitlement policy at the National Association of Manufacturers, September 25, 2002

Jim Cooper, member of Congress and the House Budget Committee, August 23, 2002

Phil Cotterill, staff member of the Centers for Medicare and Medicaid Services, April 25, 2003

Nancy-Ann DeParle, formerly chief administrator of HCFA, November 4, 2002

Robert Dickler, senior vice president of the American Association of Medical Colleges, February 14, 2003

Allen Dobson, formerly the director of HCFA's office of research, October 11, 2002

David Durenberger, formerly member of Congress and the Senate Finance Committee, July 26, 2002

Jack Faris, president and chief executive officer of the National Federation of Independent Businesses, August 15, 2002

Clif Gaus, formerly of the staff of HCFA, December 20, 2002

Paul Ginsburg, formerly director of the Physician Payment Review Commission, July 31, 2002

Bill Gradison, formerly member of Congress and the House Ways and Means Committee, June 12, 2002

Rick Grafmeyer, formerly of the staff of the Senate Finance Committee, March 10, 2003

Stuart Guterman, formerly of the staff of ProPAC and director of research of the Centers for Medicare and Medicaid Services, September 23, 2002

Glenn Hackbarth, co-chair of MedPAC, August 26, 2002

William Hsiao, professor of economics, Department of Health Policy and Management, Harvard University, October 22, 2002

Karen Ignagni, president and chief executive officer of the American Association of Health Plans, September 13, 2002

Chip Kahn, formerly staff director of the House Ways and Means Committee and president of the Health Insurance Association of America, June 20, 2002

Bob Kerrey, formerly member of Congress and the Senate Finance Committee, November 15, 2002

Judith Lave, formerly of the staff of HCFA and commissioner of MedPAC, July 30, 2002

Rob Leonard, formerly chief of staff of the House Ways and Means Committee, September 26, 2002

Linda Magno, formerly director of the Division of Hospital Payment Policy of HCFA and managing director for policy development of the American Hospital Association, November 16, 2002

James Miller, formerly director of the U.S. Office of Management and Budget, August 6, 2002

James Mongan, president and chief executive officer of Partners HealthCare, October 3, 2002

Don Moran, formerly executive associate director for budget and legislation at OMB, October 28, 2002

Jack Owen, formerly executive vice president of AHA, October 1, 2002

Leon Panetta, formerly member of Congress and the House Budget Committee, director of OMB, and White House chief of staff for President Clinton, August 13, 2002

Julian Pettengill, formerly of the staff of HCFA and research director of MedPAC, October 29, 2002

Rick Pollack, senior vice president of AHA, December 27, 2002

Lisa Potetz, formerly of the staff of the House Ways and Means and Senate Finance Committees and the Congressional Budget Office, July 24, 2002

Robert Reischauer, formerly director of the CBO, August 16, 2002

Alice Rivlin, former director of OMB, August 12, 2002

Dan Rostenkowski, former chair of the House Ways and Means Committee, June 25, 2002

Robert Rubin, M.D., formerly assistant secretary for planning and evaluation, Department of Health and Human Services, August 23, 2002

Robert Rubin, formerly secretary of the Treasury, November 12, 2002

John Salmon, formerly chief counsel of the House Ways and Means Committee, June 28, 2002

Tom Scully, formerly president and chief executive officer of FAH and chief administrator of CMS, October 25, 2002

Pete Stark, member of Congress and the House Ways and Means Committee and formerly chair of the Subcommittee on Health of the Ways and Means Committee, June 5, 2002

Laura D'Andrea Tyson, formerly chair of the President's Council of Economic Advisors and chair of the National Economic Council, September 30, 2002

Bruce Vladeck, formerly chief administrator of HCFA, August 14, 2002

Henry Waxman, member of Congress and formerly chair of the House Commerce Committee, September 3, 2002

Gail Wilensky, formerly chief administrator of HCFA, August 7, 2002

Robert Winters, formerly chairman and chief executive officer of Prudential Insurance, August 28, 2002

Donald Young, formerly president of HIAA and executive director of ProPAC, October 11, 2002

Full citations for interviews by Rick Mayes are given in the appendix.

Introduction

1. See Medicare Boards of Trustees, *2006 Annual Report.*
2. Abernethy interview with Mayes.
3. See Medicare Payment Advisory Commission, *Report to the Congress* (2002): 4.
4. Quadagno and Street, "Ideology and Public Policy," 64.
5. See Starr, *Social Transformation of American Medicine.*
6. See Vladeck, "Political Economy of Medicare," 27. "Medicare is the largest single source of income for the nation's hospitals, physicians, home care agencies, clinical laboratories, durable medical equipment suppliers, and physical and occupational therapists, among others, and all of those groups work energetically to protect and advance their interests through the political process."
7. D. Smith, *Paying for Medicare,* 212.
8. Abernethy interview.
9. See Wilensky and Newhouse, "Medicare," 92–106.
10. Medicare Boards of Trustees, *2005 Annual Report.*
11. See Pierson, "Not Just What, but When," 72–92.
12. Ibid., 72.
13. Ibid.
14. Ibid., 84.
15. Pierson, "Big, Slow-Moving, and . . . Invisible," 5–6. "*Causal Chains.* We often think of causal processes involving a straightforward, temporally-linked connection where x directly yields y. Yet in many cases the story runs more like the following: 'x triggers the sequence $a,b,c,$ which yields y' (Mahoney 2000, Pierson 2000). To the extent that a, b, and c take some time to work themselves out there is likely to be a substantial lag between x and y . . . Causal chain arguments raise some tricky issues. A key challenge is to show that the links in such chains are strong ones ("tightly-coupled" as Mahoney 2000 puts it). The persuasiveness of a causal chain argument declines quickly if there are many stages, or if the probabilities associated with any particular stage are not high (Lieberson 1997; Fearon 1996). Even if a chain has only three links,

and the probability that each link will hold is 80%, there is less than a fifty-fifty chance that the entire chain will operate."

16. See Pierson, "Increasing Returns, Path Dependence, and the Study of Politics," 251–267; Hacker, "Historical Logic of National Health Insurance," 57–130.

17. See Rueschemeyer, Stephens, and Stephens, *Capitalist Development and Democracy*, 387; Pierson, "When Effect Becomes Cause," 595–628.

18. Hacker, *Divided Welfare State*, 26.

19. Pierson, *Dismantling the Welfare State?* 40.

20. Gray, *Profit Motive and Patient Care*, 3.

21. D. Smith, *Paying for Medicare*, 3–4. Smith's book provides the definitive account of the political and technical details of Medicare's prospective payment system for hospitals and fee schedule for physicians. His companion book, *Entitlement Politics*, provides a superb account of Medicare and Medicaid politics in the latter half of the 1990s. Our work endeavors not to tread the same ground and duplicate his books. Rather, our intent is to provide an analysis of how Medicare payment reforms have transformed the U.S. health care system, largely in unintended ways.

22. Altman interview with Mayes.

23. See Reinhardt, "Columbia/HCA," 32.

24. Thanks to Joseph White for noting the semantic problems surrounding the term *managed care.*

25. Gray, *Profit Motive and Patient Care*, 6.

26. Reinhardt, "Calm before the Storm."

27. Guterman, "Putting Medicare in Context," 2; Biles, Nicholas, and Cooper, "The Cost of Privatization," 6.

28. U.S. Census Bureau, *Income, Poverty and Health Insurance Coverage.*

29. See Stuart, Simoni-Wastila, and Chauncey, "Assessing the Impact of Coverage Gaps," W5: 167–179.

30. Iglehart, "Medicare," W5–R4. "Generally, health spending has been outstripping the gross domestic product by about 3 percent per year for decades. Unless there are dramatic changes in Medicare, if not the entire system, this differential might only grow as the baby-boom generation moves toward retirement and the proportion of active workers who will pay for their care diminishes."

31. See J. Bayot, "Greenspan Warns That Deficits Are Unsustainable," *New York Times*, April 21, 2005.

32. Readers interested in books that explain the history, politics, structure and future of Medicare would benefit greatly from Oberlander, *Political Life of Medicare;* Marmor, *Politics of Medicare;* Moon, *Medicare: Now and in the Future;* Kingson and Berkowitz, *Social Security and Medicare;* White, *False Alarm.*

33. Cohen, "Politics and Realities of Medicare," 37–39.

34. Vladeck, "Political Economy of Medicare," 27–28. "Medicare accounts for as much as 40 percent of the income of the average U.S. hospital, but the hospital community is increasingly heterogeneous and internally fractious. Medicare spends so much money on hospitals—more than half of its total outlays, if all hospital-delivered services are included—that at the highest levels of aggregation, hospital politics becomes indistinguishable from macrobudgetary politics, to the dis-

advantage of the hospital community . . . A little more broadly, PPS increasingly tilts toward particular classes of hospitals, especially teaching hospitals and those in rural communities. Teaching hospitals benefit from the American love of medical technology and the popular fascination with science, especially medical science. Rural hospitals play an important role in their communities and are especially dependent on Medicare as a share of their total revenues, but the basic Madisonian formula for representation in the U.S. Senate does them no harm, either."

35. Potetz interview with Mayes. "After its implementation, you now had a system in place where you had a lot of levers that you could pull in order to generate a tremendous amount of savings. What I would say about all of the [annual] budget exercises was that if you had a kind of pure bill that consisted *only* of tax increases and budget cuts to meet deficit reduction targets, everyone [in Congress] would have been miserable. But these bills—partly because they were operating under expedited rules, which in the Senate is extremely helpful—offered the opportunity to legislate in other areas [of the budget] as part of a bigger package. So there was a lot of legislation that was done in addition to budget-cutting, and there was even quite a bit of increased spending. We did a lot to increase Medicaid coverage in those years. And a lot of that was done by saying, "Well, if you have to cut x dollars out of Medicare['s rate of expenditure growth], why not cut $x +$ something and do some good things that you'd want to vote *for*."

36. Medicare Boards of Trustees, *2006 Annual Report*, 1–3.

37. See Goldman et al., "Consequences of Health Trends," W5: R5–R17; J. Lubitz, "Health, Technology, and Medical Care Spending," W5: R81–R85; Vladeck, "Accounting for Future Costs in Medicare," W5: R94–R96.

Chapter One • Origins and Policy Gestation

1. See Marmor, *Political Analysis and American Medical Care*, 61–75.

2. Starr, *Social Transformation of American Medicine*, 379.

3. Brown, *Politics and Health Care Organization*, 12–13.

4. Starr, *Social Transformation of American Medicine*, 385.

5. Ibid.

6. See Somers and Somers, *Medicare and the Hospitals*, 32–34.

7. Goldsmith, "Death of a Paradigm," 7.

8. See McGinley, "Beyond Health Care Reform," 141–142.

9. Sloan, "Regulation and the Rising Cost of Hospital Care"; Conover and Sloan, "Removing Certificate-of-Need Regulations," 455–456.

10. Marmor, *Understanding Health Care Reform*, 22.

11. See Whetsell, "History and Evolution of Hospital Payment Systems," 1–4.

12. Hsiao interview with Mayes.

13. Bromberg interview with Mayes.

14. See Marmor, *The Politics of Medicare*, 108–119; Oberlander, "Medicare and the American State," 188–208; Patashnik, *Putting Trust in the U.S. Budget*, chap. 5; Hacker, *Divided American Welfare State*.

15. Hacker, *Divided American Welfare State*, 94, 137.

16. Patashnik and Zelizer, "Paying for Medicare," 11.

17. Quoted in Demkovich, "Devising New Medicare Payment Plan," 1981.

18. Ball, "Medicare's Roots," 8–9.

19. Cohen to the Secretary, and Cohen to the President, March 8, 1967, both Box 91, Cohen Papers, as cited in Berkowitz, "Historical Development of Social Security," 36.

20. U.S. House of Representatives, "Medicare: A Fifteen-Year Perspective," *Hearings before the Select Committee on Aging*, 96th Cong., 2d sess., July 30, 1980, comm. pub. no. 96-258, 14. "We didn't fund it properly to begin with; that is, Part A. We've had some troubles with Part A ever since the first funding. We started off with I believe 0.5 funding, combined tax on employer-employee. It should have been about 0.9. Within 3 years we found the costs had risen much faster than we had anticipated. So, we were in trouble then and we remained in trouble for some time with the fund, and I assume that we are still in trouble of financing it." For more on Medicare and Medicaid's financial problems, see Department of Health, Education, and Welfare, "Rising Costs of the Medicare and Medicaid Programs."

21. For more on the origins of DRGs and how New Jersey's plan became the national model, see Fetter, Brand, and Gamache, *DRGs: Their Design and Development*; Health Care Financing Administration, *Prospective Reimbursement System*; Health Care Financing Administration, *Diagnosis-Related Groups*; Curtin and Zurlage, *DRGs: The Reorganization of Health*; Gargand Barzansky, *Medicare System of Prospective Payment*; Smith and Fottler, *Prospective Payment*.

22. Stevens, *In Sickness and in Wealth*, 284–293.

23. Gornick et. al., "Thirty Years of Medicare," 184.

24. Oberlander, "Medicare and the American State," 219–243.

25. The monthly premiums of participating senior citizens contributed only 50 percent of Part B's total costs. Moreover, the elderly's share of Part B's costs dropped to 25 percent by 1983, because the increase in their premium rate was limited to the percent increase in OASI benefits, which rose much slower than increases in medical costs.

26. Marmor, *Politics of Medicare*, 96–99; Starr, *Social Transformation of American Medicine*, 374–376.

27. Marmor, *Politics of Medicare*, 374–376.

28. Feder, "The Social Security Administration and Medicare," 19.

29. Starr, *Social Transformation of American Medicine*, 385.

30. West, "Five Years of Medicare," 21.

31. Stevens, *In Sickness and in Wealth*, 284.

32. Clif Gaus, former associate administrator of policy, planning and research, HCFA, email message to author, February 11, 2003.

33. Executive Office of the President, Council on Wage and Price Stability, 9–11.

34. For more information on these dynamics, see Feldstein, *Hospital Costs and Health Insurance*, 176, 306. See also Congressional Budget Office, *Expenditures for Health Care*, 5; Feder, *Medicare*, 143. "The Medicare law promised to pay for medical care for the elderly without interfering in its delivery. But this promise ignored a basic economic fact: How care is paid for significantly influences the quantity and quality of care delivered. Thus a payment program necessarily interferes in the practice of medicine. If an agreement to pay for care has no strings attached, it removes any fiscal constraints on physicians' and hospitals' development and delivery of medical services."

35. Arrow, "Uncertainty and the Welfare Economics of Medical Care," 948–953. For more on Arrow's seminal article and its influence, see Hammer et al., *Uncertain Times*.

36. Arrow, "Uncertainty and the Welfare Economics of Medical Care," 951.

37. Senate Committee on Finance, "Medicare and Medicaid," 4.

38. U.S. Congress, House Committee on Ways and Means, *Summary of Major Provisions of P.L. 89-97*," part F "Statistical Data," 20–21. See also, U.S. House of Representatives, "Administration of Medicare Cost-Saving Experiments," *Hearings before the Subcommittee on Oversight, Committee on Ways and Means,* 94th Cong., 2nd sess., May 14–17, 1976; Department of Health, Education, and Welfare, *History of the Rising Costs of the Medicare and Medicaid Programs.*

39. U.S. Congress, House Committee on Ways and Means, "Summary of Major Provisions of P.L. 89-97." See also Executive Office of the President, *The Budget of the United States Government, Fiscal Year 1981,* 245; Senate Report 89-404, 85, n1.

40. Oberlander, "Medicare: The End of Consensus," 4.

41. Berkowitz, *Robert Ball,* 205.

42. "Nixon's Grand Design for the Economy," 4–14.

43. Gold et al., "Effects of Selected Cost-Containment Efforts," 183–225.

44. Ibid.

45. Altman interview with Mayes.

46. M. Sulvetta, "Achieving Cost Control in the Hospital Outpatient Department," 95–106.

47. Mongan interview with Mayes.

48. Altman interview with Mayes.

49. See D. Smith, *Paying for Medicare,* 32–35.

50. See Hackey, "Groping for Autonomy," 625–632.

51. Gaus interview with Mayes.

52. Hackey, "Groping for Autonomy," 625–632.

53. Dowling, "Prospective Reimbursement of Hospitals." See also Dowling, "Prospective Rate Setting," 8.

54. Oral history interview with John Thompson by Lewis E. Weeks Jr. (July 1989), in W. White, *Compelled by Data,* 46.

55. Ibid., 46–47.

56. Ibid., 47.

57. Averill interview with Mayes.

58. W. White, *Compelled by Data,* 72, 85.

59. Oral history interview with Thompson, 45.

60. Mills et al., "AUTOGRP," 603–615.

61. Oral history interview with Thompson, 48.

62. Ibid., 49.

63. Ibid.

64. See Dunham and Morone, *Politics of Innovation.*

65. Morone and Dunham, "The Waning of Professional Dominance," 74–76. This section of the chapter draws heavily from this excellent article.

66. Ibid.

67. Office of Technology Assessment, *Diagnosis Related Groups (DRGs) and the Medicare Program,* 6.

68. Ibid.

69. Morone and Dunham, "The Waning of Professional Dominance," 76.

70. Center for the Analysis of Public Issues, *Bureaucratic Malpractice.*

71. Morone and Dunham, "The Waning of Professional Dominance," 76.

72. Ibid.; Dunham and Morone, *Politics of Innovation,* 15–18.

73. See Fetter et al., "Case Mix Definition by Diagnosis-Related Groups," vii–53.

74. Ibid., 33.

75. Office of Technology Assessment, *Diagnosis Related Groups (DRGs) and the Medicare Program,* 6.

76. Ibid.

77. Fetter et al., "Case Mix Definition by Diagnosis-Related Groups," 33–34. "The SHARE methodology was not equipped to address the problems of 1) defining and measuring hospital case mix, productivity and effectiveness; 2) providing incentives for better management; 3) avoiding business gamesmanship; 4) fostering communications between the hospital financial systems and physicians."

78. Morone and Dunham, "The Waning of Professional Dominance," 77.

79. Ibid.

80. Office of Technology Assessment, *Diagnosis Related Groups (DRGs) and the Medicare Program,* 34.

81. Morone and Dunham, "The Waning of Professional Dominance," 80.

82. Ibid.

83. Oral history interview with Thompson, 51.

84. Office of Technology Assessment, *Diagnosis Related Groups (DRGs) and the Medicare Program,* 34–35.

85. Ibid., 12. By as early as March 1977 every hospital in New Jersey had received a profile from the state's Department of Health of all of its cases within each of the new system's 383 DRGs. The profiles had been constructed using more than 500,000 patient discharge filings from the first half of 1976.

86. Starr, *The Social Transformation of American Medicine,* 406.

87. Gold et al. "Effects of Selected Cost-Containment Efforts," 189.

88. Ibid.

89. Congressional Quarterly, *CQ Almanac, 1977,* 499–500.

90. Hackey, "Groping for Autonomy," 628–629.

91. Iglehart, "Hospitals, Public Policy, and the Future," 26; Moran interview with Mayes.

92. Quoted in Stevens, *In Sickness and in Wealth,* 309.

93. Iglehart, "Hospitals, Public Policy, and the Future," 25.

94. Gold et al., "Effects of Selected Cost-Containment Efforts," 190.

95. Rostenkowski interview with Mayes.

96. Gold et al., "Effects of Selected Cost-Containment Efforts," 191.

97. Ibid., 192.

98. Ibid., 191.

99. Feldstein, *Politics of Health Legislation,* 153.

100. Starr, *Social Transformation of American Medicine,* 414.

101. Gold et al., "Effects of Selected Cost-Containment Efforts," 192.

102. See Demkovich, "Who Can Do a Better Job of Controlling Hospital Costs?" 219–223; Hackey, "Groping for Autonomy."

103. Iglehart, "Hospitals, Public Policy, and the Future," 25.

104. Ibid., 26.

Chapter Two • Development, Growing Appeal, and Passage of Prospective Payment

1. Starr, *Social Transformation of American Medicine,* 380.

2. Congressional Budget Office, *Hospital Cost Containment Model.*

3. Iglehart, "Hospitals, Public Policy, and the Future," 25–26.

4. Oberlander, *Political Life of Medicare,* 123.

5. Ibid.

6. Dobson interview with Mayes, October 11, 2002.

7. Oberlander, *Political Life of Medicare,* 123.

8. Demkovich, "Relying on the Market," 194.

9. Rubin interview with Berkowitz, 4.

10. Ibid.

11. Pettengill interview with Mayes.

12. Davis interview with Berkowitz.

13. Oberlander, *Political Life of Medicare,* 122.

14. Pettengill interview with Mayes.

15. Iglehart, "Health Policy Report: Medicare's Uncertain Future," 1308.

16. Dole, quoted in ibid. "Our current fiscal crisis, which is, I assure you, a real, not a ficti-
tious crisis, is *forcing* us to examine very carefully what health services we pay for, and how we
pay for them. The problem becomes even more evident when we look down the road to a nation with a growing population of elderly citizens and a Medicare trust fund which is sure to go
broke within a short period of time if we don't take appropriate action. In fact, the entirety of
the Social Security system is in real trouble."

17. Burke interview with Mayes.

18. Rettig interview with Berkowitz.

19. Ibid.

20. Morone and Dunham, "The Waning of Professional Dominance," 80.

21. Oral history interview with Thompson, 50.

22. Averill interview with Mayes.

23. Ibid.

24. New Jersey's DRG system had been revised into 467 categories (from the original 383).
The revision of the original 383 DRGs arose with the promulgation, in 1979, of a revised diagnostic coding scheme, known as the International Classification of Diseases, 9th Revision, Clinical Modification, or ICD-9 for short. The introduction of the ICD-9 coding convention was
designed in part to increase precision in diagnosis and procedure coding. Its introduction meant
that the two previous coding systems (known as ICDA-8 and HICD-2), in which the 383 DRGs
had been defined, would be superseded in hospitals' medical records departments. As the ICD-9
system could be related back to the earlier coding schemes (though with some loss of information), the implementation of the new system did not in itself cause the 383 DRGs to become ob-
solete. However, the original DRGs were defined from a less refined coding system and thus
could not benefit from the increased precision of ICD-9 unless they were redefined.

25. See Morone and Dunham, "The Waning of Professional Dominance," 82. "The point was vividly demonstrated when DRGs actually went into effect. A finger broken in a softball game cost $6,000 to treat. Since a pin had been placed in the finger, the patient fell into a diagnostic group dominated by costly hip replacements. Technically, this was not a difficult problem to solve. In a system based on average costs, some patients would cost less than the average. The different extremes could simply be left to average out, or the outliers that were this far from the mean could be kicked out of the system and reimbursed in a traditional manner. Politically, however, the case was dynamite. The press had a difficult time unraveling the complications of DRGs. Now, they had something everyone could understand—a government cost-control program that yielded $6,000 fingers. The press had a field day. Proponents were embarrassed; critics derived some comfort."

26. Vladeck interview with Mayes.

27. Hsiao et al., "Lessons of the New Jersey DRG Payment System," 34.

28. Ibid., 38–40.

29. Office of Technology Assessment, *Diagnosis Related Groups (DRGs) and the Medicare Program,* 90–92.

30. Ibid.

31. Henderson and May, "The Business Community Looks at DRG-Based Hospital Reimbursement," 44.

32. Ibid.

33. Ibid., 45.

34. Hsiao et al., "Lessons of the New Jersey DRG Payment System," 41.

35. Ibid., 40.

36. Ibid., 41.

37. Averill interview with Mayes.

38. Social Security Administration, *Summary of the 1982 Annual Reports.*

39. Iglehart, "Health Policy Report: Medicare's Uncertain Future," 1309.

40. Social Security Administration, *Summary of the 1982 Annual Reports.*

41. Davis interview with Berkowitz.

42. Medicare Board of Trustees, *1983 Annual Report,* 19–20.

43. Iglehart, "Medicare Begins New Prospective Payment of Hospitals," 1428–1429.

44. P.L. 97-248.

45. Palazzolo, *Done Deal?* 27.

46. Office of Technology Assessment, *Diagnosis Related Groups (DRGs) and the Medicare Program,* 23.

47. Ginsburg interview with Berkowitz.

48. Iglehart, "New Era of Prospective Payment for Hospitals," 1288.

49. Hackey, "Groping for Autonomy," 625–635.

50. Office of Technology Assessment, *Medicare's Prospective Payment System,* 71; Iglehart, "New Era of Prospective Payment for Hospitals," 1289–1290.

51. D. Smith, *Paying for Medicare,* 30. This is the definitive account of the development, passage and implementation of Medicare's PPS, on which we have relied heavily for this chapter.

52. Ginsburg interview with Berkowitz.

53. Rubin interview with Mayes.

54. Vladeck interview with Mayes.

55. Oberlander, *Political Life of Medicare,* 124.

56. Iglehart, "New Era of Prospective Payment for Hospitals," 1292.

57. Owen interview with Mayes.

58. Pollack interview with Mayes.

59. Section 101(c) of P.L. 97–248.

60. U.S. Department of Health and Human Services, *Hospital Prospective Payment for Medicare,* 1.

61. Lave interview with Mayes.

62. U.S. Department of Health and Human Services, *Hospital Prospective Payment for Medicare,* 40.

63. Lave interview with Mayes.

64. D. Smith, *Paying for Medicare,* 36.

65. Ibid., 43.

66. Dobson interview with Mayes.

67. Rubin interview with Mayes.

68. D. Smith, *Paying for Medicare,* 33.

69. Ibid., 44.

70. Ibid., 44–45.

71. Gold et al., "Effects of Selected Cost-Containment Efforts" 193–194.

72. Rubin interview with Berkowitz. "DRGs were an example of [using] financial or economic incentives for getting people to do the correct thing versus coercing them, the difference between the carrot and the stick."

73. Ibid. See also Averill and Kalison, "Prospective Payment by DRG," 12–16; Averill and Sparrow, "TEFRA's Two-Part Strategy," 72–77.

74. Iglehart, "New Era of Prospective Payment for Hospitals," 1292.

75. Bromberg interview with Mayes.

76. Dobson interview with Mayes.

77. U.S. Department of Health and Human Services, *Hospital Prospective Payment for Medicare.*

78. Moran interview with Mayes.

79. Demkovich, "Who Says Congress Can't Move Fast?" 704.

80. Iglehart, "Medicare Begins New Prospective Payment of Hospitals," 1430.

81. Salmon interview with Mayes.

82. D. Smith, *Paying for Medicare,* 50.

83. Paul Rettig interview with Edward Berkowitz (August 14, 1995), 13.

84. Iglehart, "Medicare Begins New Prospective Payment of Hospitals," 1430.

85. Owen interview with Mayes.

86. Ibid.

87. Rubin interview with Mayes; Pollack interview with Mayes; Owen interview with Mayes.

88. Owen interview with Mayes.

89. Demkovich, "Who Says Congress Can't Move Fast?" 705.

90. Ibid.

91. Iglehart, "Medicare Begins New Prospective Payment of Hospitals," 1429.

92. D. Smith, *Paying for Medicare*, 52.

93. Rubin interview with Mayes. See also American Association of Medical Colleges, "Medicare Indirect Medical Education (IME) Payments." "In December 1982, when the Secretary of Health and Human Services proposed a new Medicare payment system, the resident-to-bed adjustment to the TEFRA cost limits was converted to a PPS payment, called the IME adjustment, to recognize the higher costs of teaching hospitals . . . The DHHS Secretary estimated that Medicare inpatient operating cost per case increased approximately 5.79 percent with each 10 percent increase in the number of residents per hospital bed. However, two months after the Secretary's report, the Congressional Budget Office (CBO) presented an impact analysis showing the proposed DRG-based payment system would have adversely affected 71 percent of teaching hospitals if the IME adjustment were set at 5.79 percent. The Administration proposed to double the adjustment to 11.59 percent for each 10 percent increase in the IRB. Congress supported this modification of the empirical estimate and included the IME adjustment in the prospective payment legislation."

94. Dobson interview with Mayes.

95. Rubin interview with Mayes.

96. D. Smith, *Paying for Medicare*, 55.

97. Clark, "Congress Avoiding Political Abyss," 611–615. See also Light, *Still Artful Work*, 1. "This is a story about a legislative miracle. Under extreme time pressure in 1983 (and largely because of it), Congress and the President finally passed a Social Security rescue bill. Two years in the making, the legislation arrived just moments before the Social Security trust fund was to run dry. Without the $170-billion package of tax increases and benefit cuts, millions of checks would have been delayed."

98. Iglehart, "Medicare Begins New Prospective Payment of Hospitals," 1429.

99. For more on the Social Security crisis, see White and Wildavsky, *Deficit and the Public Interest*, 310–330; Light, *Artful Work*.

100. Rettig interview with Berkowitz.

101. Iglehart, "Medicare Begins New Prospective Payment of Hospitals," 1430.

102. P.L. 98-21.

103. D. Smith, *Paying for Medicare*, 57.

104. Davis interview with Berkowitz.

105. See D. Smith, *Paying for Medicare*, 57–61.

106. Burke interview with Mayes.

107. Morone and Dunham, "The Waning of Professional Dominance," 74.

Chapter Three • The Phase-In Years and Beginning of "Rough Justice" for Hospitals

1. U.S. Department of Health and Human Resources, *Report to the Congress*, 1–2.

2. Office of Technology Assessment, "Medicare's Prospective Payment System," 3.

3. U.S. Department of Health and Human Resources, *Report to the Congress*, 1–4.

4. Pettengill interview with Mayes.

5. Magno interview with Mayes. "One way of looking at DRGs is really the way in which they were developed—as internal management tools. When you look at them as an internal management tool, you want to know not how the whole hospital's doing, but ought you to be

doing certain types of surgeries? Ought you to be doing certain types of cases, given your cost structure? And what I saw from both my experience at HCFA and then at the American Hospital Association was different. There are hospitals today who continue to believe that it costs the same to provide care in rural America as it does in urban areas. They say it costs them the same to hire nurses and so on and so forth. And they've been arguing about the wage index since the very beginning. The data don't support them and you can show them the data. But what do you do when people don't believe the data? If hospitals in rural parts of the country are paying lower wages, then they say, 'Well, there should be an occupational mix adjustment.' But in fact, it's not clear—while that would change things at the margin—it wouldn't change them significantly. And so hospitals routinely go back to look for political solutions, because they don't like what the data tells them.

"When I say that I think a lot of hospitals never really put the effort into understanding the DRGs at that level—at a much more detailed level—I mean, everybody and his brothers tried to reduce staff and become more efficient at the margins. But how many people have looked and said, 'No, we actually need to increase staff here because it's more efficient for us to deliver this kind of service with this kind of staffing if we're going to deliver it at all.' How many hospital executives have really used DRGs as a clinical and cost-management tool? Very few. From that standpoint, what struck me when we got comments on DRG classifications is that it was virtually never from hospitals that we got comments suggesting that this or that DRG was broken. It was from physicians who knew what was going on clinically. It was the gynecologists who wrote talking about female reproductive systems and ovarian cancers and other cancers as distinct from other reasons for hysterectomies. That's the person who was paying attention. It wasn't hospital executives who were looking at that data. Hospitals in general did not comment extensively on DRG classification changes that HCFA ended up proposing from year to year."

6. Ibid.

7. Physician Payment Review Commission, *Medicare and the American Health Care System*, 90.

8. Coulam and Gaumer, "Medicare's Prospective Payment System," 46.

9. Mongan interview with Mayes.

10. U.S. Department of Health and Human Resources, *Report to the Congress*, 1–11.

11. Vladeck interview with Mayes.

12. Ashby interview with Mayes.

13. See Rettig et al., "Medicare's Prospective Payment System," 173–188.

14. Burda, "What Have We Learned From DRGs?" 44.

15. Applegate, Mason, and Thorpe, "Design of a Management Support System," 79–95.

16. See Assaf et al., "Possible Influence of the Prospective Payment System," *New England Journal of Medicine* 931–935.

17. Whetsell, "History and Evolution of Hospital Payment Rates," 6–9.

18. Ibid.

19. See Hsia et al., "Medicare Reimbursement Accuracy," 896–899.

20. See Goldfarb, "Change in the Medicare Case-Mix Index," 385–415.

21. Coulam and Gaumer, "Medicare's Prospective Payment System," 46.

22. Ibid.

23. Guterman interview with Mayes.

24. U.S. Department of Health and Human Resources, *Report to the Congress*, 1–10.

25. U.S. Senate, "Health Care Cost Containment Strategies," *Hearing Before the Committee on Labor and Human Resources*, 98th Cong., 2nd sess., June 21, 1984, 192. "The change in behavior, not to have too many people employed per hospital simply because they are cost reimbursed, not to give extraordinary wage and benefit increases above the national average because [they are] cost reimbursed, to consider capital expenditures for the first time because they do increase operating costs and those are fixed for the first time, all the way down the line to trying to persuade the physicians to cooperate in lowering length of stay, doing more out-patient work, having arrangements with nursing homes and home health agencies and others for less expensive sites, and seeking discounts on supplies, all suddenly became real incentives for the first time . . . The most important point I can make today is that those incentives that I just outlined, every one of them, helps non-Medicare payers. In fact, those who predicted that we would simply take Medicare's price, absorb it, and raise our charges to everyone else were wrong."

26. U.S. House of Representatives, "Issues Relating to Medicare Hospital Payments," *Hearing Before the Subcommittee on Health of the Committee on Ways and Means*, 99th Cong., 1st sess., May 14, 1985, 158.

27. Whetsell, "History and Evolution of Hospital Payment Rates," 6–9.

28. Iglehart, "Early Experience with Prospective Payment," 1462.

29. "Hospital Industry's Margin Soared in '84," 1.

30. Rother interview with Berkowitz.

31. See H. Mahoney, "Discharging Elderly Patients Quicker and Sicker," *New York Times*, June 25, 1985.

32. See Guterman et al., "First Three Years of Medicare Prospective Payment," 67–77; Kahn et al., "Effects of the DRG-Based Prospective Payment System," 1956–1961.

33. Kosecoff et al., "Prospective Payment System and Impairment at Discharge," 1980–1983.

34. Guterman interview with Mayes. "I remember sitting at home watching *Nightline*, and one of Ted Koppel's staff was interviewing a sixty-eight-year-old woman whose ninety-two-year-old mother had died after being discharged from the hospital. And she was saying, 'They killed my mother!' And the whole show was this big thing on how Medicare was forcing patients out of hospitals. They were interviewing doctors who said, 'They forced me to discharge my patient before I was ready to.' There was a lot of controversy about this issue. In fact, an interview during that show indicated that that patient was terminally ill, so I couldn't believe that they didn't pick up on it. In any case, my response would have been, 'Well, you're her doctor, and you're supposed to take care of her. If you weren't comfortable with her being discharged, you should say, "I'm not comfortable with her being discharged."'

But I can tell you a little anecdote about that. David Schulke was on Senator Heinz's staff. I believe he was on Senator Heinz's staff on the Special Committee on Aging in the Senate at the time. When we produced our first impact report (it had been mandated by the Social Security amendments of '83), there was some controversy over when it was due . . . The report just took a long time to sort of go through the process. And Senator Heinz ended up subpoenaing the report, which was quite a feather in my cap. I mean, this was my first ever report for the government and it was subpoenaed! To my knowledge, and I would know, there was no effort to suppress the report. It was just that the process was incredibly unwieldy. It took a long time to get through the review process. And it is not unusual for a report to Congress to be late. And there was nothing in the report that indicated any problems, so there was no sensitive political nature of the report. In fact, if anything, it interested the administration to get it out there because it basically said, 'Hospitals are making tons of money and nobody seems to be particularly adversely affected. To the extent that quality is hurt, we're not going to really be able to see it. But looking around, we don't see any smoke.'

At any rate, David Schulke called me up after they had subpoenaed the report. The way things were in the federal government at the time—this was at the end of Reagan's first term—the non-defense federal workforce was shrinking, so resources were tight. Basically, I ended up typing a lot of the report myself, including typing the page numbers where the tables were on these little peel-off stickers and sticking the page numbers on it and having to keep track of the table numbers and stuff like that. And so Senator Heinz's staff got a copy of this report that they had subpoenaed and there was the table 4 and 4.4 and then table 4.6. The natural question was, 'Where is 4.5 and what does it have in it?' My response was, 'I'm really sorry, it was a typo. I literally typed the table numbers and I skipped a table number.' Well, Schulke didn't buy that at all. He absolutely didn't buy it at all. So I had to try my best to sort of say, 'Look . . .' And, besides, the missing figure was in the chapter on the PPS's impact on Medicare beneficiaries, so it was a terrible typo to make. But it was literally my typo. It was unbelievable. He [Schulke] totally didn't buy the fact that there was no missing table."

35. See Sloan, Morrissey, and Valvona, "Effects of the Medicare Prospective Payment System," 191–220.

36. Office of Technology Assessment, *Medicare's Prospective Payment System*, 37.

37. See Friedman and Shortell, "The Financial Performance of Selected Investor-Owned and Not-for-Profit System Hospitals," 237–267.

38. See Sabin, "Hospital Cost Accounting and the New Imperative," 52–57.

39. Dobson interview with Mayes.

40. Burda, "What Have We Learned from DRGs?" 44.

41. See Rayburn, "Study Suggests PPS Creates Job Tension," 48–52.

42. Dougherty, "Ethical Perspectives on Prospective Payment," 5–11.

43. See Kalison and Averill, "The Challenge of 'Real' Competition in Medicare," 47–57; Devers, Brewster and Casalino, "Changes in Hospital Competitive Strategy," 447–469; Robinson and Luft, "Competition and the Cost of Hospital Care," 3241–3245.

44. See Freed, "The Hospital Manager as Enthusiast," 20–23.

45. Dobson et al., "Evaluation of Winners and Losers Under Medicare's Prospective Payment System."

46. See Long et al., "The Effect of PPS on Hospital Product and Productivity," 528–538.

47. Burda, "What Have We Learned From DRGs?" 42.

48. Ibid.; See also Williams, Hadley, and Pettengill, "Profits, Community Role, and Hospital Closure," 174–187.

49. See Fisher, "Hospital and Medicare Financial Performance under PPS," 171–183.

50. Prospective Payment Assessment Commission, *Medicare and the American Health Care System*, (1994), 58; Prospective Payment Assessment Commission, *Medicare and the American Health Care System* (1996), 68.

51. Dobson interview with Mayes.

52. See C. Smith, "Hospital Management Strategies for Fixed-Price Payment," 21–26.

53. See Weil, "Changes in Physician and Non-Physician Relationships," 19–24.

54. Stevens, *In Sickness and in Wealth*, 304.

55. Weil, "Changes in Physician and Non-Physician Relationships," 20.

56. See Glandon and Morrissey, "Redefining the Hospital-Physician Relationship," 166–175; Berki, "Changes in Hospital-Doctor Relations," 114–116, 119.

57. See McKinlay and Stoeckle, "Corporatization and the Social Transformation of Doctoring," 191–205.

58. See Long, Chesney, and Fleming, "Reassessment of Hospital Product and Productivity," 69–77.

59. See Berenson, "Do Physicians Recognize Their Own Best Interest?" 185–193.

60. Mongan interview with Mayes.

61. See Campbell and N. Kane, "Physician-Management Relationships at HCA," 591–605.

62. See Patel, "Physicians and DRGs," 487–505.

63. See Margrif, "Controller's Role in Monitoring Prospective Payment," 24, 64; Barry, "Medical Staff Bylaws," 40–42; Plant, "PPS Invades the Boardroom," 13–15.

64. Young interview with Mayes.

65. Russell, *Medicare's New Hospital Payment System*, 81.

66. See Gay et al., "Appraisal of Organizational Response to Fiscally Constraining Regulation," 41–55; Morrissey, Sloan, and Valvona, "Medicare Prospective Payment and Posthospital Transfers," 685–698.

67. See Cromwell and Butrica, "Hospital Department Cost and Employment Increases," 147–165.

68. See Davis and Rhodes, "Impact of DRGs on the Cost and Quality of Health Care," 117–131.

69. See Rosko and Broyles, "Short-Term Responses of Hospitals to the DRG Prospective Pricing," 88–99.

70. Ibid.; Long et al., "Effect of PPS on Hospital Product and Productivity," 528–538; Long, Chesney, and Fleming, " Reassessment of Hospital Product and Productivity," 69–77.

71. See Ashby and Altman, "Trend in Hospital Output and Labor Productivity," 80–91; Guterman, Ashby, and Greene, "Hospital Cost Growth Down," 134.

72. Burda, "What Have We Learned from DRGs?" 42.

73. See Ippolito, *Uncertain Legacies*, chaps. 6 and 7; White and Wildavsky, *Deficit and the Public Interest*, chaps. 19 and 21.

74. U.S. House of Representatives, "1987 Medicare Budget Issues," *Hearing Before the Subcommittee on Health of the Committee on Ways and Means*, 99th Cong., 2nd sess., March 6, 1986, 338–339.

75. Reischauer interview with Mayes. "Remember, we were just at the end of phasing in the PPS system and there was a lot of evidence that the payment mechanisms that were adopted were initially excessive and that the hospitals and other providers, with time, were learning how to game the system. There was a lot of "upcoding" going on, so you had DRG-creep. And then on top of that, there was (and still is) a general feeling that hospitals were horrendously inefficient—the not-for-profit hospitals in particular . . . I, for one, was not particularly sympathetic to the hospital industry's complaints. I mean, it'd be one thing if we were talking about a truly

competitive industry, but we aren't. We're dealing with a set of administered prices that not only the government takes, but also large insurers."

76. Reischauer interview with Mayes; Gradison interview with Mayes; Potetz interview with Mayes.

77. Iglehart, "Early Experience with Prospective Payment of Hospitals," 1463–1464.

78. Altman interview with Mayes.

79. Panetta interview with Mayes.

80. Potetz interview with Mayes.

81. Pollack interview with Mayes.

82. Reischauer interview with Mayes.

83. Congressional Budget Office, *The Economic and Budget Outlook*, 58.

84. See Russell and Manning, "Effect of Prospective Payment on Medicare Expenditures," 439–444.

85. See U.S. House of Representatives, "Status of the Medicare Hospital Prospective Payment System," *Hearing Before the Subcommittee on Health of the Committee on Ways and Means*, 100th Cong., 2nd sess., March 1, 1988, 83–84.

86. See U.S. House of Representatives, "Medicare Hospital DRG Margins," *Hearing Before the Subcommittee on Ways and Means*, 100th Cong., 1st sess. February 26, 1987, 52–60.

87. See Baldwin, "Hospital Leaders Fear First-Year Profits," 30.

88. Rettig interview with Berkowitz.

89. Gradison interview with Mayes. "I should say that we had a feeling that we were not getting the best professional advice from HCFA on the issues before us. Before they could give us their opinions, they had to clear them through their department level and OMB [Office of Management and Budget]. So we felt that OMB was seeing things unnecessarily through the budget lens, which is understandable. It's not a Republican or Democrat thing. It's an institutional problem. That really concerned us, so the development of ProPAC was a direct effort to try to bring together some knowledgeable individuals that didn't have to clear anything through OMB. This way we could work with their advice on the issues that we had to deal with."

90. Burke interview with Mayes.

91. D. Smith, *Paying for Medicare*, 54–55. This section on ProPAC relies heavily on Smith's excellent account of the passage of Medicare's PPS.

92. Durenberger interview with Mayes. "So the idea of ProPAC, and I can't say I can remember exactly where it originated—could have been Sheila [Burke] for all I know—but my involvement in it was principally that we needed to learn from the experience we were going to get very quickly about how prospective payment was working. You know, 'What is the consequence of this? What does it tell us about Medicare payment? And what should we be doing about it?' And in order to get the best judgment on it, I thought we ought to have people like Stuart [Altman] and a bunch of other people who are either health economists or who made their name in health services research. You don't want a bunch of lobbyists or organization representatives."

93. Abernethy interview with Mayes.

94. Cotterill interview with Mayes.

95. D. Smith, *Paying for Medicare*, 82.

96. Pettengill interview with Mayes.

97. Altman interview with Mayes.

98. D. Smith, *Paying for Medicare*, 84.

99. Pollack interview with Mayes. "Back then the victories were determined by how much you were able to limit the cuts. And each of those deficit-reduction packages ended up being a bipartisan effort that was very hard to oppose. You would go through the budget process at a macro-level trying to limit the amount the committees of jurisdiction would be asked to extract. Then once you got into the committees of jurisdiction, they had to come up with this savings number. And the way the budget system worked, if that savings number wasn't achieved, then there would be this sequestration kick-in. So if you didn't play ball in trying to come up with a policy that was damage control, you were going to get hit with an automatic cut that could be much worse than the damage control effort."

100. D. Smith, *Paying for Medicare*, 54.

101. Iglehart, "Early Experience with Prospective Payment of Hospitals," 1462.

102. D. Smith, *Paying for Medicare*, 116.

103. Guterman, Altman and Young, "Hospitals' Financial Performance in the First Five Years of PPS," 131.

104. Ibid., 131–132.

105. See Gianfrancesco, "Fairness of the PPS Reimbursement Methodology," *Health Services Research*, 1–23.

106. See Guterman et al., "First Three Years of Medicare Prospective Payment," 67–77.

107. See Sheingold, "Unintended Results of Medicare's National Prospective Payment Rates."

108. O'Dougherty et al., "Medicare Prospective Payment without Separate Urban and Rural Rates," 31–32. "The data showed that average rural hospital costs per case were about 40 percent lower than the average urban hospital costs per case (as a percentage of the urban costs). After accounting for differences in case mix, labor costs, and indirect teaching costs, a difference of more than 20 percent remained."

109. Ibid.

110. Lave interview with Mayes.

111. See D. Smith, *Paying for Medicare*, 117–118.

112. Pollack interview with Mayes; Magno interview with Mayes.

113. Magno interview with Mayes.

114. See Lillie-Blanton et al., "Rural and Urban Hospital Closures," 332–344.

115. Abernethy interview with Mayes.

116. Thanks to Joseph White for helping us understand the importance of this point.

117. Pollack interview with Mayes.

118. D. Smith, *Paying for Medicare*, 117. "Targeting could be described as calling a spade a spade and then making one to do the job; but there is more. It represent[ed] a significant accommodation in ProPAC's advisory role. Targeting developed because of a recognition that some existing formulas, such as the disproportionate share and indirect teaching adjustments, weren't working as intended, i.e., to compensate hospitals for their added expenses. Despite various subsidies, moreover, inner city and rural hospitals were still going broke. ProPAC's analysis revealed some inadequacies in the existing formulas and documented unmet need—need

created especially by cost-shifting and demographic trends. Congress corrected its aim and fired for effect, substantially increasing its subsidies to these hospitals in 1990 and 1991.

What is notable about targeting is the decline in importance assigned to PPS numbers and system integrity and an increased emphasis upon an instrumental, means-ends conception of rationality: helping Congress to discern its own objectives more clearly and adapt various PPS formulas to reach them. A second important point about this process is that it puts the inner city and rural hospitals on an independent basis, making it easier to justify their preservation in terms of beneficiary access and economic circumstance . . . Targeting has led not just to increased subsidies for some hospitals but also to the discontinuance of the separate updates, so that getting clear about means and ends can be important in influencing policy. Yet there is a saying that he who sups with the devil needs a long spoon. This development brings ProPAC closer to political activities and a step farther from the original analytical discipline and some of the pro-competition objectives of PPS."

119. Altman interview with Mayes.

120. Guterman, Altman, and Young, "Hospitals' Financial Performance in the First Five Years of PPS," 133.

121. Rosko, "Comparison of Hospital Performance," 48–51; Dobson et al., "Evaluation of Winners and Losers Under Medicare's Prospective Payment System."

Chapter Four • Medicare Policy's Subordination to Budget Policy,
Increased Hospital Cost Shifting, and the Rise of Managed Care

1. See Drake, "Managed Care," 560–564.

2. Shi and Singh, *Delivering Health Care in America,* 299.

3. For more on this common government approach to fiscal policy, see Howard, *Hidden Welfare State.*

4. See Zelman and Berenson, *Managed Care Blues,* 33–34.

5. See Guterman, Ashby, and Greene, "Hospital Cost Growth Down," 134–139.

6. Bodenheimer, "Not-So-Sad History of Medicare Cost Containment," W89, exhibit 1.

7. See Boccuti and Moon, "Comparing Medicare and Private Insurers," 230–237.

8. Magno interview with Mayes; Scully interview with Mayes; Guterman interview with Mayes; Abernethy interview with Mayes; Ginsburg interview with Mayes.

9. Magno interview with Mayes.

10. Guterman interview with Mayes.

11. Rovner, "Reader's Guide to the 'Game,'" 967. "As lawmakers have gained experience with the budget-reconciliation process, they have also become adept at 'gaming' it. Following are some of the most common techniques used to achieve required budget 'savings' and to add new spending: Savings—The 'Golden Goose,' a provision that Congress extends only as long as required to achieve savings in a particular budget cycle—usually a single year. If such a cut was permanent, it would be factored into the 'baseline,' and could not be used to show savings in future years. Thus the nickname, which comes from the ability to lay annual 'golden eggs' of savings . . . [Another example is] the 'non-cut cut,' the practice of holding inflation increases for doctors and hospitals below the predicted inflation rate. For example, in fiscal 1989, large urban hospitals received boosts of 'market basket minus 2 percentage points.' Translated, that means

that instead of receiving a full inflation increase tied largely to the hospital inflation rate (the market-basket index), which was 4.4 percent, those hospitals received increases of 2.4 percent. Overall, holding hospital payments below inflation was scored as savings of $1.3 billion for fiscal 1989."

12. Thanks to Joseph White for highlighting this observation.

13. Kahn interview with Mayes.

14. Waxman interview with Mayes.

15. Dobson interview with Mayes.

16. See Wennberg et al., "Use Of Medicare Claims Data."

17. Biles interview with Mayes. "In the 1980s, we had these intense macro-level budget debates about how much the deficit needed to be reduced with the next year's budget and then how the deficit reduction was going to be allocated. And it was allocated between taxes and savings [or revenue and spending]. And then usually 'savings' was separated between entitlements and appropriations, which at that point was almost all defense . . . We would see these budget numbers kind of coming down from "the top," so to speak, as part of macro-level budget discussions between congressional leaders and the administration. And when they came to us, they involved substantial reductions. And in the context of big deficits and the bipartisan concerns about the deficits, there was a macro number for Medicare that came to Ways and Means and then straight to the Health Subcommittee. The Health Subcommittee then had to basically work backwards and solve to that number . . . So there was a Medicare number that, again, was sort of externally generated, albeit with the participation of some senior Ways and Means members. But year after year, people went back to the hospital side of Medicare, because you didn't get very much by reducing the Part B physician update. It was pretty hard to get much out of physicians . . .

So the budget played almost an exclusive role in driving hospital reimbursement rates. Remember it was in '86, '87, '89, and '90, the years in which there was a budget reconciliation process, that we had these agreements. The budget numbers came down politically to Ways and Means and then to the Health Subcommittee. And the subcommittee produced the savings, a very broad package of savings. But the foundation of the savings each time was the Medicare hospital payments. It really was sort of 'the devil made me do it,' and it was a bipartisan devil at that."

18. Leonard interview with Mayes.

19. Reischauer interview with Mayes; Pollack interview with Mayes. Pollack: "Medicare was viewed as a deficit reduction device in a *big* way. Providers, particularly hospitals, were always viewed as an easier target than doing anything that would have ever affected Medicare beneficiaries. I don't know how many people on the Hill would be up front in admitting this, but they would sort of have a hole in the budget target to reconciliation . . . and they'd save the PPS update factor to be the last thing to be determined and say, 'Okay, we gotta save a billion bucks over three years, so let's just make this tweak to Medicare's payment system or that tweak.' It was legislated in the back rooms and it was all a budget number . . . So it was all damage control on our part."

20. See White and Wildavsky, *The Deficit and the Public Interest: The Search for Responsible Budgeting in the 1980s* (Berkeley: University of California Press and Russell Sage Foundation, 1989).

21. See J. White, "Budgeting and Health Policymaking," 53–69.

22. Ibid., 59–60.

23. Ibid., 60–61.

24. Ibid., 58–61.

25. Bromberg interview with Mayes. "They didn't keep their promises. Although I was still happy, I just complained. Lobbyists do that, they complain. At any rate, Congress's promises were several. When the law passed, we were promised, number one and most important, that if we were efficient and kept our costs below the rate, we could make a profit. Number two, DRGs would be simpler; Congress would get rid of things like cost reports, which to this day they haven't gotten rid of. And a lot of other promises weren't kept. And then they started diddling around with the market basket. We were supposed to get an inflation adjustment and in the first year or two we did.

First thing they do is publish all these studies that showed somehow that we were making these 15 percent profits. So they cut the annual [DRG payment rate] increase. Well that was the whole point of the law . . . to let you make a profit. So I was unhappy that the basic concept of the law was being turned around and used against us. The point was that we were supposed to be rewarded for being more efficient. But, of course, the politicians had to protect all the high-cost hospitals and take it out on us [the for-profit, investor-owned hospitals]. So they basically didn't keep their promises, but the PPS is still a very good system and much better than cost-reimbursement."

26. U.S. House of Representatives, "Status of the Medicare Hospital Prospective Payment System," *Hearing Before the Subcommittee on Health of the Committee on Ways and Means,* 100th Cong., 2nd sess., March 1, 1988, 83–84:

Representative Stark (D-CA): I suspect that based on the [hospitals'] inability, supposed inability, to provide data, that they are way behind all the other industries in this country that provide us data. The railroads provide us better data than the hospitals. Think about that one for a minute!

Jack Owen (AHA): I think the record will show that we have provided you with data in your committees whenever we could, on the basis of what is proprietary and what is not from the standpoint of the hospitals themselves.

Stark: There is *no* such thing as proprietary when you are asking for Federal dollars, my friend. That is when, as I say, if you do not like the system, you can drop out . . .

Owen: I think the basic problem is that it is not that no one wants to divulge data or let it go; it is just as you said earlier, you had some concern about the lack of trust, I guess. And I think there is a lack of trust in what has happened in this program well before you became chairman of the subcommittee. [The PPS] started out in one fashion, and we hadn't even gone a year, and it was changed. There is a feeling by hospitals that all you really want data for—not you, personally, but all Congress wants data for—is so that they can take out more money to offset the budget deficits on the other side; and we are left with a patient who is lying in the hallway or who is bleeding and needs to be taken care of. That is a legitimate, I think, reason for being very cautious. If you want more data, then let's see something that indicates that we will be recognized for it, not rewarded for it, but recognized for it. It hasn't happened.

Stark: I suspect that is the concern, and if we were not providing the funds that concern would bother me. But when we are constantly pressured by the same [hospital] folks for more money—and you have seen the letters in my office, mostly from California hospitals, they just lie. They tell us they are going broke, and you and I both know that is just an unvarnished fabrication.

So you go in the same door you came out. The hospitals are concerned that we may use this data to cut funds. We are concerned that they may, in the most unconscionable way, use the data to create and fabricate situations which do not exist, in an effort to get more of the taxpayer's dollar.

27. U.S. House of Representatives, "Fiscal Year 1990 Budget Issues Relating to Hospital Payment Under Part A of the Medicare Program," *Hearing Before the Subcommittee on Health of the Committee on Ways and Means,* 101st Cong., 1st sess. March 1, 1989, 159–160 (italics added):

Representative Van Hook: I have to say that it sounds suspiciously like the AHA is cooking the numbers . . .

Carol McCarthy (AHA): I would not cook a number for you. I would be pleased to get you all of the information that is behind this [hospital] closure data and get it to you as promptly as I possibly can.

Representative Stark: Let us assume for a minute that your staff could have misled you. But let us talk about the cuts in Medicare payments. Now was there a cut in payments to hospitals in 1989?

McCarthy: There was a . . .

Stark: Yes or no?

McCarthy: There was a reduction in the planned expenditures.

Stark: No, that is *not* the question. Would you listen just for a moment, please, to my question? In 1989, was there a cut in Medicare payments to hospitals, yes or no?

McCarthy: An absolute cut? No.

Stark: In 1988, was there a cut or an increase in the total dollars paid by Medicare to hospitals in this country?

McCarthy: There has been, as you know, an increase in the total dollars in the PPS program.

Stark: In every year in the past 10 years, I believe; is that not correct?

McCarthy: Unfortunately, there has also been an increase in the cost of caring for the patients.

Stark: But that is *not* what I asked, because your testimony says, "There should be no further cuts in Medicare payments." That is what I am suggesting to you is misleading. You are flim-flamming us and the public with these numbers. Now if you want us to pay any attention to your testimony, which is getting difficult to do, do not kid us! Do *not* come out with this public relations poppycock when it cannot be delivered. That does your association *no* good and it certainly is of *no* use to this committee.

28. Altman interview with Mayes.

29. Clarke, "Altman Sees Industry Unwilling to Control Costs, 14–20. "I think it's fair to say that the data suggest that profit margins for hospitals have come down, both PPS margins and total margins. The issue is whether it is because of inadequate reimbursement or because of an inability or the unwillingness of the hospital industry to gain control over its costs. [The greatest frustration] of PPS—if not the last eight years—is the fact that hospital costs just continue to go up almost as fast as before on an inflation-adjusted per-admission or per-unit basis. The so-called discipline that we expected to come into the industry does not appear to have materialized. What the hospital industry is asking the Medicare program, if not the American people, to do is to continue to essentially support it at rates of growth that were going on before PPS. And that's a tall order . . . I sense an unwillingness on the part of the industry as a whole to really grapple with changing the cycle. Instead the policy has been, 'Let's scream. Let's pound on our Congressional delegation. Let's demand more money.'"

30. Clarke, "Wilensky Seeks Dialogue with Providers," 22–25. See also Sheingold and Richter, "Are PPS Payments Adequate?" 165–175.

31. See Manheim and Feinglass, "Hospital Cost Incentives in a Fragmented Health Care System," 56–63; Cromwell and Butrica, "Hospital Department Cost and Employment Increases," 147–165; Wagner, "No Slowdown in Capital Expenditures," 50.

32. See Chirikos, "Further Evidence that Hospital Production is Inefficient," 408–416.

33. L. Foderaro, "Half-Empty Hospitals in a Shrinking City," *New York Times,* April 25, 2005.

34. See Anderson and Ginsburg, "Prospective Capital Payments to Hospitals," 52–63.

35. See Cotterill, "Prospective Payment for Medicare Hospital Capital," 77–79; Coffey, "Retroactive Reimbursement under HCFA's PPS for Capital," 60–63.

36. Scully interview with Mayes.

37. Guterman, Ashby, and Greene, "Hospital Cost Growth Down," 136.

38. See Guterman, Altman, and Young, "Hospitals' Financial Performance," 125–134; Altman and Ashby, "The Trend in Hospital Output and Labor Productivity," 80–92.

39. See Matherlee, "Margins as Measure," 2–4.

40. See D. Smith, *Paying for Medicare,* 117.

41. Dobson interview with Mayes. "You know what that was? That was $16 billion worth of DSH [disproportionate share hospital] payments. DSH flooded the hospital industry. Medicaid is only about 11 percent of all hospitals' revenue, but you throw $16 billion at the industry and it's going to be noticeable."

42. See OBRA 1989, Sec. 6003 (c); and OBRA 1990, Sec. 4002 (b).

43. Goody, "Medicare Dependent Hospitals," 97–105.

44. Kahn interview with Mayes. "To say, 'Look at Medicare's PPS margins back then and, wow, those hospital guys were suckers and they really took it on the chin every year . . . ,' well that's not accurate. I don't buy that. The late 1980s was an intensive period of reform. If we went back and looked at them closely, we would say, 'Oh, let me look at this mark-up. It was 'market-basket minus X,' but they increased the disproportionate-share adjustment. Or in another year it was 'market-basket minus X,' but they increased the urban hospital adjustment. Or it was

'market-basket minus X,' but they increased the reimbursement of hospitals' capital costs that year.' So if you go back and look at all of those individual bills, it was always a balancing act and the hospitals had many balls in the air."

45. See Guterman, Altman, and Young, "Hospitals' Financial Performance"; Altman and Ashby, "Trend in Hospital Output and Labor Productivity," 80–92; Grassmuck, "Financial Pressures Prompt Teaching Hospitals to Cut Costs," 27–29.

46. Altman interview with Mayes. See also Needleman, "Cost Shifting or Cost-Cutting"; Morrissey, *Cost Shifting in Health Care*; Walker, "Cross-Sectional Analysis of Hospital Profitability," 121–138.

47. Reinhardt, "Health Care Spending and American Competitiveness," 19. See also Maarse, Rooijakkers, and Duzijm, "Institutional Responses to Medicare's Prospective Payment System," 255–270.

48. C. Fisher, "Hospital and Medicare Financial Performance," 171–183.

49. Johnson and Aquilina, "The Cost Shifting Issue," 101.

50. Meyer and Johnson, "Cost Shifting in Health Care," 20–35.

51. Guterman, Ashby, and Greene, "Hospital Cost Growth Down," 136.

52. Ibid.

53. Owen interview with Mayes. "It's not cost shifting; the private payers just have a 'price differential' that they are stuck with."

54. Guterman interview with Mayes. "I think part of the problem may be semantics. Cost shifting is a bad term because hospitals are not really shifting costs; they are shifting the responsibility for covering their costs. The key is how the flow of money from different payer sources flows together to cover the cost of hospital services. But I disagree with my colleagues who claim there is no such thing as cost shifting, because I think their model of hospital pricing is wrong. It doesn't describe what really happens. I think hospitals have a notion of what services they would like to provide and what it will cost them to provide those services. They then set about trying to figure out how to raise the money to cover those services. And what they do is they look around and they say, 'Well, where are we now financially?' And if they are not where they want to be, then they look at how they can get where they want to be. And there's going to be a variation in the resistance of payers to pay higher rates.

But in those days, the federal government would set the rates and they were sort of firmed up by the budget problems that the federal government was having. The state governments weren't really good sources of extra money . . . From 1986 to 1992, it was apparent that the part of the health care system that was 'giving' was the private sector payers. And from about 1993 to 1997, it was apparent that that part of the system no longer gave. And so what happened was that the costs backed up onto the hospitals and the hospitals eventually had to make a decision to reduce their cost growth."

55. Morrissey, "Hospital Cost Shifting, a Continuing Debate."

56. Ibid., p. 12.

57. Zwanziger, Melnick, and Bamezai, "Can Cost Shifting Continue in a Price Competitive Environment?" 211–225; Clement, "Dynamic Cost Shifting in Hospitals," 340–350.

58. M. Morrissey, "Cost Shifting: New Myths," W3–489.

59. Chip Kahn, quoted from "The Policymakers' Perspective." "Hospitals can sword-rattle, but basically they can't walk away. It is possible for some physician specialties to really margin-

alize their Medicare business, but that is a rare thing for a hospital to be able to do regardless of where it's located."

60. Ibid.

61. Young, interview with Mayes. "So call it cost-shifting or cross-subsidization, but on average it accounts for about 6 percent of hospital costs that go to the uninsured. Hospitals have to pay for that somehow and the way they pay for it is to either cross-subsidize, if you want to call it that, or through cost shifting. In that sense, there are cross-subsidies. It sure is a real phenomenon, but it's just not a clean kind of thing."

62. See Roberts et al., "Distribution of Variable vs. Fixed Costs of Hospital Care," 644–649.

63. See Feldstein, *Health Policy Issues*, 187–197.

64. Mann et al., "Uncompensated Care: Hospitals' Response to Fiscal Pressures," 263.

65. Roberts et al., "Distribution of Variable vs. Fixed Costs of Hospital Care," 647.

66. Ibid.

67. Ibid. See also Meyer and Johnson, "Cost Shifting in Health Care," 20–35; Johnson and Aquilina, "The Cost Shifting Issue," 101–106.

68. Mongan interview with Mayes. "You can take a malignant view of this and say that hospitals are just 'sitting there spending every dollar as fast as it comes in' . . . Or you can take a more benign view. I've been in this business a long time and we try very hard to put together as tight a budget as we can. You negotiate with the nurses, you cut what costs you can, etc. Then you see that your costs have gone up 5 percent, and you see Medicare's [payment rates are] going up only 2 percent. So you're either going to go under or you're going to get it from your private payers."

69. See C. Fisher, "Hospital and Medicare Financial Performance Under PPS," 171; Dobson and Clarke, "Shifting No Solution to Problem of Increasing Costs," 24–31; U.S. House of Representatives, "Options for Health Insurance," *Hearing Before the Subcommittee on Health of the Committee on Ways and Means*, 102nd Cong., 2nd sess., April 8, 1992, 56–57; Guterman, Altman, and Young, "Hospitals' Financial Performance in the First Five Years of PPS"; U.S. General Accounting Office, "Health Insurance."

70. U.S. Senate, "Health Care Cost Containment Strategies," *Hearing Before the Committee on Labor and Human Resources*, 98th Cong., 2nd sess. June 21, 1984, 187:

Senate Finance Committee: How do hospitals finance uncompensated care?

(AHA): The vast bulk of under-and uncompensated care is financed through charges paid by private insurers and individual patients . . . A substantial part of the "cost shift" is the private sector's contribution to the cost of treating those individuals not covered—or inadequately covered—by public programs.

71. Bromberg interview with Mayes. "Hospitals absolutely cost shift, but HMOs took that away from us. Before HMOs, you could cost shift, sure, and insurance companies would just pass it on to employers. But when HMOs came into the picture and started squeezing, then you couldn't cost shift anymore."

72. Pettengill interview with Mayes. "That's the funny part about it, the sort of ironic part about it, because it was not Medicare officials saying, 'I know that the private sector isn't paying attention, so I can just hold down the rates of increase and I'll saw off this burden on someone

else, you know, I'll force the hospital staffs to shift costs on private insurance.' That's not what happened at all. What happened was that the hospitals were allowing their costs to increase, and ProPAC repeatedly made the judgment that costs were going up much faster than they should have and that Medicare shouldn't pay those increases. In other words, Medicare should hold those increases to those that were the legitimate results of changes in technology and real changes in case mix and changes in input prices in hospitals and not to increase payment rates to accommodate the cost increases that hospitals were allowing to occur.

Nevertheless, the hospitals didn't stop raising their costs, because the insurers in the private world simply were not paying attention. Actually, it's a little odd and it mischaracterizes the situation to say that the insurers weren't paying attention, because consider what the private insurance world looked like. It was some private insurers who were selling insurance to employers who were providing it to their employees and their families. But a lot of it was that they were doing the administrative work for employers who, under ERISA, were self-insured. So it wasn't just the private insurers selling traditional indemnity insurance, and so forth, who weren't paying attention. It was the employers who weren't paying attention too. And, indeed, why would one really expect them to? I mean, would they understand at that level what was going on? Most of them didn't."

73. U.S. Senate, "Health Care Cost Containment Strategies," 148.

74. Ibid.; see also Coddington et al., *Crisis in Health Care*, chap. 6, 103–113; Banks, Foreman, and Keeler, "Cross-Subsidization in Hospital Care," 1–35.

75. See Levit et al., "National Health Expenditures," 205–242.

76. See Drake, "Managed Care," 560–564.

77. Scully interview with Mayes. "If you're a nursing home, if you're a doctor, or you're a hospital, fundamentally a big chunk of your business is as a government contractor! And your expectation, I think, when dealing with the government, whether you're in the Pentagon or in health care . . . is boring consistency, decent margins that don't go up or down or flop around. If you're Boeing, you don't want to have a 25 percent margin one year and a negative 2 percent the next year, right? I think that's what health care providers want. Unfortunately, because health care policy is frequently driven by budget deals, and the policy is so complicated, for many years it was driven by "how much money do we need to save for the budget" and not by what the right health policy is. Thus, you get these huge up and down roller coasters, which I think is unfortunate.

It's like the managed care plans that are all jumping out of Medicare + Choice because it's totally unpredictable. Margins are unpredictable. You don't know what's going to come from year to year. The doctors have to stay in, the hospitals have to stay in; but they go crazy with these big fluctuations up and down. So I will argue that the doctors have a huge problem that we've got to fix. But I've argued with the hospitals: 'Look, your margins are reasonably good, you come in this year and say, "The sky is falling," and you want to get a bunch of money back. It's short sighted! Because you know what? If your margins go back up, Congress is going to come back and whack you in two or three years!' What hospitals need to do is to figure out what a good healthy margin is and try to stick with it, because the typical reaction of hospital lobbyists or anyone else is that you get paid every year to come in and it's like Pavlov's bell . . . yell and scream and say we need more money."

78. Fein, *Medical Care, Medical Costs*, 95.

79. Fein, "The Academic Health Center," 2436.

80. See U.S. General Accounting Office, *Private Health Insurance.*

81. See Cooper and Schone, "More Offers, Fewer Takers for Employment-Based Health Insurance," 142; Fronstin and Snider, "Examination of the Decline in Employment-Based Health Insurance," 317–325; Holahan, Winterbottom, and Rajan, "Shifting Picture of Health Insurance Coverage"; Gabel, Ginsburg, and Hunt, "Small Employers and Their Health Benefits," 103–110.

82. See O'Brien and Feder, "How Well Does the Employment-Based Health Insurance System Work?"

83. Ibid.

84. See Whetsell, "History and Evolution of Hospital Payment Systems," 9–15.

85. Burda and Tokarski, "Hospitals Are Under Pressure to Justify Cost Shifting," 28–36.

86. "1990 National Executive Poll," 26.

87. Reinhardt, "Predictable Managed Care *Kvetch*," 902–903. See also U.S. House of Representatives, "Payroll Taxes, Health Insurance, and SBA Budget Proposals," *Hearing Before the Committee on Small Business*, 101st Cong., 2nd sess. March 29, 1990, 4–9.

88. See Coddington et al., *Crisis in Health Care*, 103; G. Ruffenach, "Health Insurance Premiums to Soar in '89," *Wall Street Journal*, October 23, 1989.

89. Frieden, "Health Care Costs," 52.

90. Ibid., 49. "'Cost shifting stinks, and it's getting worse,' says Richard Smith, director of public policy for the Washington Business Group on Health, an organization of employers concerned about health care costs. 'Large payers—like governments—with market share and legislative power can use their power to shift costs to the private sector instead of operating more efficiently or raising taxes. That makes it difficult for private payers to operate fairly in the marketplace.' Michael Baroody, senior vice-president of the National Association of Manufacturers (NAM), says U.S. manufacturers spent about $11.5 billion in 1991 on extra health care costs as a result of cost shifting by both government and other employers."

91. See Geisel, "Solution Proposed for N.J. Cost Shifting," *Business Insurance* 3–5; Dobson and Clarke, "Shifting No Solution to Problem of Increasing Costs," 24–30; Shalowitz, "Hospitals Shift Costs to Cover Costs," 14; McGarvey, "Challenge of Containing Health Care Costs," 34–40; Clarke, "Cost Shifting Merits an Explanation," 12.

92. Canner interview with Mayes.

93. Bowlin interview with Mayes.

94. Schiller, "Human Flap," 34. See also Johnsson, Hudson, and Anderson, "CEOs," 26–33.

95. McFadden, "Legacy of the $7 Aspirin," 38–41. "The accounting practice of cost shifting in the hospital industry has been a significant contributor to the rapid increase in health care costs . . . Cost shifting spreads around, and in some cases hides, the charges for certain items. To stay within the guidelines of reasonable and customary charges for such things as room rates, operating rooms, and intensive care units, hospitals have been breaking those charges into smaller units that can be regularly multiplied across the entire patient population under the category of ancillary charges. The price of an innocuous item such as aspirin can include a portion of hospital costs for such things as labor, supplies, and shared and shifted costs."

96. M. Gladwell, "Insurance System Squeezes Some Hospitals; Payments Drop as Governments Cut Reimbursements, Private Insurers Fight Cost-Shifting," *Washington Post*, March 29, 1992. "The difficulty for many hospitals comes in large part from the bulk of patients who are

insured by Medicare or Medicaid. In most cases, government insurers do not bargain with hospitals over prices; they dictate prices to hospitals. And in recent years, in the face of rapidly rising budgets, government payers have become increasingly thrifty. While it was once common for hospitals to make money treating Medicare patients, a recent federal report estimated that, on average, every U.S. hospital now loses more than $1 million a year treating the elderly. Medicaid provides even less . . . The hospital industry has responded to this steady decrease in reimbursement in part by becoming leaner . . . The second step the industry has taken is raising its prices for private patients. In the early 1980s, hospitals charged private insurance companies an average of 10 percent above costs; now, that figure has climbed to 40 percent or more. This practice of cost-shifting is one of the biggest reasons health insurance premiums to employers continue to rise every year by as much as 25 percent."

97. Dobson and Clarke, "Shifting No Solution to Problem of Increasing Costs," 24–30.

98. Ibid, 28. "Employers in their role as health insurance purchasers fund the cost shifting. (Employees also fund cost shifting through higher cost-sharing requirements; business customers pay their share through higher product prices.) Employers cover not only the healthcare costs of their employees, but also a portion of the costs of the uninsured and of public payers whose payments do not meet costs. This is a major reason private sector employer premium payments rise faster than underlying healthcare costs. Hewitt Associates has estimated that 27 percent of insurance costs increases are due to cost shifting. Governments are perhaps the major beneficiaries of cost shifting. As Medicare and Medicaid pursue policies of marginal (variable) cost payment (as opposed to average cost payment), the costs of treating government beneficiaries are shifted to private pay patients. This paper has shown that this "sick tax" is increasing. The politics of cost shifting may become the politics of health care as remaining payers resist government underpayment policies."

99. See www.businessroundtable.org.

100. Winters interview with Mayes.

101. Reinhardt, "Predictable Managed Care *Kvetch*," 903.

102. Starr, *Social Transformation of American Medicine*, 320–327.

103. See Zelman and Berenson, *Managed Care Blues*, 49.

104. Ibid., 51.

105. Starr, *Social Transformation of American Medicine*, 395.

106. See O. Anderson et al., *HMO Development: Patterns and Prospects* (Chicago: Health Administration Studies, 1985).

107. Zelman and Berenson, *Managed Care Blues*, 52.

108. See Brown, *Politics and Health Care Organizations*.

109. See Martin, "Nature or Nurture?" 898–914.

110. Feldstein, *Health Policy Issues*, 197. "Previously, when insurance premiums were paid almost entirely by the employer and managed care was not yet popular, hospitals were probably less interested in making as much money as possible. Many hospitals were reimbursed according to their costs, and they could achieve many of their goals without having to set profit-maximizing prices. However, as occupancy rates declined and left hospitals with excess capacity, price competition increased, HMOs and PPOs entered the market, and hospitals could no longer count on having their costs reimbursed regardless of what those costs were. Hospital

profitability declined. Those hospitals that did not price to make as much money as possible began to do so. Some cost shifting occurred during this transition period."

111. See Swenson and Greer, "Foul Weather Friends," 622–623.

112. See Titlow and Emanuel, "Employer Decisions and the Seeds of Backlash," 943–944.

113. Wholey et al., "HMO Market Structure and Performance," 75–84.

114. Gold, "DataWatch," 189–206.

115. Gabel, "Ten Ways HMOs Have Changed During the 1990s," 136.

116. Ibid., 134–145.

117. Pauly and Nicholson, "Adverse Consequences of Adverse Selection," 925.

118. Ibid.

119. Pauly and Nicholson, "Adverse Consequences of Adverse Selection," 924.

120. See Gold, "DataWatch," 192–193.

121. See Hoy, Curtis, and Rice, "Change and Growth in Managed Care," 18–36.

122. Halvorson, "Health Plans' Strategic Responses," 28–29.

123. Ruggie, "The Paradox of Liberal Intervention," 919–944.

124. Ibid.

125. *Chain causation:* your car hit mine and knocked it into the car in front of me; *causal network*: affecting one part of a related network, such as an intrusion into an environment or habitat; and *contributing causes* (common in tort cases), such as environmental pollution, in which several factors converge and lead to global warming, for example, but it is impossible to determine how much each factor contributed and which factors were partly due to other factors.

126. D. Smith, email exchange with the authors, August 13, 2005.

127. See Thorpe, "Managed Care as Victim or Villain?" 950.

Chapter Five • The Resource-Based Relative-Value Scale Reforms for Physician Payment

1. See Ginsburg, "Physician Payment Policy in the 101st Congress," 5–20; Epstein and Blumenthal, "Physician Payment Reform," 193–215.

2. See Delbanco, Meyers, and Segal, "Paying the Physician's Fee," 1314–1320.

3. Roe, "Sounding Board," 41–44.

4. Congressional Budget Office, *Physician Reimbursement under Medicare*, 26.

5. Hadley, "Theoretical and Empirical Foundations," 103.

6. Ibid., 104.

7. Antos, "The Policy Context for Physician Payment," 40.

8. Ibid., 40.

9. U.S. Government Accountability Office, *Medicare Physician Payments*, 1.

10. Prospective Payment Review Commission, *Annual Report to the Congress, 1992*.

11. Ibid., 5.

12. Altman interview with Mayes; Carey, "Cost Allocation Patterns," 275–292.

13. See Kay, "Volume and Intensity of Medicare Physicians' Services,"133; Newhouse, "Medicare," 6.

14. See Oliver, "Analysis, Advice, and Congressional Leadership," 113–174.

15. Hsiao interview with Shuster. "This view was expressed by all specialists—surgeons, internists, pathologists . . . I interviewed about 20 physicians, I recall, and most of them told me the fee was not fair. They thought some prices were too high, some were too low. So I asked the obvious question, 'If you say something is not fair, then tell me what is fair?' . . . Remember this was in the 1970s. The government was paying physicians based on what they were charging. So physicians had the right to set charges and to receive payments based on that; and the government's only control was to say, 'You cannot charge more than what 90% of what [your colleagues] are charging.'"

16. See Hsiao and Stason, "Toward Developing a Relative Value Scale," 23–38.

17. See Congressional Budget Office, *Physician Reimbursement under Medicare*, 31.

18. See Roe, "Sounding Board," 42.

19. See Congressional Budget Office, *Physician Reimbursement Under Medicare*, 32.

20. Hsiao and Dunn, "Resource-Based Relative Value Scale," 223.

21. Blumberg, "Rational Provider Prices," 49.

22. See Lasker et al., "Medicare Surgical Global Fees," 255–262.

23. See Berenson, "Editorial: Physician Payment Reform" 929–931.

24. Hsiao interview with Mayes. "Jim Todd [AMA President] and a handful of his colleagues saw a benefit to pumping up the income of general practitioners as part of an effort to [engineer] some kind of 'reunited medicine.'"

25. See "Reimbursement for Physicians," 1–4.

26. See Riddick and Hartfield, "Medicine Prepares for Battle," 32.

27. See Hsiao et al., "Results and Policy Implications," 881–888.

28. Hsiao interview with Mayes. See also Peck and Anderson, "William Hsiao," 18–22.

29. Gawande, "Piecework," 46.

30. Oberlander, *Political Life of Medicare*, 127.

31. See Iglehart, "Health Policy Report: Payment of Physicians Under Medicare," 863–869.

32. Consolidated Omnibus Reconciliation Act of 1985, P.L. 99-272, § 9305.

33. For the best summary and analysis of the PPRC, see Oliver, "Analysis, Advice, and Congressional Leadership."

34. D. Smith, *Paying for Medicare*, 20.

35. Ginsburg interview with Mayes.

36. Prospective Payment Review Commission, *Annual Report to the Congress, 1988,* 7 and 11–13. To assess whether a procedure was overvalued by Medicare relative to other procedures, the PPRC compared Medicare relative values to relative values from several other sources that had some of the attributes of the anticipated Hsiao-based relative value scale for Medicare.

37. See D. Smith, *Paying for Medicare*, 174–175.

38. For explanation of "balance billing," see Feldstein, *Health Policy Issues,* 103–104. "When Medicare was enacted in 1965, Part B was included, which paid for physician and out-of-hospital services. Physicians were paid fee-for-service for Medicare patients and were given the choice of whether to be a participating physician, or whether to participate for some medical claims but not others. When physicians participated, they agreed to accept the Medicare fee for that service. The patient was responsible for 20 percent of that fee after they paid their annual deductible. If the physician was not a participating physician, the patient would have to pay the

physician's entire charge, which was higher than the Medicare fee, and apply for reimbursement from Medicare. When the government reimbursed the patient, however, it would only pay the patient 80 percent of the Medicare-approved fee for that service. Thus, a patient going to a non-participating physician would have to pay 20 percent of the physician's Medicare-approved fee, plus the difference between the approved fee and the physician's actual charges. The difference is referred to as balance billing. Medicare patients going to nonparticipating physicians also were burdened by the paperwork of sending their bills to Medicare for reimbursement."

39. Omnibus Budget Reconciliation Act of 1986, P.L. 99-509, October 21, 1986, § 9331.

40. D. Smith, *Paying for Medicare*, 174.

41. Ibid, 175.

42. Iglehart, "Medicare's Declining Payments to Physicians," 1924.

43. Hsiao interview with Mayes. "So what the RBRVS was trying to do was to mimic a set of methods that determine what the cost is of a particular physician's service, and that requires decomposition of the cost into three parts. One part is the work that a physician has to do. The second part is the practice costs that a physician incurs. And the third part is the amount of professional training a physician needs to do that procedure. Then the work part is further decomposed into two components, and [one of those is] time. But time is not equal. Twenty minutes for a pediatrician to do a well-baby checkup versus the same pediatrician spending twenty minutes to resuscitate a newborn baby in the emergency room are not the same amount of work. So there's a difference in what we call 'intensity of work.' . . . And we found that the most difficult part of our work was to measure this variation in intensity."

44. Ibid. "I've worked closely enough with Congress to know what drives congressional decisions related to Medicare, which is cost. When the program is in financial difficulty, then Congress has to sit up and pay attention . . . But when it comes to considering an increase in the [payroll] tax rate or something along those lines, they don't want to touch it. They are also not particularly keen on changing payment systems unless they have to, because Medicare just about touches every hospital and physician."

45. See D. Smith, *Paying for Medicare*, 208, 212–213.

46. See U.S. General Accounting Office, *Health Care Spending Control*.

47. See Physician Payment Review Commission, *Annual Report to Congress: 1989*.

48. Ibid.

49. Epstein and Blumenthal, "Physician Payment Reform," 199.

50. See Physician Payment Review Commission, *Annual Report to Congress: 1989*, 159–161.

51. Hsiao et al., "Results and Policy Implications," 881.

52. See Iglehart, "Health Policy Report: New Law on Medicare's Payments to Physicians," 1247–1252.

53. See Riddick and Hartfield, "Medicine Prepares for Battle," 32.

54. Ibid. "James Sammons, M.D., Executive Vice President of the AMA, took the podium to announce the AMA's campaign against ET's [expenditure targets] . . . He cited the failures of the Canadian system and expressed concern over the primacy given to cost savings over provision of care."

55. D. Smith, *Paying for Medicare*, 212.

56. Scully interview with Mayes.

57. Waxman interview with Mayes.

58. Iglehart, "Health Policy Report: Payment of Physicians Under Medicare," 866–867.

59. Iglehart, "Recommendations of the Physician Payment Review Commission," 1160.

60. Scully interview with Mayes.

61. Ibid.

62. Ibid. "Now this was at the very end, as the bill was passing in the House in October '89. And I remember sitting in the Legislative Council on the House side looking at the bill along with Waxman's staffers. Bill [Roper] and I really wanted tighter targets for budget purposes, for inflation. And we said we weren't going to go for it; we were going to blow the whole thing up if it didn't have tighter [expenditure] targets. Waxman's staffers said, 'Well, that's too bad because it's going to the [House] floor.'

And I remember Leon Panetta's chief of staff walked in, John Angel, who is now chief of staff in the Senate Finance Committee. He walked in with Rostenkowski's chief of staff, Wendell Primus, and they pulled me outside and said, 'You don't like those expenditure numbers, do you?' And I said, 'No, we don't and we're thinking of opposing it. We're really unhappy; this wasn't the deal.' And they said, 'Well, you know what? If you put $600 million in for teaching hospitals, we'll agree to give you tougher expenditure targets.' I said, 'How can you do that? They [Waxman's staffers] are all looking at the bill!' And they said (chuckling), 'Well, actually, there's two bills.' These were all Democratic staffers, by the way, and they said to me, 'Those guys in there reading the bill don't really make a difference; it's a diversion. The real bill is in the other room.' I said, 'I don't believe you can pull it off.' And they said, 'Yes we can. If you'll agree to put $600 million in for teaching hospitals, we'll agree to ratchet down the doctors.' This [extra money] was a big deal for Rostenkowski in Chicago. So I called up [Richard] Darman [at OMB] and I offered him the deal and he said, 'Go for it!' So that's what we did.

The bill went to the floor and I've never seen Waxman's people more upset. They just absolutely got sandbagged. They spent all this time editing their bill, and the one that went to the floor came from the Budget Committee, which controlled the process because they had the [House] Speaker on board. So in the end, while the Commerce Committee guys were marking up one bill, the other bill went to the House floor with our deal in it . . . The bottom line is that the ultimate expenditure targets on Part B were tougher by about a point and a half, because we swapped them for $600 million for teaching hospitals."

63. D. Smith, *Paying for Medicare,* 210.

64. P.L. 101-239. President George H. W. Bush signed the legislation into law on December 19, 1989.

65. A completely separate process had to be created for developing the resource-based practice expenses that make up almost half of the total costs of providing physician services overall. Because it was also subject to bickering among the various specialties, which stood to benefit or lose from substituting resource-based practice expenses for charge-based practice expenses, it took a full ten years, until 2002, to fully implement the RBRVS system.

66. Medicare Payment Advisory Commission, "MedPAC Brief: Physician Services Payment System." Established by the Omnibus Budget Reconciliation Act of 1989 (OBRA 89), the volume-performance-standard system set the first performance standard in 1990, with all physicians working under the same standard for the first year. Separate performance standards for surgical services and nonsurgical services were used for the next two years. A third category for primary care services, that is, evaluation and management services performed by any physician,

was added under OBRA 93, applicable in 1994. See Physician Payment Review Commission, *Annual Report to Congress, 1995,* 59. Under three separate performance standards, the actual conversion factors that determined payment amounts diverged because of differential volume increases. In 1997, the conversion factor for surgical services was $40.96, compared to $35.77 for primary care services and $33.85 for other nonsurgical services. Under pressure from physicians who were not surgeons, Congress in the Balanced Budget Act created the new Sustainable Growth rate method for setting expenditure limits, and as part of this reform reverted to having a single conversion factor. It was set at $36.69 for 1998. See Medicare Payment Advisory Commission, *Report to the Congress* (1998): 96.

67. Wilensky interview with Mayes. "DRGs had been worked on for a very long time before the legislation was passed [and also tested at the state level]. There were 5,000 hospitals and, at the time, 467 DRGs, so I don't want to make light of what was a major change. But that still pales in comparison to what was very much a "work in progress" in terms of the research on RBRVS and the 9,000 medical codes and the 600,000 or so physicians who, as individuals, are primarily in the private practice of medicine, as opposed to major institutions like hospitals, that—for the most part—are set up to respond to major policy changes in a different way. The RBRVS activity was contracted out and done jointly with the AMA and Bill Hsiao at Harvard. So HCFA was not actually responsible for calculating the relative values, but taking them and having them implemented instead. There were a variety of things that had to happen once the relative values were in place to convert that to dollars. Among other things, there were (initially) multiple conversion factors, because there were separate payments for the specialist physicians and for the primary care physicians."

68. See Hsiao et al., "Overview of the Development and Refinement of the Resource-Based Relative Value Scale," NS1–12; Hsiao et al., "Results and Impacts of the Resource-Based Relative Value Scale," NS61–79.

69. See Starr, *Social Transformation of American Medicine.*

70. See Laugesen and Rice, "Is the Doctor In?" 289–316.

71. GAO analysis of data from CMS and the Boards of Trustees of the Federal HI and SMI Trust Funds, 2004.

72. See Iglehart, "Health Policy Report: American Health Care System," 330, table 1.

73. Dyckman and Hess, "Survey of Health Plans," 13–15.

74. See Hadley et al. "Alternative Approaches to Constructing a Relative Value Schedule."

75. Dyckman and Hess, "Survey of Health Plans," 15.

76. For more information on the role of the AMA in the RBRVS system, see www.ama-assn .org/ama/pub/category/10559.html (accessed May 1, 2005).

77. D. Smith, *Paying for Medicare,* 270.

78. Writing in 1980, John Holahan identified the problems with the approach that Medicare would adopt a decade later. See Holahan, "Physician Reimbursement," 73–128.

79. Ibid, 85.

80. For example, see Rosenthal et al., "Paying for Quality," 127–141.

81. See Hadley and Berenson, "Seeking the Just Price," 461–466.

82. See E. Fisher et al., "Implications of Regional Variations in Medicare Spending," 273–298; Wennberg, Fisher, and Skinner, "Geography and the Debate over Medicare Reform," W3:586–602.

83. Results of a recent Urban Institute Study to be published soon.

84. For more on the effect of Medicare's new fee schedule on physicians and how they compare to private payers, see Miller, Zuckerman, and Gates, "How Do Medicare Physician Fees Compare with Private Payers?" 25–39.

85. See Hagland, "RBRVS and Hospitals," 24–27.

86. Holahan, "Physician Reimbursement," 107.

87. U.S. Government Accountability Office, *Medicare Physician Payments*, 4.

88. Holahan, "Physician Reimbursement," 107.

89. See Physician Payment Review Commission, *Annual Report to Congress*: (1989), 207–217.

Chapter Six • *The Calm before the Storm*

1. Social Security Administration, "Actuarial Status of the Social Security and Medicare Programs," 58–64.

2. See Kahn and Kuttner, "Budget Bills and Medicare Policy," 37–47.

3. Oberlander, *Political Life of Medicare,* 172–176.

4. Ibid., 176.

5. Marmor, *The Politics of Medicare,* 139–140.

6. See Palazzolo, *Done Deal?* 36–54.

7. Waxman interview with Mayes.

8. See Medicare Payment Advisory Commission, *Report to the Congress* (2002): 5–32.

9. See O'Sullivan et al., *Medicare Provisions in the Balanced Budget Act of 1997*; Congressional Budget Office, *Budgetary Implications of the Balanced Budget Act.*

10. Oberlander, *Political Life of Medicare,* 183.

11. See Casalino, "Physicians and Corporations," 869–883; Bazzoli, "Corporatization of American Hospitals," 885–905.

12. Ibid.

13. See Pauly, "Medicare Drug Coverage and Moral Hazard," 113–114. "Health insurance causes people to behave differently, in terms of use of medical care and total spending, than they would behave without insurance. Insurance does more than just pay bills; it changes the amount and composition of bills. This is true even if the person has a reasonably high income and the potentially insured medical expense is small relative to a person's wealth. People generally use more, and more costly, medical goods and services when insurance covers their cost than when it does not. To the extent that this increase in use or spending arises from the lower user price that health insurance brings about, it is called "moral hazard."

14. Feldstein, *Health Policy Issues,* 209–210.

15. L. Brown and Eagan, "The Paradoxical Politics of Provider Reempowerment," 1046.

16. See Bodenheimer and Grumbach, "Reconfiguration of U.S. Medicine," 85–90.

17. Thorpe, "Managed Care as Victim or Villain?" 951.

18. See Hacker and Marmor, "Misleading Language of Managed Care," 1033–1043.

19. McLaughlin, "The Who, What, and How of Managed Care," 1045–1049.

20. Ibid., 1047.

21. See Halvorson, "Health Plans' Strategic Responses to a Changing Marketplace," 28–29.

22. Thorpe, "Managed Care as Victim or Villain?" 951.

23. Ibid.

24. See Nichols et al., "Are Market Forces Strong Enough?" 8–21.

25. See Bodenheimer and Sullivan, "How Large Employers Are Shaping the Health Care Marketplace," 1004.

26. See KPMG Peat Marwick, *Health Benefits in 1996*; Thorpe, "Managed Care as Victim or Villain?" 951.

27. See Gold, "Changing U.S. Health Care System," 6–7.

28. See Morrissey, "Hospital Cost Shifting"; Gardner, "Drop in Hospital Cost Shifting," 24.

29. Ibid.

30. With low marginal costs and public patients as half of their revenue base, hospitals' expenses have often chased their revenues. In other words, when Medicare payments increase, hospitals frequently increase their purchase of new technologies and other capital investments and, thereby, increase their operating expenses in the long run. For instance, according to former president of the Federation of American Hospitals and former CMS administrator Tom Scully, Medicare's generous rate of reimbursement—especially of capital expenses prior to 2001— often encouraged hospitals to expand their resources (sometimes unnecessarily):

> *Mayes:* Others I've interviewed have said that hospitals will cry, cry, cry [about their financial status and Medicare reimbursement], but that you have take it with a grain of salt sometimes.

> *Scully:* Oh, they're doing great! I'll tell you, go find me a hospital that hasn't built a giant new bed-tower in the last few years. They've actually slowed down, because the government has phased out Medicare capital (reimbursement) . . . We used to pay for capital in Medicare; it was a DRG add-on for capital expenditures. Well, if you're getting 40 percent of your revenues from Medicare and you want to build a new building and Medicare will pay for 40 percent of it, right? Then, why not? So what you were getting all through the 1980s was a massive building spree up into the early 1990s and even through the '90s, because it was a ten-year phase out. If you wanted to build a new hospital wing in 1990—even if you didn't have any patients for it—if you budgeted $100 million, Medicare would write you a check for $40 million! So what do you get? You got a hell of a lot of big new hospital wings, need them or not. This is one of the reasons we've had such massive overcapacity . . . You'd have to be an idiot *not* to put up a new building every couple of years, because Medicare paid for such a big part of it. That is slowing down now and you're starting to see the demand catch up on capacity in a lot of markets.

31. Pollack interview with Mayes.

32. Ibid.

33. See Bamezai et al., "Price Competition and Hospital Cost Growth," 233–243; Gaskin and Hadley, "The Impact of HMO Penetration," 205–216.

34. See Guterman, "Putting Medicare in Context," 10–11. "Another way of looking at this situation is to compare explicitly the pattern of cross-subsidies across sources of revenue over time. In 1992, hospitals received payments from private payers that exceeded their costs by $29 billion. This more than offset the $26 billion by which payments for Medicare and other patient

care fell short of costs. Combined with $8.8 billion in net revenues from other sources (including philanthropy, revenues from assets, etc.), hospitals realized $11.8 billion in total net revenues, for a total margin of 4.6 percent. In 1997, despite considerably slower cost growth, the surplus from private payers had fallen to $20.3 billion—still substantial, to be sure, but a drop of $8.7 billion from five years before. Medicare, however, had gone from a $10.8 billion shortfall to a $4.2 billion surplus. Therefore, although the private payer surplus still was much greater, the $15 billion improvement in Medicare net revenue was crucial in offsetting the falling private payer surplus."

35. Iglehart, "Support for Academic Medical Centers," 302.

36. See Bellandi, "The Quiet Restructuring," 2–3, 16.

37. See Buerhaus and Staiger, "Trouble in the Nurse Labor Market?" 214–222.

38. Ibid.

39. Ibid.

40. Ibid., 216.

41. See Johnson, "Home Health, Nursing Homes," 2–3.

42. See Guterman et al., "First Three Years of Medicare Prospective Payment," 67–77.

43. See Medicare Payment Advisory Commission, *Report to Congress: Context for a Changing Medicare Program,* 89.

44. Hospitals that owned post-acute care facilities discharged patients one day sooner on average than those that did not and use some type of post-acute care about 10 percent more frequently. Prospective Payment Review Commission, *Medicare and the American Health Care System.*

45. See Medicare Payment Advisory Commission, *Report to Congress: Context for a Changing Medicare Program,* 91.

46. Cotterill and Gage, "Overview: Medicare Post-Acute Care," 1–6.

47. A fiscal intermediary is a Medicare contractor that determines and makes payments for Part A benefits and performs related administrative functions.

48. See Medicare Payment Advisory Commission, *Report to Congress: Context for a Changing Medicare Program,* 108.

49. See Gage, "Medicare's Home Health Interim Payment System," 1–13.

50. See Medicare Payment Advisory Commission, *Report to Congress: Context for a Changing Medicare Program,* 108.

51. Newhouse, "Medicare," 11.

52. See Freeman, "Home-Sweet-Home Health Care," 1; E. Mauser, "Medicare Home Health Initiative," 275–281.

53. Mauser, "Medicare Home Health Initiative," 276.

54. Scully interview with Mayes.

55. SNF payments rose from $2.5 billion to $11.7 billion between 1990 and 1996, while home health payments grew from $3.9 billion to over $18.3 billion during the same period. ProPAC, *Report and Recommendations to the Congress,* 1997.

56. The figures actually overstate the growth in inpatient spending and understate growth in post-acute care because hospital spending for rehabilitation and long-term care were then included in the hospital inpatient category. See Wiener, Stevenson, and Goldenson, "Controlling the Supply of Long-Term Care Providers," 1–7.

57. See Cotterill and Gage, "Overview: Medicare Post-Acute Care," 2.

58. See Wickham, "Future Developments," 193–196; Herzlinger, "Quiet Health Care Revolution," 72–90.

59. See Medicare Payment Advisory Commission, *Report to Congress: Context for a Changing Medicare Program*, 59.

60. Ibid.

61. Ibid. Over a dozen different payment methods could then apply to hospital outpatient services, depending on the service, the location and type of hospital, and the hospital's cost and charge structure.

62. Ibid. Most Medicare beneficiaries have supplemental insurance that usually covers their co-insurance obligation, so much of the financial burden of this excess was being picked up by third parties.

63. Ashby interview with Mayes; MedPAC, *Report to the Congress: Context for a Changing Medicare Program*.

64. Guterman, "Putting Medicare in Context," 7.

65. See Weissenstein, "Medicare Margins Climb through Cost Cutting," 2.

66. See Wilensky and Newhouse, "Medicare," 95.

67. Ibid.

68. Weissenstein, "Changing Tunes," 30–34.

69. Bellandi, "Hospitals, Look Within," 2–3.

70. See Stanton, "Fraud-and-Abuse Enforcement in Medicare," 32; Ruhnka, Gac, and Boerstler, "Qui Tam Claims," 283–308.

71. Iglehart, "Pursuing Health Care Fraud," 6.

72. See Weil, *Health Networks*, 28–82.

73. See Kuttner, "Columbia/HCA," 362–367.

74. See Kleinke, "Deconstructing the Columbia/HCA Investigation," 7–26.

75. See Japsen, "The Rise and Fall," 30–36.

76. See Sparrow, *License to Steal*, 87–95.

77. See U.S. General Accounting Office, "Civil Fines and Penalties Debt," 24; Centers for Medicare and Medicaid Services, "Fighting Fraud."

78. See Fogel, "Reforming Home Health Care," 82–84; Dugan, "Federal Government Expands Compliance Initiatives," 54–58; Anderson and Sadoff, "Home Health," 48–51.

79. See Hedges, "New Face of Medicare," 46–51; Saphir, "Leaving Home," 42–44; J. Scott, "Feds Discover Home Health Care," 26–29.

80. Hedges, "New Face of Medicare," 46.

81. See Komisar, "Rolling Back Medicare Home Health," 33–54.

82. Ibid.

83. PBS Online News Hour, "Medicare Fraud."

84. See Flower, "Rick Scott and the Columbia/HCA Healthcare System," 71–78.

85. Kuttner, "Columbia/HCA," 364.

86. M. Gottlieb and K. Eichenwald, "A Hospital Chain's Brass Knuckles, and the Backlash," *New York Times*, May 11, 1997.

87. See Sellers, "No. 1 Health-Care Company," 26.

88. Goldsmith, "Columbia/HCA: A Failure of Leadership," 27.

89. Snow, "Home Health Heats Up," 28–33; K. Eichenwald, "Columbia/HCA's Use of Special Medicare Units Under Scrutiny," *New York Times*, September 26, 1997; K. Eichenwald, "Columbia/HCA Discussions on Cost Shifting were Secretly Taped by U.S. Informants," *New York Times*, September 2, 1997.

90. See Reinhardt, "Columbia/HCA: Villain or Victim?" 35.

91. See M. Gottlieb and K. Eichenwald, "For Biggest Hospital Operator, A Debate Over Ties that Bind," *New York Times*, April 6, 1997; Reinhardt, "Columbia/HCA: Villain or Victim?" 33.

92. Goldsmith, "Columbia/HCA: A Failure of Leadership," 28.

93. K. Eichenwald, "U.S. Contends Billing Fraud Was 'Systemic,'" *New York Times*, October 7, 1997.

94. K. Eichenwald, "Columbia/HCA Inquiry Is Said to Produce Evidence of Fraud," *New York Times*, July 18, 1997.

95. Gottlieb and Eichenwald, "A Hospital Chain's Brass Knuckles."

96. K. Eichenwald, "He Blew the Whistle, and Health Giants Quaked," *New York Times*, October 18, 1998; K. Eichenwald, "More Details Seen in Health Care Inquiry: U.S. Affidavit on Columbia/HCA Describes Cheating Allegations," *New York Times*, February 11, 1998; K. Eichenwald, "Health Care's Giant: Artful Accounting," *New York Times* December 18, 1997. The suit was filed in 1993 by James Alderson, a financial officer with a Montana hospital. He was fired after he refused to file "aggressive" claims that the company knew were not reimbursable. Keeping two sets of books is not in itself illegal, because there are gray areas in billing procedures that are open to different interpretations. But it is illegal to do so with claims that a hospital administrator knows are not permissible.

97. See Schneidman, "PATH (Physicians at Teaching Hospitals) Audits," 6–10.

98. K. Eichenwald, "For Hospitals, a New Prognosis on Fraud-Charge Exposure," *New York Times*, August 1, 1997.

99. Oberlander, *Political Life of Medicare*, 177–189.

100. Social Security Administration, *Summary Trust Fund Reports: 1995*.

101. Hager, "Medicare is Targeted for Large Cuts," 1013.

102. Marmor, *Politics of Medicare*, 141–147.

103. See D. Smith, *Entitlement Politics*, 39–146.

104. Rushefsky and Patel, *Politics, Power and Policy Making*, 208–209, 237–238.

105. Ibid.

106. Oberlander, *Political Life of Medicare*, 172–178.

107. Iglehart, "American Health Care System," 328.

108. D. Smith, *Entitlement Politics* 192. "Over half of the total [$115 billion], nearly $60 billion, would come from hospitals, cuts in the physician fee schedule, and leaving the Part B premium contribution at 25 percent. Net savings from managed care plans were scored by the CBO at $18 billion, with almost 90 percent of that expected to result from lower growth rates in FFS Medicare, from which the capitation rates would be calculated."

109. Iglehart, "American Health Care System," 328.

110. Waxman interview with Mayes. "I voted against the Balanced Budget Act and there weren't too many of us who did that. It sounded so popular to balance the budget, but the budget was going to be balanced even if we didn't pass any legislation. The only reason that deep cuts were made in the Medicare program was to pay for a tax cut. And that was to satisfy the Re-

publicans who wanted the tax cut and the Clinton administration that wanted to say that they passed legislation, so they were going to triangulate the issue and get this balanced budget issue off the table."

111. Quoted from "The Policymakers' Perspective" (symposium).

112. Ashby interview with Mayes; Guterman interview with Mayes; Young interview with Mayes. "And that's where ProPAC played a very important role in looking at the options: 'Well, if we did this, what would happen to the margins? If we titrate the teaching adjustments at this level and do the DSH changes, what would happen to different groups of hospitals?' We even got into things like the New York delegation wanting to know what would happen to New Jersey hospitals and those kinds of things. So ProPAC played a big role. The Hill [Congress] had budget numbers that they wanted to get and they were back and forth with CBO in scoring the various proposals. In looking at their options, they had us do a lot of the simulations of what the impact would be for this and that change. There was not only PPS for hospitals; it was also SNF [skilled nursing facilities] and home health and rehab and all of these other parts."

113. Ibid.

114. Guterman interview with Mayes.

115. See Medicare Payment Advisory Commission, *Report to Congress: Context for a Changing Medicare Program*, 5.

116. Cotterill and Gage, "Overview: Medicare Post-Acute Care," 3; Kahn and Kuttner, "Budget Bills and Medicare Policy," 44.

117. D. Smith, *Paying for Medicare*, 246.

118. Ibid., 282.

119. Medicare Payment Advisory Commission, "How Medicare Pays for Services," 3–33.

120. Biles et al., "Medicare + Choice after Five Years."

121. Durenberger interview with Mayes. "Because of Senator John Heinz's Amendment to create the TEFRA 'risk contracts' for Medicare and HMOs, we had a huge explosion of Medicare reform across the northern part of the United States in 1985, '86, '87, and so forth. In other words, this was the privatization of Medicare. It worked beautifully except for the fact that we in Washington kept all of the savings gained from the changed behavior of the doctors and the hospitals. And without rewards for good behavior, the HMOs ran out of money and they said, 'The hell with it.' And it just went back to where managed care, then, tried to beat up on the hospitals and doctors. But they [the managed care organizations] lost, so we're now back to the future. But that was really critical. It was Minnesota; Portland, Oregon; Rochester, New York; Utah; Hawaii, places all the way across the country where they grabbed these HMO-like contracts, made them work in their communities to spill over onto fee-for-service and then drive down costs. But instead of allowing the health plans to keep the savings and put them into something else, we took it all back.

But it all began with Medicare's HMO demonstration projects, which got approved, I think, in the late '70s and I know for sure in the early '80s, because places like the Marsh Field clinic, Intermountain, people up here in group health in Minnesota, got risk contracts to deliver Medicare via HMOs. At the same time, four places in the country were experimenting with social HMOs, which are combinations of Medicare and Medicaid for the elderly or disabled. And so [Senator John Heinz's] amendment in '82, in effect, required HCFA to move those from demonstrations to just opening them up across the country, or at least the HMOs for Medicare.

It put them at risk for 95 percent of the AAPCC [adjusted average per capita cost], and that's why they're called Medicare risk contracts."

122. Biles et al., "Medicare + Choice after Five Years," vii, 21 app. A.

123. Scully interview with Mayes.

124. Berenson and Dowd, "Future of Private Plan Contracting in Medicare," 13–14. "This was accomplished through a formula establishing: (1) a floor payment rate, representing a minimal payment level that all plans were guaranteed, even if actual county FFS spending was lower; (2) a minimum update guarantee applied to the previous year's rate, which, in most subsequent years, has been 2 percent; and (3) a blended rate combining a national rate and the local rate, representing the county-level 1997 payment rate trended forward by a national update factor."

125. Thanks to Joseph White for this observation.

126. For more on the BBA's Medicare + Choice program to dramatically increase the number of beneficiaries enrolled in managed care plans, see Oberlander, *Political Life of Medicare,* 182–183.

127. Ibid.

128. Ibid., 183.

129. See Murtaugh et al., "Trends in Medicare Home Health Use," 146–156; Meara, White, and Cutler, "Trends in Medical Spending by Age," 176–183; Levit et al., "Health Spending in 1998," 124–132.

130. Berenson, "Medicare + Choice," W65-W82.

131. See Enthoven, "Employment-Based Health Insurance Is Failing."

132. See Grossman and Ginsburg, "As the Health Insurance Underwriting Cycle Turns," 91–102. "Higher profits attract new entrants and drive more intense price competition, which in turn leads to losses as premiums fall below costs. As plans exit the market, the remaining plans raise premiums above costs, driving a return to higher profits and a repeat of the cycle. In the 1990s, though, something else happened, which sparked uncertainty about future industry profitability. Managed care's ascendance suppressed prices in unexpected ways, but the consumer backlash and the market's reactions made for unpredictable price increases later in the decade."

133. See Havighurst, "Starr on the Corporatization and Commodification of Health Care," 947–967.

134. See Mayes, "Causal Chains and Cost Shifting," 144–174.

135. See Swartz, "Death of Managed Care," 1201–1205. "In the fee-for-service world of health insurance that existed before managed care organizations had a large proportion of the U.S. population as enrollees, consumer trust in physicians was based on three mechanisms. First, the consumer recognized that the physician had no financial incentive to ration medical care. To the contrary, a doctor, like a mechanic, had financial incentives to do more than might be absolutely necessary. But the second mechanism at work in fostering consumer trust in a physician was the insurance system, which diffused the doctor's charges among all policyholders. Hence, the individual consumer paid less attention to the possibility of physician overcharging or overprescribing of tests and visits. Last, the consumer lived in a world of free choice of providers. If a patient feared that a particular provider was advising too many diagnostic tests or unnecessary invasive surgery, he or she could seek out a different physician or other health care provider. Together, these three mechanisms—no incentive for underprovision of medical care,

no fear of overcharging, and the option to change providers—were enough to counter the information asymmetry inherent in health care transactions and maintain consumer trust in providers and health insurance."

136. Ibid.

137. See Feldstein, *Health Policy Issues,* 178, fig. 15.2.

Chapter Seven • The Reckoning and Reversal

1. Heffler et al., "Health Spending Growth Up in 1999," 193–203.

2. Kaiser Family Foundation, "Trends and Indicators in the Changing Health Care Marketplace."

3. See Stone, "Bedside Manna."

4. See Hurley, Strunk, and White, "Puzzling Popularity of the PPO," 56–68.

5. See Mayes, *Universal Coverage,* 147–155.

6. See Holahan and Wang, "Changes in Health Insurance Coverage," W4:31–42.

7. See Families USA, "One in Three."

8. See Vladeck, "Struggle for the Soul of Medicare," 410–415.

9. Senate Budget Committee chairman Judd Gregg (R-NH) voted against the Medicare reform bill in 2003. Moffit, "Fixing the New Medicare Law #1."

10. See Blumenthal, "Controlling Health Expenditures," 766–769; Bodenheimer, "American Health Care System," 584–588.

11. Selis, "Just Say No," 1–5.

12. See Feldstein, *Health Policy Issues,* 222–224.

13. HMO Industry Report 7.2 (Minneapolis: InterStudy Publications, 1998); Serb, "Another Vicious Cycle?" 24–28.

14. See Medicare Payment Advisory Commission, *Report to the Congress: Medicare Payment Policy* (2004): 80, fig. 3A-8; Medicare Payment Advisory Commission, *Report to the Congress: Medicare Payment Policy* (2001): 59–72.

15. Medicare Payment Advisory Commission, *Report to the Congress: Medicare Payment Policy* (2002): 62, table 2B-4.

16. According to Nancy-Ann DeParle, HCFA's administrator from 1997 to 2000, "I am proud of what [HCFA] was able to achieve during the three years I was there, particularly in view of the difficult environment in which we were operating. The BBA reduced Medicare payments to virtually every hospital, physician, nursing home, home health agency, and other health care provider in the country." www.gao.gov/medpac/medpac02.pdf (accessed October 1, 2002). Nancy-Ann DeParle, prepared witness testimony, U.S. House of Representatives, *Hearing Before the Subcommittee on Health of the Committee on Energy and Commerce,* 107th Cong., 1st sess., May 10, 2001.

17. Medicare Payment Advisory Commission, *Report to the Congress: Medicare Payment Policy* (2003): 6, table 1-1.

18. C. White, "Rehabilitation Therapy in Skilled Nursing Facilities," 214–222.

19. See Newhouse, "Medicare," 26–27.

20. Foster, "Trends in Medicare Expenditures," 50.

21. J. Scott, "BBA Bad News Gets Worse," 24–25.

22. See U.S. General Accounting Office, "Medicare Home Health Agencies"; Fishman, Penrod, and Vladeck, "Medicare Home Health Utilization in Context," 107–112; Office of the Inspector General, "Results of the Operation Restore Trust Audit."

23. Medicare Payment Advisory Commission, *Report to the Congress: Medicare Payment Policy* (2003): 6.

24. Ibid., 10, fig. 1-6.

25. Medicare Payment Advisory Commission, *Report to the Congress: Medicare Payment Policy* (2004): 70–71, fig. 3A-2.

26. See Guterman, "Putting Medicare in Context," 13–14; Iglehart, "Support for Academic Medical Centers," 299–304.

27. See Gardner, "Lawmakers Changed Tune about '97 BBA," 2.

28. Newhouse, "Medicare," 27.

29. Foster, "Trends in Medicare Expenditures," 50–51. "These specific behavioral changes alone had a substantial impact on Medicare expenditures (roughly $3 billion in 1999)."

30. See K. Eichenwald, "How One Questionable Hospital Benefited on Questionable Operations," *New York Times,* August 12, 2003.

31. Healthcare Financial Management Association, "Improper Medicare Home Care Payments Drop," 21. "The Office of the Inspector General found that the percentage of Medicare payments for improper or highly questionable home health care services fell from 40 percent in 1995 to 19 percent by 1998."

32. Newhouse, "Medicare," 27n66. See also statement of Paul N. Van de Water, "The Impact of the Balanced Budget Act on the Medicare Fee- for-Service Program," CBO Testimony before the Senate Finance Committee, 106th Cong., 1st sess., June 10, 1999.

33. Cunningham, "Hospital Finance," 233.

34. See Cowan et al., "National Health Expenditures, 2002," 143–166.

35. Scully interview with Mayes. "I think you also have to look at it from 'What's the right margin for a provider to make? not 'How much money do we need to save this year in the budget?' Because frequently what happens when you use budget deals is that the Budget Committee would say, 'We need this much money from Medicare,' and then the committees would go back and backfill on how to get to that number, rather than, 'What's the right margin and how do you get there?' They should be looking at the hospitals and saying, 'What's the right margin to make a hospital run right?' 'What's the right margin for a physician practice?' 'What's the right margin for a home health agency?' Instead, the Budget Committee would say, "We need $200 billion dollars; go back and figure out how to do it.' They were coming up with [Medicare payment] policies to meet budget targets that weren't realistic. That's what happened in '97 with the BBA."

36. Newhouse, "Medicare," 36.

37. See Reed and Ginsburg, "Behind the Times."

38. Ibid.

39. Dickler and Shaw, "Balanced Budget Act of 1997," 820.

40. Ibid.

41. See Harris, Ripperger, and Horn, "Managed Care at a Crossroads," 157–163.

42. See Feldstein, *Health Policy Issues,* 209–226.

43. Kertesz, "HMO Enrollment Soars," 10.

44. Gold, "Changing U.S. Health Care System," 7–8.

45. See Titlow and Emanuel, "Employer Decisions and the Seeds of Backlash," 945.

46. Iglehart, "From the Editor," 7–8.

47. Blendon et al., "Understanding the Managed Care Backlash," 80–94.

48. See L. Scott, "Maternity-Stay Rule Sparks Backlash," 8.

49. See Kertesz, "Backlash Continues," 33.

50. See Mayes, *Universal Coverage*, 122–131.

51. Reinhardt, "The Predictable Managed Care *Kvetch*," 908.

52. Lesser and Ginsburg, "Update on the Nation's Health Care System," 208.

53. Draper et al., "Changing Face of Managed Care," 17.

54. Lesser, Ginsburg, and Devers, "End of an Era," 344.

55. See Bloche and Studdert, "Quiet Revolution," 29–30; Kesselheim and Brennan, "Over-billing vs. Downcoding," 855–857.

56. See M. Freudenheim, "Medical Insurers Revise Cost-Control Efforts," *New York Times,* December 3, 1999.

57. See Fox, "Strengthening State Government through Oversight," 1185–1190.

58. Sorian and Feder, "Why We Need a Patients' Bill of Rights," 1137–1144.

59. Ibid.

60. See Dudley and Luft, "Health Policy in 2001," 1090–1091, table 4.

61. Ibid.; Sorian and Feder, "Why We Need a Patients' Bill of Rights."

62. See Greenwald, "HMO Industry Continues Battle for Profitability," 1–2.

63. See Grossman, "Health Plan Competition in Local Markets," 17–35.

64. See Hansen, "Healthcare," 20–21.

65. See Ginsburg, "1998 Annual Report."

66. "Health-Care Costs," 65.

67. Grossman, "Health Plan Competition in Local Markets," 32.

68. "Health-Care Costs," 65.

69. M. Freudenheim, "Humana Sued in Federal Court over Incentives for Doctors," *New York Times,* October 5, 1999.

70. Cutler, *Your Money or Your Life,* 94.

71. See Ginsburg, "Managed Care Woes."

72. Christianson and Trude, "Managing Costs, Managing Benefits," 357–373.

73. See Christianson, "Role of Employers in Community Health Care Systems," 158–164.

74. Lesser, Ginsburg, and Devers, "End of an Era," 343–344.

75. Robinson, "End of Managed Care," 2623.

76. "HMO Hell: The Backlash."

77. Bodenheimer and Casalino, "Executives with White Coats," 1945–1948, 2029–2031; Weber, "Managed Care Medical Directors Under Fire," 12–18.

78. See Wooten, *Employee Retirement Income Security Act of 1974.*

79. See Hacker, *Divided Welfare State,* 147–153.

80. See M. Freudenheim, "Under Legal Attack, H.M.O.'s Face a Supreme Court Test," *New York Times,* January 4, 2000; Kilberg, "Impending Collision between HMOs and ERISA," 1–5.

81. Bloche and Studdert, "Quiet Revolution," 9–10. "The class action alleged that widely used cost control rewards, including refusal to cover medically necessary prescribed treatments

and financial rewards to doctors for frugal practice, violated the federal laws that govern employees' fringe benefits. Within hours of the complaint's filing, managed care industry share prices dropped by as much as 10 percent . . . The lawyers who brought the class actions against Humana and other plans spoke openly of their hope that market pressures would push the industry to settle. This hope went unrealized. But during the two years after the suit against Humana was filed, much of the managed care industry moved away from the practices by the suit."

82. Ibid.

83. Kesselheim and Brennan, "Overbilling vs. Downcoding," 856. "Among the stipulations, Aetna pledged, for example, to decrease administrative hassles such as preauthorizations and denials based on technicalities, pay claims more promptly, end automatic downcoding, and make the claim-adjudication procedure more open and user-friendly. To improve its relations with physicians, Aetna established an advisory committee of physicians to help implement the proposed changes, based its definition of medical necessity on an AMA standard, and removed contractual provisions such as gag clauses that limited communication between physicians and patients."

84. See Draper et al., "Changing Face of Managed Care," 11–23.

85. See Dranove, Simon, and White, "Is Managed Care Leading to Consolidation?" 573–594.

86. See Bazzoli, "Corporatization of American Hospitals," 885–905.

87. Kohn, "Organizing and Managing Care," 37–52.

88. See Capps and Dranove, "Hospital Consolidation and Negotiated PPO Prices," 175–181.

89. See Cuellar and Gertler, "Trends in Hospital Consolidation," 77–87; Bazzoli, "Corporatization of American Hospitals," 889–890.

90. Lesser and Ginsburg, "Update on the Nation's Health Care System," 214–215.

91. Ibid., 214.

92. See Center for Studying Health System Change, "Community Report: Boston, Massachusetts."

93. See Reilly, "Riding High," 16; Medicare Payment Advisory Commission, *Report to the Congress: Medicare Payment Policy* (2001): 60–61.

94. See Strunk, Devers, and Hurley, "Health Plan-Provider Showdowns." "After years of low payments and less volume than expected under commercial contracts, providers have had to deal with Medicare payment reductions and other problems, including higher labor costs because of nursing and other staff shortages. These financial pressures, coupled with greater sophistication in managed care contracting strategies and tactics, have spelled the end of a period when some providers uncritically accepted contract terms. Emboldened by the managed care backlash, providers are testing the waters to see just how far they can push their emerging bargaining power. As a result, contentious negotiations between providers and plans are becoming more common across the country."

95. See Medicare Payment Advisory Commission, *Report to the Congress: Medicare Payment Policy* (2004): 204–211.

96. Jaklevic, "What Hospitals 'See' They Get," 60–62.

97. Strunk, Devers, and Hurley, "Health Plan-Provider Showdowns."

98. See Devers et al., "Hospitals' Negotiation Leverage with Health Plans," 419–446.

99. Draper et al., "Changing Face of Managed Care," 13–14.

100. M. Freudenheim, "A Changing World is Forcing Changes on Managed Care," *New York Times*, July 2, 2001.

101. See Strunk and Reschovsky, "Kinder and Gentler."

102. See Hall, "Death of Managed Care," 447–451.

103. Grossman and Ginsburg, "As the Health Insurance Underwriting Cycle Turns," 97.

104. See Robinson, "Consolidation and the Transformation of Competition," 11–24.

105. Draper et al., "Changing Face of Managed Care," 17–18.

106. See Gold, "Can Managed Care and Competition Control Medicare Costs?" W3–177.

107. Medicare Payment Advisory Commission, *Report to the Congress: Medicare Payment Policy* (2004): 205–209.

108. Ibid., 206, fig. 4-1.

109. See Biles, Dallek, and Nicholas, "Medicare Advantage," W4:586–597.

110. See Antos, "Medicare + Choice," W83–W85.

111. See Berenson, "Medicare + Choice," W65–W82.

112. See Grossman, Strunk, and Hurley, "Reversal of Fortune."

113. Iglehart, "Bias toward Action."

114. See Berenson, "Medicare + Choice," W65–W82.

115. Reilly, "Riding High," 16.

116. Robinson, "Consolidation and the Transformation of Competition," 18–19; Prince, "Rate Hikes Spur Managed Care Profits," 2; Benko, "Going for the Green," 6; Gonzalez, "Lower Medical Costs Aid Profits," 3; Kaiser Family Foundation, "Trends and Indicators."

117. See White, Hurley, and Strunk, "Getting Along or Going Along?"

118. See Nichols et al., "Are Market Forces Strong Enough?" 8–21.

119. See Mayes, *Universal Coverage*, 150–155.

120. See Gabel et al., "Health Benefits in 2004," 200–209.

121. See Iglehart, "Changing Health Insurance Trends," 956–962; Regopoulos and Trude, "Employers Shift Rising Health Care Costs."

122. Kaiser Family Foundation, "Retiree Health Benefits in 2003."

123. See Edwards, Doty, and Schoen, "Erosion of Employer-Based Health Coverage."

124. Gabel et al., "Health Benefits in 2004," 200, 206.

125. Ibid.

126. U.S. Census Bureau, *Income, Poverty and Health.*

127. See Strunk and Reschovsky, "Trends in U.S. Health Insurance Coverage, 2001–2003."

128. Holahan and Ghosh, "Understanding the Recent Growth in Medicaid Spending"; Kaiser Family Foundation, "The President's FY2005 Budget Proposal."

129. See R. Pear, "States Resist Bush's Appeal for Fast Deal on Medicaid," *New York Times*, March 1, 2005.

130. R. Pear, "Most States Cutting Back on Medicaid, Survey Finds," *New York Times*, January 14, 2003.

131. See Tu, "Rising Health Costs."

132. Warren, Sullivan, and Jacoby, "Medical Problems and Bankruptcy Problems."

133. R. Abelson and C. Dean, "Study Ties Bankruptcy to Medical Bills," *New York Times*, February 2, 2005.

134. Himmelstein et al., "Illness and Injury as Contributors to Bankruptcy," W5-70–W5-72.

135. This subsection of the chapter draws extensively on Oberlander, *Political Life of Medicare,* 183–189; D. Smith, *Entitlement Politics,* 350–355; Marmor, *Politics of Medicare,* 147–149.

136. D. Smith, *Entitlement Politics,* 350.

137. See Wilensky, "Medicare Reform," 458–462.

138. See Serafini, "If It's Good Enough for Congressmen," 340–341.

139. See Aaron and Reischauer, "The Medicare Reform Debate," 8–30.

140. See Wilensky and Newhouse, "Medicare," 92–106.

141. Oberlander, *Political Life of Medicare,* 185.

142. National Bipartisan Commission on the Future of Medicare. "We believe a premium support system is necessary to enable Medicare beneficiaries to obtain secure, dependable, comprehensive high quality health care coverage comparable to what most workers have today. We believe modeling a system on the one Members of Congress use to obtain health care coverage for themselves and their families is appropriate. This proposal, while based on that system, is different in several important ways in order to better meet the unique health care needs of seniors and individuals with disabilities. Our proposal would allow beneficiaries to choose from among competing comprehensive health plans in a system based on a blend of existing government protections and market-based competition."

143. See Schlesinger, "On Values and Democratic Policy Making," 889–925.

144. Oberlander, *Political Life of Medicare,* 187.

145. D. Smith, *Entitlement Politics,* 352.

146. See Serafini, "Quest for Medicare Compromise Challenges Congress," 3–10.

147. See Tyson, "Healing Medicare," 32–37.

148. See Vladeck, "Plenty of Nothing," 1503–1506.

149. J. Scott, "Saving Medicare," 30.

150. See Serafini, "Medicare's Challenge," 1602–1604.

151. D. Smith, *Entitlement Politics,* 354.

152. J. Scott, "Line in the Sand," 24–25; Reinhardt, "Churchill's Dictum," 38–51.

153. P.L. 108-173, December 8, 2003.

154. A major scandal erupted over the cost of Medicare's new prescription drug benefit. During legislators' deliberation, the CBO estimated the benefit's cost to be approximately $395 billion over ten years. After the MMA's passage, however, Congress learned that Medicare's chief actuary (Richard S. Foster) had previously estimated the cost of the new drug plan to be $534 billion. Foster's boss, CMS administrator Thomas Scully, threatened to fire him during Congress's deliberations if he told Congress of the higher (and more accurate) estimate. For more information on this affair, see R. Pear, "Inquiry Proposes Penalties for Hiding Medicare Data," *New York Times,* September 8, 2004; R. Pear, "Inquiry Confirms Top Medicare Official Threatened Actuary over Cost of Drug Benefits," *New York Times,* July 7, 2004; Government Accountability Office, "Department of Health and Human Services."

155. For the best comprehensive account of the history and political evolution of Medicare's new prescription drug benefit, see Oliver, Lee, and Lipton, "Political History of Medicare and Prescription Drug Coverage," 283–354.

156. "Medicare Drug Folly," editorial in the *Wall Street Journal,* June 16, 2003.

157. See Sambamoorthi, Shea, and Crystal, "Total and Out-of-Pocket Expenditures for Prescription Drugs," 345–359.

158. Iglehart, "New Medicare Prescription-Drug Benefit," 826.

159. Ibid.

160. Ibid., 828–829.

161. N. Ornstein, "[Malaise] . . . and Mischief," *Washington Post*, November 26, 2003.

162. Iglehart, "New Medicare Prescription-Drug Benefit," 828.

163. See Oliver, Lee, and Lipton, "Political History of Medicare and Prescription Drug Coverage," 284–285.

164. Vladeck, "Struggle for the Soul of Medicare," 410–415.

165. Iglehart, "New Medicare Prescription-Drug Benefit," 826–827.

166. R. Pear, "Bush Vows Veto of Any Cutback in Drug Benefit," *New York Times*, February 12, 2005.

167. Hacker and Schlesinger, "Good Medicine."

168. See National Academy of Social Insurance, *Medicare and the American Social Contract*, 71–73. "One version of managed competition models proposed for Medicare is based on a 'premium support model' in which Medicare could pay a defined proportion of the cost of an insurance policy or health plan premium. Premium support models include elements of both a defined benefit and defined contribution approach. The federal payment would be pegged to a specified percentage of the cost of health plans providing a statutorily-defined Medicare benefit package . . . This model differs significantly from voucher models in which Medicare would provide a specific dollar contribution that individuals could use toward the payment of premiums for a wide range of insurance products with different benefit designs . . . Rather than continuing to guarantee a defined benefit to be provided by any health plan enrolling Medicare beneficiaries, [under a voucher approach] Medicare would simply provide a defined 'cash' amount toward the cost of health coverage . . . The differences between the two defined contribution models are very important. In the premium support model, there is a standard Medicare benefits package defined in law, and Medicare guarantees to pay a fixed proportion of the market cost of these defined benefits provided by some set of qualified plans in each market area . . . This stands in contrast to defined contribution models using the voucher approach, without a defined benefit. Vouchers can guarantee the reduction in the rate of spending in Medicare, but cannot guarantee that Medicare will continue to pay most of the cost of a comprehensive benefits package over time, at prices beneficiaries can afford. Maintaining the comprehensiveness of the coverage offered to beneficiaries would depend on explicit political decisions about whether to maintain budgets or preserve benefits."

169. See Scully, "All Seniors Gain Benefits," 22.

170. R. Pear, "Bush May Link Drug Benefit in Medicare to Private Plans," *New York Times*, January 24, 2003.

171. R. Pear, "Bush Medicare Proposal Urges Switch to Private Payers," *New York Times*, March 5, 2003.

172. Oberlander, *Political Life of Medicare*, 192.

173. Iglehart, "New Medicare Prescription-Drug Benefit," 829–930.

174. Ibid.

175. Pauly, "Means-Testing in Medicare," W4–547.

176. Moon, "Medicare Means-Testing," W4–559.

177. Geisel, "Medicare Advantage Federal Funding Boost," 3–4.

178. See Pizer, Feldman, and Frakt, "Defective Design," W5:399–409.

179. Medicare Payment Advisory Commission, *Report to the Congress: Medicare Payment Policy* (2003): 195–197.

180. Biles, Dallek, and Nicholas, "Medicare Advantage," W4–594.

181. Berenson, "Medicare Disadvantaged," W4–577.

182. Biles, Nicholas, and Cooper, "Cost of Privatization," 6; Doherty, "Assessing the New Medicare," 391.

183. See Kennedy and Thomas, "Dramatic Improvement or Death Spiral," 749–751.

184. See U.S. General Accounting Office, "Medicare Demonstration PPOs"; Congressional Budget Office, "CBO's Analysis of Regional Preferred Provider Organizations under the Medicare Modernization Act," (Washington, D.C.: October 2004); Biles, Nicholas, and Cooper, "Cost of Privatization."

185. See Altman et al., "Escalating Health Care Spending," W3:1–14.

186. See Mayes, "Universal Coverage and the American Health Care System."

187. H. Clinton, "Now Can We Talk About Health Care?" *New York Times Sunday Magazine,* April 18, 2004.

188. Cohen, "Politics and Realities of Medicare."

189. See Medicare Boards of Trustees, *2005 Annual Report.*

190. Ibid., 2–3.

Conclusion • How Medicare Does and Should Shape U.S. Health Care

1. "Give It Back Now," editorial in the *Wall Street Journal,* June 30, 1999.

2. See Arrow, "Uncertainty and Welfare Economics," 941–973.

3. Fuchs, "'Competition Revolution,'" 22.

4. Berenson, "Which Way for Competition?" 1536–1542.

5. Porter and Teisberg, "Redefining Competition in Health Care," (July 2004): 73.

6. Berk and Monheit, "Concentration of Health Care Expenditures," 9–18.

7. See Wennberg and Wennberg, "Addressing Variations"; E. Fisher et al., "Implications of Regional Variations," 273–298; Wennberg, Fisher, and Skinner, "Geography and the Debate over Medicare Reform," W3: 586–602; E. Fisher et al., "Variations in Longitudinal Efficiency," 1127–1137; Wennberg et al., "Use of Medicare Claims Data," VAR5–VAR18.

8. Enthoven and Tollen, "Competition in Health Care," 426.

9. K. Davis et al., "Medicare Extra."

10. Enthoven, "Consumer-Choice Health Plan: Inflation and Inequity," 650–658; Enthoven, "Consumer-Choice Health Plan: National Health Insurance Proposal," 709–720.

11. See Enthoven and Tollen, *Toward a Twenty-First Century Health System.*

12. Enthoven and Tollen, "Competition in Health Care," 420–433.

13. Kronick, "Financing Health Care," 1253.

14. See Reinhardt, "Can Efficiency in Health Care Be Left to the Market?" 126; Berenson and Dowd, *Future of Private Plan Contracting,* 5. The National Academy of Social Insurance has ex-

plained the difference between a social insurance program and a social welfare program. Social insurance (1) is paid, at least in part, through mandatory contributions from individuals and/or employers according to a formula established in law; (2) provides benefits that come from a fund earmarked for this purpose; and (3) pays out these benefits under the same set of rules for all qualified individuals, who regard the benefits that they will receive as "insurance" to which they have contributed over time. As a social insurance program, Medicare provides a set of benefits, defined by law, to all eligible individuals as an earned right, irrespective of health condition and without the requirement of a means test. See the National Academy of Social Insurance, 31. Note that nothing in the description implies that fee-for-service or complete patient choice of provider are integral to social insurance.

15. Enthoven and Tollen, "Competition In Health Care," 429–430.

16. Fuchs, "Competition Revolution in Health Care," 7. "A . . . practical approach to the question of competition emphasizes the following conditions: (1) a large number of buyers and sellers, no one of whom is so big as to have a significant influence on the market price; (2) no collusion among the buyers and sellers to fix prices or quantities; (3) relatively free and easy entry into the market by new buyers and sellers; (4) no governmentally imposed restraints on prices and quantities; and (5) reasonably good information about price and quality to buyers and sellers."

17. Nichols et al, "Are Market Forces Strong Enough?" 12.

18. Ibid., 12.

19. Robinson, "Consolidation and Transformation of Competition," 11–24.

20. See U.S. Government Accountability Office, *Federal Employees Health Benefits Program.*

21. See Medicare Payment Review Commission, *Report to Congress, Medicare Payment Policy* (2005), 9.

22. Berenson and Harris, "Using Managed Care Tools," 139–168.

23. Berenson, "Medicare Disadvantaged," W4: 580–581.

24. See Angell, "Placebo Politics."

25. B. Vobejda, "Democrats Pounce on GOP Medicare Comments," *Washington Post,* October 27, 1995.

26. Berenson, "Medicare Disadvantaged," W4:572–585.

27. Lee et al., "Does Cost Shifting Matter," W3:480–488.

28. Harris, "Beyond Beneficiaries," 1290–1297.

29. See National Academy of Social Insurance, *Medicare and the American Social Contract,* 23. "A National Academy of Social Insurance study panel identified two main reasons for using Medicare to subsidize broader social goals. First, Medicare can use its reimbursement policies to assure the availability of providers for its own beneficiaries and to support providers in communities that would be unable to support the existence of necessary services on their own. Second, as the largest health insurer in the country, the United States can use Medicare to perform functions and accomplish goals that other nations assign to their national health insurance systems. NASI argued that Congress may use Medicare to accomplish other public goals simply because 'it is there.'"

30. Harris, "Beyond Beneficiaries," 1299–1303.

31. 529 U.S. 667 (2000).

32. Nichols, et al., "Are Market Forces Strong Enough?" 19.

33. See Medicare Payment Review Commission, *Report to the Congress: Issues in a Modernized Medicare Program,* 159–174.

34. See Anderson et al., "It's the Prices, Stupid," 89–105.

35. See Medicare Payment Review Commission, *Report to Congress, Medicare Payment Policy* (2005), 72–73.

36. See U.S. Government Accountability Office, *Medicare Physician Payments,* 16–17.

37. The Physician Payment Review Commission reaffirmed its recommendations to link the volume performance standard to the national economy in 1995, stating that had been its position since 1990. The linkage was enacted as part of the SGR formula in the BBA. PPRC argued "projected GDP growth is used because it represents the economy's capacity to grow. Historical trends are avoided because they reflect business cycles." Physician Payment Review Commission, *Annual Report to Congress, 1995,* 65.

38. See U.S. Government Accountability Office, *Medicare Physician Payments,* 4.

39. See Iglehart, "Medicare's Declining Payments to Physicians," 1924–1930.

40. See Iglehart, "Health Policy Report: The New Law," 1247–1252.

41. Medicare Payment Review Commission, *Report to Congress: Medicare Payment Policy* (2005), 171.

42. Kuhn letter to Hackbarth.

43. See Medicare Payment Advisory Commission, *Report to the Congress: Medicare Payment Policy* (2005): 143–175.

44. Medicare Boards of Trustees, *2006 Annual Report,* 21.

45. See U.S. Government Accountability Office, *Medicare Physician Payments,* 14. The factor used to increase or decrease the update relative to the MEI is subject to annual limits. This performance adjustment factor is set such that it may not cause the update to be more than 3 percent above MEI or 7 percent below MEI.

46. Ibid., 21.

47. Ibid., 171.

48. Kaiser Family Foundation, "Medicare Part B Premiums to Rise."

49. Medicare Boards of Trustees, *2004 Annual Report,* 70–75.

50. See Wennberg and Wennberg, "Addressing Variations," W3:614–617.

51. See E. Fisher, "Implications of Regional Variations in Medicare Spending," 273–298; Wennberg, Fisher, and Skinner, "Geography and the Debate over Medicare Reform," W3:586–602.

52. Pettengill interview with Mayes.

53. See Wilensky and Newhouse, "Medicare," 94.

54. See Ginsburg and Grossman, "When The Price Isn't Right," W5:186–194.

55. See Iglehart, "Emergence of Physician-Owned Specialty Hospitals," 1405–1407.

56. See Medicare Payment Review Commission, *Report to Congress: Physician-Owned Specialty Hospitals* (2005).

57. See Mitchell, "Effects of Physician-Owned Limited-Service Hospitals," W5:481–490.

58. See also Iglehart, "Uncertain Future of Specialty Hospitals," 1405–1407; Iglehart, "Emergence of Physician-Owned Specialty Hospitals," 78–84.

59. See Devers, Brewster, and Ginsburg, "Specialty Hospitals."

60. See Medicare Payment Review Commission, *Report to Congress: Physician-Owned Specialty Hospitals* (2005), 29.

61. See Devers, Brewster, and Casalino, "Changes in Hospital Competitive Strategy," 465.

62. See Akerlof, "Behavioral Macroeconomics," 411–433.

63. Medicare Payment Review Commission, "Review of CMS's Preliminary Estimate," 205.

64. See Medicare Payment Review Commission, "Defining Long-term Care Hospitals," 122. "To qualify as long-term care hospitals for Medicare payment, facilities must meet conditions of participation for acute hospitals. Currently, the only other requirement is that LTCHs must have an average Medicare length of stay greater than twenty-five days. In the ten years from 1993 to 2003, the number of LTCHs increased from 105 to 318 and growth continues."

65. See Gage, "Medicare's Home Health Payment System"; Wiener, Stevenson, and Goldenson, "Controlling the Supply of Long-Term Care Providers."

66. Medicare Payment Advisory Commission, "Assessing Payment Adequacy and Updating Payments for Ambulatory Surgical Center Services," in *Report to the Congress: Medicare Payment Policy* (2003): 133–149.

67. Kronick, "Financing Health Care-Finding the Money Is Hard and Spending It Well Is Even Harder," 1253

68. See U.S. General Accounting Office, *Medicare Physician Payments: Medical Settings and Safety of Endoscopic Procedures* (Washington, D.C.: GPO, GAO-03-179).

69. Coleman and Berenson, "Lost in Transition," 533–536.

70. Partnership for Solutions, "Medicare: Cost and Prevalence of Chronic Conditions."

71. Berenson and Horvath, "Clinical Characteristics of Medicare Beneficiaries."

72. See National Academy of Social Insurance, *Medicare in the Twenty-first Century.*

73. Kronick "Financing Health Care," 1253.

74. Vladeck, "The Political Economy of Medicare," 30.

75. See Atlas, "Role of PBMs," W4:504–515.

76. Ibid., 30

77. E. Fisher et al., "Implications of Regional Variations in Medicare Spending," 273–298.

78. Berenson, "Getting Serious about Excessive Medicare Spending," W3:586–602; Fox, "Medicare Fee-For-Service System," 185–206.

79. Berenson and Harris, "Using Managed Care Tools in Traditional Medicare," 141–144.

80. Berenson, "Getting Serious about Excessive Medicare Spending," 590.

81. Berenson and Harris, "Using Managed Care Tools in Traditional Medicare," 139–167.

82. See www.cms.hhs.gov/researchers/demos/ (accessed October 28, 2005).

83. Berenson and Harris, "Using Managed Care Tools in Traditional Medicare—Should We? Could We?" 146.

84. Medicare Boards of Trustees, *2005 Annual Report.*

85. Foote, "Why Medicare Cannot Promulgate a National Coverage Rule," 707–730.

86. Neumann et al., "Medicare's National Coverage Decisions," 246.

87. R. Weiss, "A Tale of Politics: PET Scans' Change in Medicare Coverage," *The Washington Post,* October 14, 2004.

88. Jost, "Methodological Introduction," 11–15.

89. Kinney, "Medicare Coverage Decision-Making," 1501–1505.

90. See Fuchs, "Medicare Reform," 57–70.

91. Chernew et al., "Barriers to Constraining Health Care Cost Growth," 122–128.

92. Berenson, Bodenheimer, and Pham, "Specialty Service Lines."

93. *World Health Report 2000.*

94. Ibid., 117.

95. Ibid.

96. Nichols et al, "Are Market Forces Strong Enough?" 8–21.

Aaron, H., and R. Reischauer. 1995. "The Medicare Reform Debate: What is the Next Step?" *Health Affairs* 18 (January/February): 92–106.

Akerlof, G. 2002. "Behavioral Macroeconomics and Macroeconomic Behavior." *American Economic Review* 92 (June): 411–433.

Altman, S., C. Tompkins, E. Eilat, and M. Glavin. 2003. "Escalating Health Care Spending: Is It Desirable or Inevitable?" *Health Affairs* (web exclusive, January 8): W3:1–14.

American Association of Medical Colleges. "Medicare Indirect Medical Education (IME) Payments." www.aamc.org/advocacy/library/gme/gme0002.htm (accessed October 27, 2005).

American Society of Internal Medicine. 1981. "Reimbursement for Physicians; Cognitive and Procedural Services: A White Paper." *Internist* 22 suppl (January): 1–4.

Anderson, G., and P. Ginsburg. 1983. "Prospective Capital Payments to Hospitals." *Health Affairs* 2 (Fall): 52–63.

Anderson, G., U. Reinhardt, P. Hussey, and V. Petrosyan. 2003. "It's the Prices, Stupid: Why the United States Is So Different from Other Countries." *Health Affairs* 22 (May/June): 89–105.

Anderson, O., T. Herold, B. Butler, C. Kohrman, and E. Morrison. 1985. *HMO Development: Patterns and Prospects* Chicago: Health Administration Studies.

Anderson, T., and J. Sadoff. 1999. "Home Health, Long-Term Care, and Other Compliance Activities." *Healthcare Financial Management* 53 (April): 48–51.

Angell, M. 2000. "Placebo Politics." *American Prospect* 11, November.

Antos, J. 2001. "Medicare + Choice: Where did the Scorekeepers Go Wrong?" *Health Affairs* (web exclusive, November 28): W83–W85.

Antos, J. 1991. "The Policy Context for Physician Payment." In *Regulating Doctors' Fees: Competition and Controls Under Medicare,* ed. H. Frech III. Washington, D.C.: AEI Press.

Applegate, L., R. Mason, and D. Thorpe. 1986. "Design of a Management Support System for Hospital Strategic Planning." *Journal of Medical Systems* 10 (February): 79–95.

Arrow, K. 1963. "Uncertainty and the Welfare Economics of Medical Care." *American Economic Review.* 53 (December): 941–973.

Ashby, J., and S. Altman. 1992. "The Trend in Hospital Output and Labor Productivity: 1980–1989." *Inquiry* 29 (Spring): 80–91.

Assaf, A., K. Lapane, J. McKenney, and R. Carleton. 1993. "Possible Influence on the Prospective

Payment System on the Assignment of Discharge Diagnoses for Coronary Heart Disease." *New England Journal of Medicine* 329 (September 23): 931–935.

Atlas, R. 2004. "The Role of PBMs in Implementing the Medicare Prescription Drug Benefit." *Health Affairs* (web exclusive, October 28): W4:404–415.

Averill, R., and M. Kalison. 1983. "Prospective Payment by DRG." *Healthcare Financial Management* 13: 12–16.

Averill, R., and D. Sparrow. 1983. "TEFRA's Two-Part Strategy Will Reduce Medicare's Financial Liability to Hospitals." *Healthcare Financial Management* 13: 72–77.

Baldwin, M. 1986. "Hospital Leaders Fear First-Year Profits Will Trigger Medicare Payment Freeze." *Modern Healthcare* 16 (March 14): 30.

Ball, R. 1995. "Perspectives on Medicare: What Medicare's Architects Had in Mind." *Health Affairs* 14 (Winter): 62–72.

Bamezai, A., J. Zwanziger, G. Melnick, and J. Mann. 1999. "Price Competition and Hospital Cost Growth in the United States." *Health Economics* 8 (May): 233–243.

Banks, D., S. Foreman, and T. Keeler. 1999. "Cross-Subsidization in Hospital Care." *Health Matrix Journal of Law-Medicine* 9 (Winter): 1–35.

Barry, D. 1986. "Medical Staff Bylaws: Protecting Hospitals' Financial Viability." *Healthcare Financial Management* 40 (September): 40–44.

Bazzoli, G. 2004. "The Corporatization of American Hospitals." *Journal of Health Politics, Policy and Law* 29 (August-October): 885–905.

Bellandi, D. 1997. "Hospitals, Look Within: HHS Memo Recommends In-House Anti-Fraud Programs." *Modern Healthcare* 27 (September 22): 2–3.

Bellandi, D. 1998. "The Quiet Restructuring: Blaming Feds, Hospitals Shed Workers, Facilities in Droves." *Modern Healthcare* 28 (December 14): 2–16.

Benko, L. 2003. "Going for the Green: As Higher Premiums and Stable Medical Costs Fuel Health Plans' Profits, Providers Say Time is Right to Win Bigger Reimbursement." *Modern Healthcare* 33 (August 18): 6–7, 14–15.

Berenson, R. 1994. "Do Physicians Recognize Their Own Best Interest?" *Health Affairs* 13 (Spring): 185–193.

———. 1987. "Editorial: Physician Payment Reform: Finally." *Annals of Internal Medicine*. (December): 929–931.

———. 2003. "Getting Serious about Excessive Medicare Spending: A Purchasing Model." *Health Affairs* (web exclusive, December 10): W3:586–602.

———. 2004. "Medicare Disadvantaged and the Search for the Elusive 'Level Playing Field.'" *Health Affairs* (web exclusive, December 15): W4:572–85.

———. 2001. "Medicare + Choice: Doubling or Disappearing?" *Health Affairs* (web exclusive, November 28): W65–82.

———. 2005. "Which Way for Competition?: 'None of the Above.'" *Health Affairs* 24 (November/December): 1536–1542.

Berenson R., T. Bodenheimer, and H. Pham (in press). "Specialty Service Lines: Salvos in the New Medical Arms Race." *Health Affairs.*

Berenson, R., and B. Dowd. 2002. "The Future of Private Plan Contracting in Medicare." Research report, American Association of Retired Persons, Washington, D.C. http://assets.aarp.org/rgcenter/health/2002_12_medicare.pdf (accessed April 25, 2005).

Berenson, R., and D. Harris. 2002. "Using Managed Care Tools in Traditional Medicare: Should We? Could We?" *Law and Contemporary Problems* 65 (Autumn): 139–168.

Berenson, R., and J. Horvath. 2002. "The Clinical Characteristics of Medicare Beneficiaries and Implications for Medicare Reform." Prepared for Partnership for Solutions (March). www .medicareadvocacy.org/chronic_PartnerPaper_ClinChars.htm.

Berk, M., and A. Monheit. 2001. "The Concentration of Health Care Expenditures, Revisited." *Health Affairs* 20 (March/April): 9–18.

Berki, S. 1988. "Changes in Hospital-Doctor Relations." *Consultant* 28 (February): 114–119.

Berkowitz, E. 1997. "The Historical Development of Social Security in the United States." In *Social Security in the 21st Century,* ed. E. Kingson and J. Schulz. New York: Oxford University Press.

———. 2004. *Robert Ball.* Madison: University of Wisconsin Press.

Biles, B., G. Dallek, and L. Nicholas. 2004. "Medicare Advantage: Déjà vu All Over Again?" *Health Affairs* (web exclusive, November 28): W4:586–597.

Biles, B., L. Nicholas, and B. Cooper. 2004. "The Cost of Privatization: Extra Payments to Medicare Advantage Plans—2005 Update." Issue brief. Washington, D.C.: Commonwealth Fund. www.cmwf.org/usr_doc/750_Biles_costofprivatization_update_ib_pdf.pdf (accessed April 15, 2004).

Biles, B., et al. 2002. "Medicare + Choice after Five Years: Lessons for Medicare's Future, Findings from Seven Major Cities." Issue brief. Washington, D.C.: Commonwealth Fund. www .cmwf.org/usr-doc/biles/M+Cafterfiveyears_562.pdf.

Blendon, R., M. Brodie, J. Benson, and D. Altman, et al. 1998. "Understanding the Managed Care Backlash." *Health Affairs* 17 (July/August): 80–94.

Bloche, M., and D. Studdert. 2004. "A Quiet Revolution: Law as an Agent of Health System Change." *Health Affairs* 23 (March/April): 29–42.

Blumberg, M. 1978. "Rational Provider Prices: An Incentive for Improved Health Care Delivery." In *Health Handbook,* ed. G. Chacko. Amsterdam: North Holland Publishing.

Blumenthal, D. 2001. "Controlling Health Expenditures." *New England Journal of Medicine* 344 (March 8): 766–769.

Boccuti, C., and M. Moon. 2003. "Comparing Medicare and Private Insurers: Growth Rates in Spending over Three Decades." *Health Affairs* 22 (March/April): 230–237.

Bodenheimer, T. 1999. "The American Health Care System: Physicians and the Changing Medical Marketplace." *New England Journal of Medicine* 340 (February 18): 584–588.

———. 2002. "The Not-So-Sad History of Medicare Cost Containment as Told in One Chart." *Health Affairs* (web exclusive, January 23): W88–W90.

Bodenheimer, T., and L. Casalino. 1999. "Executives with White Coats—The Work and World View of Managed Care Medical Directors." *New England Journal of Medicine* 341 (December 23): 1945–1948.

Bodenheimer, T., and K. Grumbach. 1995. "The Reconfiguration of U.S. Medicine." *Journal of the American Medical Association* 274 (July 5): 85–90.

Bodenheimer, T., and K. Sullivan. 1998. "How Large Employers Are Shaping the Health Care Marketplace." *New England Journal of Medicine* 338 (April 2): 1003–1007.

Brown, L. 1983. *Politics and Health Care Organization: HMOs as Federal Policy.* Washington, D.C.: Brookings Institution Press.

———. 1985. "Technocratic Corporatism and Administrative Reform in American Medicine." *Journal of Health Politics, Policy and Law* 10 (Fall): 579–599.

Brown, L., and E. Eagan. 2004. "The Paradoxical Politics of Provider Reempowerment." *Journal of Health Politics, Policy, and Law* 29 (December): 1045–1071.

Buerhaus, P., and D. Staiger. 1999. "Trouble in the Nurse Labor Market? Recent Trends and Future Outlook." *Health Affairs* 18 (January/February): 214–222.

Burda, D. 1993. "What Have We Learned from DRGs?" *Modern Healthcare* (October 4): 44.

Burda, D., and C. Tokarski. 1990. "Hospitals are Under Pressure to Justify Cost Shifting: But Some Payers are Rejecting Hospitals' Excuses and are Demanding Data." *Modern Healthcare* (November 12): 28–36.

Campbell, P., and N. Kane. 1990. "Physician-Management Relationships at HCA: A Case Study." *Journal of Health Politics, Policy and Law* 15 (Fall): 591–605.

Capps, C., and D. Dranove. 2004. "Hospital Consolidation and Negotiated PPO Prices." *Health Affairs*. 23 (March/April): 175–181.

Carey, K. 1994. "Cost Allocation Patterns Between Hospital Inpatient and Outpatient Departments." *Health Services Research* 29 (August): 275–292.

Casalino, L. 2004. "Physicians and Corporations: A Corporate Transformation of American Medicine?" *Journal of Health Politics, Policy and Law* 29 (August-October): 869–883.

Center for the Analysis of Public Issues. 1974. *Bureaucratic Malpractice*. Princeton, N.J.: CAPI.

Centers for Medicare and Medicaid Services. 1999. "Fighting Fraud, Waste and Abuse in Medicare and Medicaid" (February 22). www.cms.hhs.gov/media/press/release.asp?Counter=349 (accessed May 6, 2005).

Center for Studying Health System Change. 2003. "Community Report: Boston, Massachusetts" (Fall). www.hschange.org/CONTENT/611/611.pdf (accessed March 4, 2005).

Chernew, M., P. Jacobson, T. Hofer, et al. 2004. "Barriers to Constraining Health Care Cost Growth." *Health Affairs* 23 (November/December): 122–128.

Chirikos, T. 1998. "Further Evidence That Hospital Production is Inefficient." *Inquiry* 35 (Winter): 408–416.

Christianson, J. 1998. "The Role of Employers in Community Health Care Systems." *Health Affairs* 17 (July/August): 158–164.

Christianson, J., and S. Trude. 2003. "Managing Costs, Managing Benefits: Employer Decisions in Local Health Care Markets." *Health Services Research* 38 (February): 357–373.

Clare, R. 1990. "Wilensky Seeks Dialogue with Providers." *Healthcare Financial Management* 44 (June): 22–25.

Clark, T. 1983. "Congress Avoiding Political Abyss by Approving Social Security Changes." *National Journal* 15 (March 19): 611–615.

Clarke, R. 1991. "Altman Sees Industry Unwilling to Control Costs." *Healthcare Financial Management* 45 (April): 14–20.

———. 1992. "Cost Shifting Merits an Explanation." *Healthcare Financial Management* 46 (July 1992): 12.

———. 1990. "Wilensky Seeks Dialogue with Providers." *Healthcare Financial Management* 44 (June): 22–25.

Clement, J. 1997–1998. "Dynamic Cost Shifting in Hospitals: Evidence From the 1980s and 1990s." *Inquiry* 34 (Winter): 340–350.

Coddington, D., D. Keen, K. Moore, and R. Clarke. 1990. *The Crisis in Health Care: Costs, Choices, and Strategies.* San Francisco: Jossey-Bass.

Coffey, S. 1993. "Retroactive Reimbursement under HCFA's PPS for Capital." *Health Care Financing Review* 47 (October): 60–63.

Cohen, E. 2004. "The Politics and Realities of Medicare and Prescription Drug Coverage." *Public Interest* (Summer): 37–50.

Coleman, E., and R. Berenson. 2004. "Lost in Transition: Challenges and Opportunities For Improving the Quality of Transitional Care." *Annals of Internal Medicine* 141 (October): 533–536.

Congressional Budget Office. 1997. *Budgetary Implications of the Balanced Budget Act of 1997.* Washington, D.C.: Government Printing Office.

———. 2004. *CBO's Analysis of Regional Preferred Provider Organizations under the Medicare Modernization Act.* Washington, D.C.: GPO.

———. 1993–1997. *The Economic and Budget Outlook: Fiscal Years.* Washington, D.C.: GPO.

———. 1977. *Expenditures for Health Care: Federal Programs and Their Effects.* Washington, D.C.: GPO.

———. 1981. *Hospital Cost Containment Model: A Technical Analysis.* Washington, D.C.: CBO.

———. 1986. *Physician Reimbursement under Medicare: Options for Change.* Washington, D.C.: CBO.

Conover, C., and F. Sloan. 1998. "Does Removing Certificate-of-Need Regulations Lead to a Surge in Health Care Spending?" *Journal of Health Care Politics, Policy and Law* 23 (June): 455–481.

Cooper, P., and B. Schone. 1997. "More Offers, Fewer Takers for Employment-Based Health Insurance: 1987 and 1996." *Health Affairs* 16 (November/December): 142–149.

Cotterill. P. 1991. "Prospective Payment for Medicare Hospital Capital: Implications of the Research." *Health Care Financing Review* 13: 77–79.

Cotterill, P., and B. Gage. 2002. "Overview: Medicare Post-Acute Care Since the Balanced Budget Act of 1997." *Health Care Financing Review* 12 (Winter): 1–6.

Coulam, R., and G. Gaumer. 1991. "Medicare's Prospective Payment System: A Critical Appraisal." *Health Care Financing Review* annual supplement.

CQ Almanac 1977. Washington, D.C: Congressional Quarterly.

Cromwell, J., and B. Butrica. 1995. "Hospital Department Cost and Employment Increases: 1980–92." *Health Care Financing Review* 17 (Fall): 147–165.

Cuellar, A., and P. Gertler. 2003. "Trends in Hospital Consolidation: The Formation of Local Systems." *Health Affairs* 22 (November/December): 77–87.

Cunningham, R. 2001. "Hospital Finance: Signs of 'Pushback' Amid Resurgent Cost Pressures." *Health Affairs* 20 (March/April): 233–240.

Curtin, L., and C. Zurlage, eds. 1984. *DRGs: The Reorganization of Health.* Chicago: S-N Publications.

Cutler, D. 2005. *Your Money or Your Life: Strong Medicine for American's Healthcare System.* New York: Oxford University Press.

Davis, C., and D. Rhodes. 1988. "The Impact of DRGs on the Cost and Quality of Health Care in the United Sates." *Health Policy* 9: 117–131.

Davis, Carolyne. 1995. Interview by Edward Berkowitz, November 8. www.cms.hhs.gov/about/history/davis.asp (accessed March 5, 2005).

Davis, K., M. Moon, B. Cooper, and C. Schoen. 2005. "Medicare Extra: A Comprehensive Benefit Option For Medicare Beneficiaries." *Health Affairs* (web exclusive, Oct 5, 2005): W5:442–454. http://content.healthaffairs.org/cgi/content/full/hlthaff.w5.442/DC1 (accessed May 11, 2006)

Delbanco, T., K. Meyers, and E. Segal. 1981. "Paying the Physician's Fee: Blue Shield and the Reasonable Charge." *New England Journal of Medicine* 301 (December 13): 1314–1320.

Demkovich, L. 1982. "Devising New Medicare Payment Plan May Prove Easier Than Selling It." *National Journal* 14 (November 20): 1981–1985.

———. 1982. "Relying on the Market—The Reagan Approach to Containing Medical Costs." *National Journal* 14 (January 30): 194–197.

———. 1979. "Who Can Do a Better Job of Controlling Hospital Costs?" *National Journal* 11 (February 10): 219–223.

———. 1983. "Who Says Congress Can't Move Fast? Just Ask Hospitals about Medicare." *National Journal* 15 (April 2): 704–707.

Devers, K., L. Brewster, and L. Casalino. 2003. "Changes in Hospital Competitive Strategy: A New Medical Arms Race?" *Health Services Research* 38 (February): 447–469.

Devers, K., L. Brewster, and P. Ginsburg. 2003. "Specialty Hospitals: Focused Factories or Cream Skimmers?" Issue brief no. 62 (April). Washington, D.C.: Center for Studying Health System Change.

Devers, K., L. Casalino, L. Rudell, J. Stoddard, L. Brewster, and T. Lake. 2003. "Hospitals' Negotiation Leverage with Health Plans: How and Why Has It Changed?" *Health Services Research* 38 (February): 419–446.

Dickler, R., and G. Shaw. 2000. "The Balanced Budget Act of 1997: Its Impact on U.S. Teaching Hospitals." *Annals of Internal Medicine* 132 (May 16): 820–824.

Dobson, A., N. Bray, et al. 1992. "An Evaluation of Winners and Losers Under Medicare's Prospective Payment System." *Lewin-ICF Report to the Prospective Payment Assessment Commission* (May 11).

Dobson, A., and R. Clarke. 1992. "Shifting No Solution to Problem of Increasing Costs." *Healthcare Financial Management* 46 (July): 24–31.

Doherty, R. 2004. "Assessing the New Medicare Prescription Drug Law." *Annals of Internal Medicine* 141 (September 7): 391–395.

Dougherty, C. 1989. "Ethical Perspectives on Prospective Payment: Cost Containment, DRGs, and the Ethics of Health Care." *Hastings Center Report* 19 (January/February): 5–11.

Dowling, W. 1974. "Prospective Reimbursement of Hospitals." *Inquiry* 11 (September): 163–180.

———. 1976. "Prospective Rate Setting." *Topics in Health Care Financing* 3 (Winter): 7–37.

Drake, D. 1997. "Managed Care: A Product of Market Dynamics." *Journal of the American Medical Association* 277 (February 19): 560–564.

Dranove, D., C. Simon, and W. White. 2002. "Is Managed Care Leading to Consolidation in Health-Care Markets?" *Health Services Research* 37 (June): 573–594.

Draper, D., R. Hurley, C. Lesser, and B. Strunk. 2002. "The Changing Face of Managed Care." *Health Affairs* 21 (January/February): 11–23.

Dudley, R., and H. Luft. 2001. "Health Policy in 2001: Managed Care in Transition." *New England Journal of Medicine* 344 (April 5): 1087–1092.

Dugan, J. 1997. "Federal Government Expands Compliance Initiatives." *Healthcare Financial Management* 51 (September): 54–58.

Dunham, A., and J. Morone. 1983. *Politics of Innovation: The Evolution of DRG Rate Regulation in New Jersey.* Princeton: Health Research and Education Trust.

Dyckman, Z., and P. Hess. 2003. "Survey of Health Plans Concerning Physician Fees and Payment Methodology." Study prepared for the Medicare Payment Advisory Commission, Washington, D.C.

Edwards, J., M. Doty, and C. Schoen. 2002. *The Erosion of Employer-Based Health Coverage and the Threat to Workers' Health Care: Findings from the Commonwealth Fund 2002 Workplace Health Insurance Survey* (August). Washington, D.C.: Commonwealth Fund.

Enthoven, A. 1978. "Consumer-Choice Health Plan (First of Two Parts). Inflation and Inequity in Health-Care Today: Alternative for Cost Control and an Analysis of Proposals for National Health Insurance," *New England Journal of Medicine* 298 (March 23): 650–658.

———. "Consumer-Choice Health Plan (Second of Two Parts). A National Health Insurance Proposal Based on Regulated Competition on the Private Sector," *New England Journal of Medicine* 298 (March 30): 709–720.

———. 2003. "Employment-Based Health Insurance is Failing: Now What?" *Health Affairs* (web exclusive, May 28): W3:237–249.

Enthoven, A. and L. Tollen. 2005. "Competition in Health Care: It Takes Systems To Pursue Quality and Efficiency" *Health Affairs* (web exclusive, September 7, 2005): W5:420–433.

———, eds. 2004. *Toward a Twenty-First Century Health System.* San Francisco: Jossey-Bass.

Epstein, A., and D. Blumenthal. 1993. "Physician Payment Reform: Past and Future." *Milbank Quarterly* 71: 193–215.

Executive Office of the President. 1981. *The Budget of the United States Government, Fiscal Year 1981.* Washington, D.C.: GPO.

Families USA. 2004. "One in Three: Non-Elderly Americans without Health Insurance, 2002–2003." Washington, D.C. www.familiesusa.org/assets/pdfs/82million_uninsured_report6fdc.pdf.

Feder, J. 1977. *Medicare: The Politics of Federal Hospital Insurance.* Lexington, Mass.: Lexington Books.

———. 1977. "The Social Security Administration and Medicare: A Strategy of Implementation." In *Toward a National Health Policy: Public Policy and the Control of Health-Care Costs,* ed. K. Friedman and S. Rakoff. Lexington, Mass.: Lexington Books.

Fein, R. 2000. "The Academic Health Center: Some Policy Reflections." *Journal of the American Medical Association.* 283 (May 10): 2436–2437.

———. 1999. *Medical Care, Medical Costs: The Search for a Health Insurance Policy.* 2nd ed. Cambridge: Harvard University Press.

Feldstein, M. 1981. *Hospital Costs and Health Insurance.* Cambridge: Harvard University Press.

———. 1977. "The Rapid Rise of Hospital Costs," *Executive Office of the President's Council on Wage and Price Stability Staff Report* (January). Washington, D.C.: GPO.

Feldstein, P. 2003. *Health Policy Issues: An Economic Perspective.* 3rd ed. Chicago: Health Administration Press.

———. 2001. *The Politics of Health Legislation: An Economic Perspective.* Chicago: Health Administration Press.

Fetter, R., D. Brand, and D. Gamache. 1991. *DRGs: Their Design and Development.* Ann Arbor, Mich.: Health Administration Press.

Fetter, R., Y. Shin, J. Freeman, R. Averill, and J. Thompson. 1980. "Case Mix Definition by Diagnosis-Related Groups." *Medical Care* 18 (February): vii–53.

Fisher, C. 1992. "Hospital and Medicare Financial Performance under PPS, 1985–90." *Health Care Financing Review* 14 (Fall): 171–183.

Fisher, E., et al. 2003. "The Implications of Regional Variation in Medicare Spending." *Annals of Internal Medicine* 138 (February 18): 273–298.

———. 2004. "Variations in the Longitudinal Efficiency of Academic Medical Centers." *Health Affairs* (web exclusive, October 7): 1127–1137.

Fishman, E., J. Penrod, and B. Vladeck. 2003. "Medicare Home Health Utilization in Context." *Health Services Research* 38 (February): 107–112.

Flower, J. 1995. "Rick Scott and the Columbia/HCA Healthcare System." *Healthcare Forum Journal* 38 (March/April): 71–78.

Fogel, L. 1998. "Reforming Home Health Care." *Healthcare Financial Management* 52 (June): 82–84.

Foote, S. 2002. "Why Medicare Cannot Promulgate a National Coverage Rule: A Case of *Regula Mortis.*" *Journal of Health Policy, Politics, and Law* 27 (October): 707–730.

Foster, R. 2000. "Trends in Medicare Expenditures and Financial Status, 1966–2000." *Health Care Financing Review* 22 (Fall): 35–51.

Fox, D. 1999. "Strengthening State Government through Oversight." *Journal of Health Politics, Policy and Law* 24 (October): 1185–1190.

Fox, P. 1999. "The Medicare Fee-For-Service System: Applying Managed Care Techniques." In *Medicare: Preparing for the Challenges of the Twenty-First Century*, ed. R. Reischauer, S. Butler, and J. Lave, 185–206. Washington, D.C.: National Academy of Social Insurance.

Freed, D. 1992. "The Hospital Manager as Enthusiast." *Health Care Supervisor* 10 (June): 20–23.

Freeman, L. 1995. "Home-Sweet-Home Health Care." *Monthly Labor Review* (March): 3–11.

Frieden, J. 1992. "Health Care Costs: The Shift Goes On." *Business and Health* 10 (March): 49–54.

Friedman, B., and S. Shortell. 1988. "The Financial Performance of Selected Investor-Owned and Not-for-Profit System Hospitals Before and After Medicare Prospective Payment." *Health Services Research* 23: 237–267.

Fronstin, P., and S. Snider. 1996–1997. "An Examination of the Decline in Employment-Based Health Insurance between 1988 and 1993." *Inquiry* (Winter): 317–325.

Fuchs, V. 1988. "The 'Competition Revolution' in Health Care." *Health Affairs* 7 (Fall): 5–24.

Gabel, J. 1997. "Ten Ways HMOs Have Changed during the 1990s." *Health Affairs* 16 (May–June): 134–145.

Gabel, J., G. Claxton, I. Gil, J. Pickreign, H. Whitmore, et al. 2004. "Health Benefits in 2004: Four Years of Double-Digit Premium Increases Take Their Toll on Coverage." *Health Affairs* 23 (September/October 2004): 200–209.

Gabel, J., P. Ginsburg, and K. Hunt. 1997. "Small Employers and Their Health Benefits, 1988–1996: An Awkward Adolescence." *Health Affairs* (September/October): 103–110

Gage, B. 2000. "Medicare Reform: The Larger Picture." *Journal of Economic Perspectives* 14: 57–70.

————. 1999. "Medicare's Home Health Interim Payment System: Is Access a Problem?" Research report (April). Urban Institute: Washington, D.C.

Gardner, J. 1995. "Drop in Hospital Cost Shifting Showing up on the Bottom Line." *Modern Healthcare* 25 (November 20): 24.

————. 2000. "Lawmakers Change Tune about '97 BBA," *Modern Healthcare* 30 (February 7): 2.

Garg, M., and B. Barzansky, eds. 1986. *The Medicare System of Prospective Payment*. New York: Praeger.

Gaskin, D., and J. Hadley. 1997. "The Impact of HMO Penetration on the Rate of Hospital Cost Inflation." *Inquiry* 34 (Fall): 205–216.

Gawande, A. 2005. "Piecework: Medicine's Money Problem." *The New Yorker*, April 4.

Gay, E., J. Kronenfeld, S. Baker, and R. Amdion. 1988. "An Appraisal of Organizational Response to Fiscally Constraining Regulation: The Case of Hospitals and DRGs." *Journal of Health and Social Behavior* 30 (March): 41–55.

Geisel, J. 2004. "Medicare Advantage Federal Funding Boost Renews Plans' Interest," *Business Insurance* 38 (February 16): 3–4.

————. 1992. "Solution Proposed for N.J. Cost Shifting," *Business Insurance* 26 (November 2): 3–5.

Gianfrancesco, F., 1990. "The Fairness of the PPS Reimbursement Methodology." *Health Services Research* 25 (April): 1–23.

Ginsburg, P. 1998. "Managed Care Woes: Industry Trends and Conflicts." Issue brief no. 31 (May). Washington, D.C.: Center for Studying Health System Change. www.hschange.com/CONTENT/68.

————. "1998 Annual Report." Center for Studying Health System Change. www.hschange.org/CONTENT/151/98arperspective.html (accessed February 10, 2005).

————. 1989. "Physician Payment Policy in the 101st Congress." *Health Affairs* 8 (Spring): 5–20.

Ginsburg, P., and J. Grossman, "When The Price Isn't Right: How Inadvertent Payment Incentives Drive Medical Care." *Health Affairs* (web exclusive, August 9, 2005): W5:186–194.

Ginsburg, Paul. 1995. Interview by Edward Berkowitz, August 22.

Glandon, G., and M. Morrissey. 1986. "Redefining the Hospital-Physician Relationship Under Prospective Payment." *Inquiry* 23 (Summer): 166–175.

Gold, M. 2003. "Can Managed Care and Competition Control Medicare Costs?" *Health Affairs* (web exclusive, April 2): W3:176–188.

————. 1999. "The Changing U.S. Health Care System: Challenges for Responsible Public Policy." *The Milbank Quarterly* 77(1): 3–37.

————. 1991. "DataWatch: HMOs and Managed Care." *Health Affairs* 10 (Winter): 189–206.

Gold, M., K. Chu, S. Felt, M. Harrington, and T. Lake. 1993. "Effects of Select Cost- Containment Efforts: 1971–1993." *Health Care Financing Review* 14 (Spring): 183- 225.

Goldfarb, M. 1992. "Change in the Medicare Case-Mix Index in the 1980s and the Effect of the Prospective Payment System." *Health Services Research* 27 (August): 385–415.

Goldman, D., et al. 2005. "Consequences of Health Trends and Medical Innovation for the Future Elderly." *Health Affairs* (web exclusive, September 26): W5:R5–R17.

Goldsmith, J. 1998. "Columbia/HCA: A Failure of Leadership" *Health Affairs* 17 (March/April): 27–29.

————. 1984. "Death of a Paradigm: The Challenge of Competition." *Health Affairs* 3: 5–19.

Gonzalez, G. 2004. "Lower Medical Costs Aid Profits: Managed Care Earnings Surge," *Business Insurance* 38 (March 15): 3–4.

Goody, B., 1992. "Medicare Dependent Hospitals: Who Depends on Them?" *Health Care Financing Review* 14 (Winter): 97–105.

Gornick, M., et al. 1996. "Thirty Years of Medicare: Impact on the Covered Population." *Health Care Financing Review* 18: 179–237. www.ssa.gov/history/pdf/ThirtyYearsPopulation.pdf.

Grassmuck, K. 1991. "Financial Pressures Prompt Teaching Hospitals to Cut Costs." *Chronicle of Higher Education* 37 (March 27): 27–29.

Gray, B. 1991. *The Profit Motive and Patient Care: The Changing Accountability of Doctors and Hospitals.* Cambridge, Mass.: Harvard University Press.

Greenwald, J. 1998. "HMO Industry Continues Battle for Profitability." *Business Insurance* 32 (August 17): 1–2.

Grossman, J. 2000. "Health Plan Competition in Local Markets." *Health Services Research* 35 (April): 17–35.

Grossman, J., and P. Ginsburg. 2004. "As the Health Insurance Underwriting Cycle Turns: What Next?" *Health Affairs* 23 (November/December): 91–102.

Grossman, J., B. Strunk, and R. Hurley. 2002. "Reversal of Fortune: Medicare + Choice Collides with Market Forces." Issue brief no. 52 (May). Washington, D.C.: Center for Studying Health System Change.

Guterman, S. 2000. "Putting Medicare in Context: How Does the Balanced Budget Act Affect Hospitals?" Research paper, Health Policy Center, The Urban Institute (July).

Guterman, S., S. Altman, and D. Young. 1990. "Hospitals' Financial Performance in the First Five Years of PPS." *Health Affairs* 9: 125–134.

Guterman, S., J. Ashby, and T. Greene. 1996. "Hospital Cost Growth Down." *Health Affairs* 15 (Fall): 134–139.

Guterman, S., P. Eggers, G. Riley, T. Green, and S. Terrell. 1988. "The First Three Years of Medicare Prospective Payment: An Overview." *Health Care Financing Review* 9 (Spring): 67–77.

Hacker, J. 2002. *The Divided Welfare State: The Battle Over Public and Private Social Benefits in the United States.* Cambridge: Cambridge University Press.

————. 1998. "The Historical Logic of National Health Insurance." *Studies in American Political Development* 12 (Spring): 57–130.

Hacker, J., and T. Marmor. 1999. "The Misleading Language of Managed Care." *Journal of Health Politics, Policy and Law.* 24 (October): 1033–1043.

Hacker, J., and M. Schlesinger. 2004. "Good Medicine." *American Prospect* (October 1). www .prospect.org/web/printfriendly-view.ww?id=8545 (accessed March 2, 2005).

Hackey, R. 1999. "Groping for Autonomy: The Federal Government and American Hospitals, 1950–1990." 33 (September): 625–632.

Hadley, J. 1991. "Theoretical and Empirical Foundations of the Resources-Based Relative Value Scale." In *Regulating Doctors' Fees: Competition and Controls Under Medicare,* ed. H. Frech III. Washington, D.C.: AEI Press.

Hadley, J., and R. Berenson. 1987. "Seeking the Just Price: Constructing Relative Value Scales and Fee Schedules." *Annals of Internal Medicine* 106 (March): 461–466.

Hadley, J., R. Berenson, D. Juba, and J. Wagner. 1986. "Alternative approaches to constructing a relative value schedule." In *Medicare Physician Payment Reform-Issues and Options,* ed. J. Holahan and L. Etheredge. Washington, D.C.: Urban Institute Press.

Hager, G. 1995. "Medicare is Targeted for Large Cuts." *Congressional Quarterly* (April 8): 1012–1014.

Hagland, M. 1991. "The RBRVS and Hospitals: The Physician Payment Revolution on Our Doorstep." *Hospitals* 65 (February): 24–27.

Hall, M. 2005. "The Death of Managed Care: A Regulatory Autopsy." *Journal of Health Care Politics, Polic, and Law* 30 (June): 447–451.

Halvorson, G. 1999. "Health Plans' Strategic Responses to a Changing Marketplace." *Health Affairs* 18 (March/April): 28–29.

Hammer, P., D. Haas-Wilson, M. Peterson, and W. Sage. 2003. *Uncertain Times: Kenneth Arrow and the Changing Economics of Health Care.* Durham: Duke University Press.

Hansen, F. 1999. "Healthcare: Trouble Ahead." *Compensation and Benefits Review* (March): 20–21.

Harris, D. 2003. "Beyond Beneficiaries: Using the Medicare Program to Accomplish Broader Public Goals." *Washington and Lee Law Review* 60 (Fall): 1290–1297.

Harris, G., M. Ripperger, and H. Horn. 2000. "Managed Care at a Crossroads." *Health Affairs* 19 (January/February): 157–163.

Havighurst, C. 2004. "Starr on the Corporatization and Commodification of Health Care, the Sequel." *Journal of Health Politics, Policy and Law* 24 (August-October): 947–967.

"Health-Care Costs: On the Critical List." 1999. *Economist,* February 13.

Health Care Financing Administration. 1984. *Diagnosis-Related Groups: The Effect in New Jersey—The Potential for the Nation.* Washington, D.C.: GPO.

Health Care Financing Administration. 1981. *A Prospective Reimbursement System Based on Patient Case-Mix For New Jersey Hospitals, 1976–1981.* Washington, D.C.: GPO.

Healthcare Financial Management Association. 1999. "Improper Medicare Home Care Payments Drop." *Healthcare Financial Management* 53 (December): 21.

Hedges, S. 1998. "The New Face of Medicare: Organized-Crime Involvement with Medicare." *U.S. News and World Report* (February 2): 46–51.

Heffer, S., K. Levit, S. Smith, C. Cowan, et al. 2001. "Health Spending Growth up in 1999; Faster Growth Expected in the Future." *Health Affairs* 20 (March/April): 193–203.

Henderson, R., and J. May. 1983. "The Business Community Looks at DRG-Based Hospital Reimbursement." *Health Affairs* 2 (Spring): 38–49.

Herzlinger, R. 1994. "The Quiet Health Care Revolution." *Public Interest* (Spring): 72–90.

Himmelstein, D., E. Warren, D. Thorne, and S. Woolhandler. 2005. "Illness and Injury as Contributors to Bankruptcy." *Health Affairs* (web exclusive, February 2): W5:63–73.

"HMO Hell: The Backlash." 1999. *Newsweek,* November 8.

"HMO Industry Report 7.2." 1998. Minneapolis: InterStudy Publications.

Holahan, J. "Physician Reimbursement." 1980. In *National Health Insurance: Conflicting Goals and Policy Choices,* ed. J. Feder, J. Holahan, and T. Marmor, 73–128. Washington, D.C.: The Urban Institute Press.

Holahan, J., and L. Etheredge, eds. 1986. *Medicare Physician Payment Reform: Issues and Options.* Washington, D.C.: Urban Institute Press.

Holahan, J., and A. Ghosh. 2005. "Understanding the Recent Growth in Medicaid Spending,

2000–2003." *Health Affairs* (January 26). http://content.healthaffairs.org/cgi/content/full/hlthaff.w5.52/DC1 (accessed March 1, 2005).

Holahan, J., and M. Wang. 2004. "Changes in Health Insurance Coverage During the Economic Downturn: 2000–2002." *Health Affairs* (web exclusive, January 28): W4:31–42.

Holahan, J., C. Winterbottom, and S. Rajan. 1995. "A Shifting Picture of Health Insurance Coverage." *Health Affairs* 14 (Winter): 253–264.

"Hospital Industry's Margin Soared in '84." 1985. *American Medical News* 28 (April 26).

Howard, C. 1997. *The Hidden Welfare State: Tax Expenditures and Social Policy in the United States.* Princeton, N.J.: Princeton University Press.

Hoy, E., R. Curtis, and T. Rice. 1991. "Change and Growth in Managed Care." *Health Affairs* 10 (Winter): 18–36.

Hsia, D., C. Ahern, B. Ritchie, L. Moscoe, and W. Krushat. 1992. "Medicare Reimbursement Accuracy under the Prospective Payment System, 1985 to 1988." *Journal of the American Medical Association* 268 (August 19): 896–899.

Hsiao, W. 1995. Interview by R. Shuster. www.ssa.gov/history/HSIAO.html (accessed May 5, 2005).

Hsaio, W., and D. Dunn. 1991. "The Resource-Based Relative Value Scale for Pricing Physicians' Services." In *Regulating Doctors' Fees: Competition and Controls Under Medicare,* ed. H. Frech III. Washington, D.C.: AEI Press.

Hsiao, W., H. Sapolsky, D. Dunn, and S. Weiner. 1986. "Lessons of the New Jersey DRG Payment System." *Health Affairs* 5 (Summer): 32–45.

Hsiao, W., and W. Stason. 1979. "Toward Developing a Relative Value Scale for Medical and Surgical Services." *Health Care Financing Review* 1 Fall: 23–38.

Hsiao, W., et al. 1992. "An Overview of the Development and Refinement of the Resource-Based Relative Value Scale." *Medical Care* 30 (November): 1–12.

Hsiao, W., et al. 1992. "Results and Impacts of the Resource-Based Relative Value Scale." *Medical Care* 30 (November): 61–79.

Hsiao, W., et al. 1988. "Results and Policy Implications of the Resource-Based Relative-Value Scale Study." *New England Journal of Medicine* 319 (September 29): 881–888.

Hurley, R., B. Strunk, and J. White. 2004. "The Puzzling Popularity of the PPO." *Health Affairs* 23 (March/April): 56–68.

Iglehart, J. 1999. "The American Health Care System: Medicare." *New England Journal of Medicine* 340 (January 28): 327–32.

———. 2001. "A Bias toward Action: A Conversation with Leonard Schaeffer." *Health Affairs* (web exclusive, August 22): W35. http://content.healthaffairs.org/cgi/reprint/hlthaff.w1.30v1 (accessed April 26, 2005).

———. 2002. "Changing Health Insurance Trends." *New England Journal of Medicine* 347 (September 19): 956–962.

———. 1986. "Early Experience with Prospective Payment of Hospitals." *New England Journal of Medicine* 314 (May 29): 1460–1464.

———. 2005. "The Emergence of Physician-Owned Specialty Hospitals." *New England Journal of Medicine.* 352 (January 6): 78–84.

———. 1997. "From the Editor: The Struggle over Public Opinion." *Health Affairs* 16 (January/February): 7–8.

———. 1982. "Health Policy Report: Medicare's Uncertain Future." *New England Journal of Medicine* 306 (May 27): 1308–1312.

———. 1990. "Health Policy Report: The New Law on Medicare's Payments to Physicians." *New England Journal of Medicine* 322 (April 26): 1247–1252.

———. 1988. "Health Policy Report: Payment of Physicians Under Medicare." *New England Journal of Medicine* 318 (March 31): 863–869.

———. 1985. "Hospitals, Public Policy, and the Future: An Interview with John Alexander McMahon." *Health Affairs* 4 (Fall): 20–34.

———. 1983. "Medicare Begins Prospective Payment of Hospitals." *New England Journal of Medicine* 308 (June 9): 1428–1432.

———. 2005. "Medicare: Identifying the Challenges That Lie Ahead." *Health Affairs* (web exclusive, September 26).

———. 2002. "Medicare's Declining Payments to Physicians." *New England Journal of Medicine* 346 (June 13): 1924–1930.

———. 1982. "The New Era of Prospective Payment for Hospitals." *New England Journal of Medicine* 307 (November 11): 1288–1292.

———. 2004. "The New Medicare Prescription-Drug Benefit—A Pure Power Play." *New England Journal of Medicine* 350 (February 19): 826–833.

———. 1998. "Pursuing Health Care Fraud and Abuse." *Health Affairs* 17 (March/April): 6.

———. 1989. "The Recommendations of the Physician Payment Review Commission." *New England Journal of Medicine* 320 (April 27): 1156–1160.

———. 1999. "Support for Academic Medical Centers: Revisiting the 1997 Balanced Budget Act." *New England Journal of Medicine* 341 (July 22): 299–304.

———. 2005. "The Uncertain Future of Specialty Hospitals." *New England Journal of Medicine* 352 (April 7): 1405–1407.

Ippolito, D. 1990. *Uncertain Legacies: Federal Budget Policy from Roosevelt through Reagan.* Charlottesville: University Press of Virginia.

Jaklevic, J. 2000. "What Hospitals 'See' They Get: Private Sector Acquiesces to Providers' Price Hikes." *Modern Healthcare* 30 (March 6): 60–62.

Japsen, B. 1997. "The Rise and Fall." *Modern Healthcare* 27 (September 8): 30–36.

Johnson, A., and D. Aquilina. 1982. "The Cost Shifting Issue." *Health Affairs* 1 (Fall): 101.

Johnson, D. 1994. "Home Health, Nursing Homes Take Patients from Hospitals." *Health Care Strategic Management* 12 (May): 2–3.

Johnsson, J., T. Hudson, and H. Anderson. 1992. "CEOs: There's No Simple Cure for Billing and Pricing Woes." *Hospitals* 66 (June 20): 26–33.

Jost, T. 2005. "Methodological Introduction." In *Health Care Coverage Determinations: An International Comparative Study,* ed. T. Jost, 11–15. London: Open University Press.

Jost, T. 2005. "The Most Important Health Care Legislation of the Millennium (So Far): The Medicare Modernization Act." *Yale Journal of Health Policy, Law and Ethics* 5 (Winter): 437–449.

Kahn, C., and H. Kuttner. 1999. "Budget Bills and Medicare Policy: The Politics of the BBA." *Health Affairs* 18 (January/February): 37–47.

Kahn, K., L. Rubenstein, D. Draper, J. Kosecoff, and W. Rogers, et al. 1990. "The Effects of the DRG-Based Prospective Payment System on Quality of Care for Hospitalized Medicare Patients." *Journal of the American Medical Association* 264 (October 17): 1956–1961.

Kaiser Family Foundation. 2004. "Medicare Part B Premiums to Rise 17% Next Year." (September 7). www.kaisernetwork.org/daily_reports/rep_index.cfm?DR_ID=25628 (accessed May 8, 2005).

Kaiser Family Foundation. 2004. "The President's FY2005 Budget Proposal." (June) Washington, D.C. www.kff.org/medicaid/7115.cfm.

Kaiser Family Foundation. 2004. "Retiree Health Benefits in 2003: Employer Survey." (January). www.kff.org/medicare/011404package.cfm (accessed March 1, 2005).

Kaiser Family Foundation. 2005. "Trends and Indicators in the Changing Health Care Marketplace." www.kff.org/insurance/7031/print-sec6.cfm (accessed February 23, 2005).

Kalison, M., and R. Averill. 1986. "The Challenge of 'Real' Competition in Medicare." *Health Affairs* 4 (Fall): 47–57.

Kay, T. 1990. "Volume and Intensity of Medicare Physicians' Services: An Overview." *Health Care Financing Review* 11 (Summer): 133–146.

Kennedy, E., and B. Thomas. 2004. "Dramatic Improvement or Death Spiral—Two Members of Congress Assess the Medicare Bill." *New England Journal of Medicine* 350 (February 19): 749–751.

Kertesz, L. 1997. "Backlash Continues: Survey Finds Managed Care is Still the Bad Guy in Many Americans' Eyes." *Modern Healthcare* 27 (November 10): 33.

———. "HMO Enrollment Soars, Profits Don't." *Modern Healthcare* 26 (October 28): 10.

Kesselheim, A., and T. Brennan. 2005. "Overbilling vs. Downcoding—The Battle between Physicians and Insurers." *New England Journal of Medicine* 352 (March 3): 855–857.

Kilberg W. 2000. "The Impending Collision between HMOs and ERISA: Can Either Emerge Unscathed?" *Employee Relations Law Journal* 25 (Spring): 1–5.

Kingson, E., and E. Berkowitz. 1993. *Social Security and Medicare.* Westport, Conn.: Auburn House.

Kinney, E. 2003. "Medicare Coverage Decision-Making and Appeal Procedures: Can Process Meet the Challenge of New Medical Technology?" *Washington and Lee Law Review* 60 (Fall): 1501–1505.

Kleinke, J. 1998. "Deconstructing the Columbia/HCA Investigation." *Health Affairs* 17 (March/April): 7–26.

Kohn, L. 2000. "Organizing and Managing Care in a Changing Health System." *Health Services Research* (April): 37–52.

Komisar, H. 2002. "Rolling Back Medicare Home Health." *Health Care Financing Review* 24 (Winter): 33–54.

Kosecoff, J., K. Kahn, W. Rogers, E. Reinisch, M. Sherwood, and L. Rubenstein, et al. 1990. "Prospective Payment System and Impairment at Discharge." *Journal of the American Medical Association* 264 (October 17): 1980–1983.

KPMG Peat Marwick. 1996. *Health Benefits in 1996.* Washington, D.C.: KPMG Peat Marwick.

Kronick, R. 2005. "Financing Health Care-Finding the Money Is Hard and Spending It Well Is Even Harder," *New England Journal of Medicine* 352 (March 24): 1252–1254.

Kuhn, H. 2005. Letter to Glenn M. Hackbarth, Medicare Payment Advisory Commission (March 31). www.healthlawyers.org/hlw/issues/050401/CMS_medpacltr.pdf (accessed May 11 2005).

Kuttner, R. 1996. "Columbia/HCA and the Resurgence of the For-Profit Hospital Business." *New England Journal of Medicine* 335 (August 1): 362–367.

Lasker, R., et al. 1990. "Medicare Surgical Global Fees: The Relationship between Included Services and Payment." *Inquiry* 27 (Fall): 255–262.

Laugesen, M., and T. Rice. 2003. "Is the Doctor In? The Evolving Role of Organized Medicine in Health Policy." *Journal of Health Politics, Policy and Law* 28 (April-June): 289–316.

Lee, J., R. Berenson, R. Mayes, and A. Gauthier. 2003. "Does Cost Shifting Matter?" *Health Affairs* (web exclusive, October 8): W3:480–488.

Lesser, C., and P. Ginsburg. 2000. "Update on the Nation's Health Care System: 1997–1999." *Health Affairs* 19 (November/December): 206–216.

Lesser, C., P. Ginsburg, and K. Devers. 2003. "The End of an Era: What Became of the 'Managed Care Revolution' in 2001?" *Health Services Research* 38 (February): 337–355.

Levit, K., C. Cowan, H. Lazenby, and A. Sensenig, et al. 2000. "Health Spending in 1998: Signals of Change." *Health Affairs* 19 (January/February): 124–132.

Levit, K., H. Lazenby, L. Sivarajan, et al. 1996. "National Health Expenditures, 1994." *Health Care Financing Review* 17 (Fall): 205–242.

Light, P. 1985. *Artful Work: The Politics of Social Security Reform*. New York: Random House.

———. 1995. *Still Artful Work: The Continuing Politics of Social Security Reform*. New York: McGraw-Hill.

Lillie-Blanton, M., S. Felt, P. Redmon, S. Renn, S. Machlin, and E. Wennar. 1992. "Rural and Urban Hospital Closures, 1985–1988." *Inquiry* 29 (Fall): 332–344.

Long, M., J. Chesney, R. Ament, and S. DesHarnais, et al. 1987. "The Effect of PPS on Hospital Product and Productivity." *Medical Care* 25 (June): 528–538.

Long, M., J. Chesney, and S. Fleming. 1990. "A Reassessment of Hospital Product and Productivity over Time." *Health Care Financing Review* 11 (Summer): 69–77.

Lubitz, J. 2005. "Health, Technology, and Medical Care Spending." *Health Affairs* (web exclusive, September 26): W5:R81–R85.

Maarse, H., D. Rooijakkers, and R. Duzijm. 1993. "Institutional Responses to Medicare's Prospective Payment System." *Health Policy* 25 (October): 255–270.

Manheim, L., and J. Feinglass. 1994. "Hospital Cost Incentives in a Fragmented Health Care System." *Health Care Management Review* 19 (Winter): 56–63.

Mann, J., G. Melnick, A. Bamezai, and J. Zwanziger. 1995. "Uncompensated Care: Hospitals' Response to Fiscal Pressures." *Health Affairs* 14 (Spring): 263–270.

Margrif, F. 1986. "Controller's Role in Monitoring Prospective Payment System." *Health Progress* 67 (May): 24, 64.

Marmor, T. 1983. *Political Analysis and American Medical Care*. Cambridge: Cambridge University Press.

———. 2000. *The Politics of Medicare*, 2nd ed. New York: Aldine de Gruyter.

———. 1994. *Understanding Health Care Reform*. New Haven, Conn.: Yale University Press.

Martin, C. 1995. "Nature or Nurture? Sources of Firm Preference for National Health Reform." *American Political Science Review* 89 (December): 898–914.

Matherlee, K. 1999. "Margins as Measure: Gauging Hospitals' Financial Health." Issue brief no. 734 (March 30). National Health Policy Forum.

Mauser, E. 1996. "Medicare Home Health Initiative: Current Activities and Future Directions." *Health Care Financing Review* 18 (Spring): 275–281.

Mayes, R., 2004. "Causal Chains and Cost Shifting: How Medicare's Rescue Inadvertently Triggered the Managed Care Revolution." *Journal of Policy History* 16 (April): 144–174.

———. 2004. "Universal Coverage and the American Health Care System in Crisis (Again)." *Journal of Health Care Law and Policy* 7 (Summer): 242–279.

———. 2005. *Universal Coverage: The Elusive Quest for National Health Insurance.* Ann Arbor: University of Michigan Press.

Mayes, R., and J. Lee. 2004. "Medicare.Payment Policy and the Controversy over Hospital Cost Shifting." *Applied Health Economics and Health Policy* 3: 153–159.

McFadden, D. 1990. "The Legacy of the $7 Aspirin." *Management Accounting* 71 (April): 38–41.

McGarvey, M. 1992. "The Challenge of Containing Health Care Costs." *Financial Executive* 8 (January/February): 34–40.

McGinley, P. 1995. "Beyond Health Care Reform: Reconsidering Certificate of Need Laws in a Managed Competition System." *Florida State University Law Review* 23 (Summer): 143–188.

McKinlay, J., and J. Stoeckle. 1988. "Corporatization and the Social Transformation of Doctoring." *International Journal of Health Services* 18: 191–205.

McLaughlin, C. 1999. "The Who, What and How of Managed Care." *Journal of Health Politics, Policy and Law* 24 (October): 1045–1049.

Meara, E., C. White, and D. Cutler. 2004. "Trends in Medical Spending by Age." *Health Affairs* 23 (July/August): 176–183.

Medicare Boards of Trustees, Federal Hospital Insurance Trust Fund. *1983 Annual Report, Federal Hospital Insurance Trust Fund,* 98th Cong., 1st sess., H. doc. 98-75.

Medicare Boards of Trustees, Federal Hospital Insurance and Federal Supplementary Medical Insurance Trust Funds. *2004 Annual Report.* www.cms.hhs.gov/ReportsTrustFunds/downloads/tr2004.pdf (accessed May 16, 2006).

Medicare Boards of Trustees, Federal Hospital Insurance and Federal Supplementary Medical Insurance Trust Funds. *2005 Annual Report.* www.cms.hhs.gov/ReportsTrustFunds/downloads/tr2005.pdf (accessed May 16, 2006).

Medicare Boards of Trustees, Federal Hospital Insurance and Federal Supplementary Medical Insurance Trust Funds. *2006 Annual Report.* Washington, D.C.: Government Printing Office. www.cms.hhs.gov/ReportsTrustFunds/downloads/tr2006.pdf (accessed May 16, 2006).

Medicare Payment Advisory Commission. 2002. "How Medicare Pays for Services: An Overview." In *Report to Congress: Medicare Payment Policy* (March): 3–33.

Medicare Payment Advisory Commission. 2004. *MedPAC Brief: Physician Services Payment System* (July 13).

Medicare Payment Advisory Commission. 1998. *Report to the Congress: Context for a Changing Medicare Program* (June).

Medicare Payment Advisory Commission. 1998–2005. *Report to the Congress: Medicare Payment Policy.*

Medicare Payment Review Commission. 2004. "Defining Long-Term Care Hospitals." In *Report to the Congress: New Approaches in Medicare* (June): 121–135.

Medicare Payment Review Commission. 2005. *Report to the Congress: Issues in a Modernized Medicare Program* (June).

Medicare Payment Review Commission. 2005. *Report to the Congress: Physician-Owned Specialty Hospitals* (March).

Medicare Payment Review Commission. 2005. "Review of CMS's Preliminary Estimate of the Physician Update for 2006." In *Report to the Congress: Issues in a Modernized Medicare Program* (June): 197–208.

Meyer, H. 1997. "Big Spender: Signs Show that Medicare, Once Considered a Skinflint by Doctors is Looking Better." *Hospitals and Health Networks* 71 (March 20): 54–56.

Meyer. J., and W. Johnson. 1983. "Cost Shifting in Health Care: An Economic Analysis." *Health Affairs* 2 (Summer): 20–35.

Miller, M., S. Zuckerman, and M. Gates. 1993. "How Do Medicare Physicians Fees Compare with Private Payers?" *Health Care Financing Review* 14 (Spring): 25–39.

Mills, R., R. Fetter, D. Riedel, and R. Averill. 1976. "AUTOGRP: An Interactive Computer System for the Analysis of Health Care Data." *Medical Care* 14 (July): 603–615.

Mitchell, J. 2005. "Effects of Physician-Owned Limited-Service Hospitals: Evidence from Arizona," *Health Affairs* (web exclusive, October 25): W5:481–490.

Moffit, R. 2004. "Fixing the New Medicare Law #1: An Agenda for Constructive Change." Backgrounder report no. 1750 (April 26). Washington, D.C.: Heritage Foundation. www.heritage.org/Research/HealthCare/bg1750.cfm (accessed 26 April 2005).

Moon, M. 1996. *Medicare: Now and in the Future,* 2nd ed. Washington, D.C.: Urban Institute Press.

Morone, J., and A. Dunham. 1984. "The Waning of Professional Dominance: DRGs and the Hospitals." *Health Affairs* 3 (Spring): 73–87.

Morone, J., and L. Jacobs, eds. 2005. *Healthy, Wealthy, and Fair: Health Care and the Good Society.* New York: Oxford University Press.

Morrissey, M. 2003. "Cost Shifting: New Myths, Old Confusion, and Enduring Reality." *Health Affairs* (web exclusive, October 8): W3:489.

———. 1994. *Cost Shifting in Health Care.* Washington, D.C.: AEI Press.

———. 1996. "Hospital Cost Shifting, a Continuing Debate." Issue brief no. 180 (December). Employee Benefit Research Institute. www.ebri.org/ibpdfs/1296ib.pdf (accessed October 1, 2004).

Morrissey, M., F. Sloan, and J. Valvona. 1988. "Medicare Prospective Payment and Posthospital Transfers to Subacute Care." *Medical Care* 26 (July): 685–698.

Murtaugh, C., N. McCall, S. Moore, and A. Meadow. 2003. "Trends in Medicare Home Health Use: 1997–2001." *Health Affairs* 22 (September/October): 146–156.

National Academy of Social Insurance. 1999. *Medicare and the American Social Contract: Final Report of the Study Panel on Medicare's Larger Social Role* (February). Washington, D.C.: NASI.

———. 2003. *Medicare in the Twenty-First Century: Building a Better Chronic Care System* (January). Washington, D.C.: NASI.

National Bipartisan Commission on the Future of Medicare. 1999. "Building a Better Medicare for Today and Tomorrow." (March 16). http://thomas.loc.gov/medicare/bbmtt31599.html (accessed April 28, 2005).

Needleman, J. 1994. "Cost Shifting or Cost-Cutting: Hospital Responses to High Uncompensated Care." (Cambridge, Mass.: Malcolm Wiener Center for Social Policy, John F. Kennedy School of Government, Harvard University).

Neumann, P., N. Divi, M. Beinfeld, et al. 2005. "Medicare's National Coverage Decisions, 1999–2003: Quality Of Evidence And Review Times." *Health Affairs* 24 (January/February): 243–254.

Newhouse, J. 2001. "Medicare." Paper prepared for the Conference on Economic Policy during the 1990s, Kennedy School of Government, Harvard University, June 27–30.

Nichols, L., P. Ginsburg, R. Berenson, J. Christianson, and R. Hurley. "Are Market Forces Strong Enough to Deliver Efficient Health Care Systems? Confidence is Waning." *Health Affairs* 23 (March/April): 8–21.

"1990 National Executive Poll on Health Care Costs/Benefits." 1990. *Business and Health* (April): 24–26, 30–31, 34–38.

"Nixon's Grand Design for the Economy." 1971. *Time* 98 (August 30), 4–14.

Oberlander, J. 1995. "Medicare and the American State" PhD diss., Yale Univ.

———. 1998. "Medicare: The End of Consensus." Paper presented at the Annual Meeting of the American Political Science Association, Boston, Mass., September 3–6.

———. 2003. *The Political Life of Medicare.* Chicago: University of Chicago Press.

O'Brien, E., and J. Feder. 1998. "How Well Does the Employment-Based Health Insurance System Work for Low-Income Families?" *Medicaid and the Uninsured,* Kaiser Commission issue paper (September).

O'Dougherty, S., P. Cotterill, S. Phillips, E. Richter, N. De Lew, B. Wynn, and T. Ault. 1992. "Medicare Prospective Payment without Separate Urban and Rural Rates." *Health Care Financing Review* 14 (Winter): 31–47.

Office of the Inspector General. 1997. "Results of the Operation Restore Trust Audit of Medicare Home Health Services in California, Illinois, New York and Texas." Washington, D.C.: U.S. Department of Health and Human Services.

Office of Technology Assessment. 1983. *Diagnosis Related Groups (DRGs) and the Medicare Program: Implications for Medical Technology.* Washington, D.C.: GPO.

Office of Technology Assessment. 1985. *Medicare's Prospective Payment System: Strategies for Evaluating Cost, Quality, and Medical Technology.* Washington, D.C.: GPO.

Oliver, T. 1993. "Analysis, Advice, and Congressional Leadership: The Physician Payment Review Commission and the Politics of Medicare." *Journal of Health Politics, Policy and Law* 18 (Spring): 113–174.

Oliver, T., P. Lee, and H. Lipton. 2004. "A Political History of Medicare and Prescription Drug Coverage." *Milbank Quarterly* 82 (June): 283–354.

O'Sullivan, J., et al. 1997. *Medicare Provisions in the Balanced Budget Act of 1997.* Washington, D.C.: Congressional Research Service.

Palazzolo, D. 1999. *Done Deal? The Politics of the 1997 Budget Agreement.* New York: Chatham House Publishers.

Partnership for Solutions. 2002. "Cost and Prevalence of Chronic Conditions" (July). www.partnershipforsolutions.org/DMS/files/Medicare_fact_sheet.pdf (accessed May 17, 2006).

Patashnik, E. 2000. *Putting Trust in the U.S. Budget: Federal Trust Funds and the Politics of Commitment.* Cambridge: Cambridge University Press.

Patashnik, E., and J. Zelizer. 2001. "Paying for Medicare: Benefits, Budgets, and Wilbur Mills's Policy Legacy." *Journal of Health Politics, Policy and Law* 26 (February): 7–36.

Patel, K. 1988. "Physicians and DRGs: Hospital Management Alternatives." *Evaluating the Health Professions* 11 (December): 487–505.

Pauly, M. 2004. "Medicare Drug Coverage and Moral Hazard." *Health Affairs* 23 (January/February): 113–114.

———. 2004. "Means-Testing in Medicare." *Health Affairs* (web exclusive): W4:546–557.

Pauly, M., and S. Nicholson. 1999. "Adverse Consequences of Adverse Selection." *Journal of Health Politics, Policy and Law* 24 (October): 921–930.

PBS Online News Hour. 1997. "Medicare Fraud," July 31. www.pbs.org/newshour/bb/medicare/july-dec97/medicare_fraud_7–31.html (accessed January 7, 2005).

Peck, P., and J. Anderson. 1992. "William Hsiao, Architect of RBRVS: What's Right, What's Wrong and What's Ahead." *Medical World News* 33 (January): 18–22.

Physician Payment Review Commission. 1989–1997. *Annual Report to Congress.* Washington, D.C.: PPRC.

———. 1991. *Medicare and the American Health Care System, Report to the Congress.* Washington, D.C.: PPRC.

Pierson, P. 2004. *Dismantling the Welfare State?* Cambridge: Cambridge University Press.

———. 2000. "Increasing Returns, Path Dependence, and the Study of Politics." *American Political Science Review* 94 (June): 251–267.

———. 2000. "Not Just What, but When: Timing and Sequence in Political Processes." *Studies in American Political Development* 14 (Spring): 72–92.

———. 1993. "When Effect Becomes Cause: Policy Feedback and Political Change." *World Politics* 45 (July): 595–628.

Pizer, S., R. Feldman, and A. Frakt. 2005. "Defective Design: Regional Competition in Medicare." *Health Affairs* (web exclusive, August 23): W5:399–409.

Plant, J. 1985. "PPS Invades the Boardroom." *Trustee* 38 (March): 13–15.

"The Policymakers' Perspective: How Has Current Policy Developed and How Can the Past Inform the Future?" 2002. *When Public Payment Declines Does Cost-Shifting Occur? Hospital and Physician Responses,* symposium sponsored by Changes in Health Care Financing and Organization (HCFO), Washington, D.C., November 13, 2002. www.kaisernetwork.org/health_cast/hcast_index.cfm?display=detail&hc=715

Porter, M., and E. Teisberg. 2004. "Redefining Competition in Health Care." *Harvard Business Review* 82 (July): 64–77.

Prince, M. 2002. "Rate Hikes Spur Managed Care Profits." *Business Insurance* 36 (August 26): 2–3.

Prospective Payment Assessment Commission. 1985–1997. *Medicare and the American Health Care System: Report to the Congress.* Washington, D.C.: ProPAC.

Quadagno, J., and D. Street. 2005. "Ideology and Public Policy: Antistatism in American Welfare State Transformation." *Journal of Policy History* 17 (Spring): 52–71.

Rayburn, L. 1986. "Study Suggests PPS Creates Job Tension for the Financial Manager." *Healthcare Financial Management* 40 (February): 48–52.

Reed, M., and P. Ginsburg. 2003. "Behind the Times: Physician Income, 1995–99." Issue Brief no. 24 (March). Washington, D.C.: Center for Studying Health System Change.

Regopoulos, L., and S. Trude. 2004. "Employers Shift Rising Health Care Costs to Workers: No Long-Term Solution in Sight." Issue Brief no. 83 (May). Washington, D.C.: Center for Studying Health System Change.

Reilly, P. 2003. "Riding High: Study Finds Hospital Margins at Five-Year Peak." *Modern Healthcare* 33 (March 3): 16.

Reinhardt, U. "Calm before the Storm. Will There Be a Second Revolution in American Health Care?" 1997. Duke University Private Sector Conference, session 1: "The Status of Managed Care and Evolutionary Trends." http://conferences.mc.duke.edu/privatesector/dpsc1997/TOC.html (accessed April 19, 2005).

———. 2003. "Can Efficiency in Health Care Be Left to the Market?" In *Uncertain Times: Kenneth Arrow and the Changing Economics of Health Care,* ed. P. Hammer, D. Haas-Wilson, M. Peterson, and W. Sage, 111–133. Durham: Duke University Press.

———. 2003. "Churchill's Dictum and the Next New Thing in American Health Care." *Business Economics* 38 (July): 38–51.

———. 1998. "Columbia/HCA: Villain or Victim?" *Health Affairs* 17 (March/April): 30–36.

———. 1989. "Health Care Spending and American Competitiveness." *Health Affairs* 8 (Winter): 5–21.

———. 1994. "The Predictable Managed Care *Kvetch* on the Rocky Road from Adolescence to Adulthood." *Journal of Health Politics, Policy and Law* 24 (October): 897–910.

Rettig, P. 1995. Interview by E. Berkowitz, August 14.

Rettig, P., G. Markus, J. Bentley, A. Dobson, et al. 1987. "Medicare's Prospective Payment System: The Expectations and the Realities." *Inquiry* 24 (Summer): 173–188.

Riddick, F., and J. Hartfield. 1989. "Medicine Prepares for Battle." *Physician Executive* (September/October): 32–34.

Roberts, R., P. Frutos, and G. Ciavarella, et al. 1999. "Distribution of Variable vs. Fixed Costs of Hospital Care." *Journal of the American Medical Association* 281 (February 17): 644–649.

Robinson, J. 2004. "Consolidation and the Transformation of Competition in Health Insurance." *Health Affairs* 23 (November/December): 11–24.

———. 2001. "The End of Managed Care." *Journal of the American Medical Association* 285 (May 23/30): 2622–2628.

Robinson, J., and H. Luft. 1987. "Competition and the Cost of Hospital Care, 1972 to 1982." *Journal of the American Medical Association* 257 (June 19): 3241–3245.

Roe, B. 1981. "Sounding Board: The UCR Boondoggle, A Death Knell for Private Practice?" *New England Journal of Medicine* 305 (July 2): 41–44.

Rosenthal, M., R. Fernandopulle, H. Song, and B. Landon. "Paying for Quality: Providers' Incentives for Quality Improvement." *Health Affairs* 23 (March/April): 127–141.

Rosko, M. 1989. "A Comparison of Hospital Performance under the Partial-Payer Medicare PPS and State All-Payer Rate-Setting Systems." *Inquiry* 26 (Spring): 48–51.

Rosko, M., and R. Broyles. 1987. "Short-Term Responses of Hospitals to the DRG Prospective Pricing Mechanism in New Jersey." *Medical Care* 25: 88–99.

Rother, J. 2002. Interview by E. Berkowitz, August 27.

Rovner, J. 1989. "A Reader's Guide to the 'Game.'" *CQ Weekly* (April 29).

Rubin, Robert. 1995. Interview by Edward Berkowitz, August 16.

Rueschemeyer, D., E. Stephens, and J. Stephens. 1992. *Capitalist Development and Democracy.* Chicago: University of Chicago Press.

Ruggie, M. 1992. "The Paradox of Liberal Intervention: Health Policy and the American Welfare State." *American Journal of Sociology* 97 (January): 919–944.

Ruhnka, J., E. Gac, and H. Boerstler. 2000. "Qui Tam Claims: Threat to Voluntary Compliance

Programs in Health Care Organizations." *Journal of Health Politics, Policy and Law.* 25 (April): 283–308.

Rushefsky, M., and K. Patel. 1998. *Politics, Power, and Policy Making: The Case of Health Care Reform in the 1990s.* Armonk, N.Y.: M.E. Sharpe.

Russell, L. 1989. *Medicare's New Hospital Payment System: Is It Working?* Washington, D.C.: Brookings Institution Press.

Russell, L., and C. Manning. 1989. "The Effect of Prospective Payment on Medicare Expenditures." *New England Journal of Medicine.* 320 (February 16): 439–444.

Sabin, P. 1987. "Hospital Cost Accounting and the New Imperative." *Health Progress* 68 (May): 52–57.

Sambamoorthi, U., D. Shea, and S. Crystal. 2003. "Total and Out-of-Pocket Expenditures for Prescription Drugs among Older Persons." *Gerontologist* 43 (June): 345–359.

Saphir, A. 1998. "Leaving Home: Home Health Survey Looks at Industry in Turmoil." *Modern Healthcare* 28 (December 21–28): 42–44.

Schiller, Z. 1991. "The Human Flap Could Make All Hospitals Feel Sick." *Business Week,* November 4: 34.

Schlesinger, M. 2002. "On Values and Democratic Policy Making: The Deceptively Fragile Consensus around Market-Oriented Medical Care." *Journal of Health Politics, Policy and Law* 27 (December): 889–925.

Schneidman, D. 1999. "PATH (Physicians at Teaching Hospitals) Audits." *Bulletin of the American College of Surgeons* 84 (August): 6–10.

Scott, J. 2003. "A Line in the Sand: The Politics of Medicare Reform." *Healthcare Financial Management* 57 (June): 24–25.

———. 1999. "BBA Bad News Gets Worse," Thanks to Flawed Calculations." *Healthcare Financial Management* 53 (September): 24–25.

———. 1997. "The Feds Discover Home Health Care." *Healthcare Financial Management* 51 (December): 26–29.

———. 1999. "Saving Medicare: What Will it Cost and Whom Will it Benefit?" *Healthcare Financial Management* 53 (February): 30–31.

Scott, L. 1996. "Maternity-Stay Rule Sparks Backlash." *Modern Healthcare* 26 (March 4): 81.

Scully, T. 2003. "All Seniors Gain Benefits." *Modern Healthcare* 33 (December 22): 22.

Selis, S. 2000. "Just Say No." *Healthcare Business* (January/February): 1–5.

Sellers, P. 1998. "The No. 1 Health-Care Company Goes Under the Knife." *Fortune* 137 (January 12): 26–28.

Serafini, M. 1999. "If It's Good Enough for Congressmen . . . ." *National Journal* 31 (February 6): 340–341.

———. 2000. "Medicare's Challenge." *National Journal* 32 (May 20): 1602–1604.

———. 1999. "Quest for Medicare Compromise Challenges Congress." *National Journal* (February 27): S8–S15.

Serb, S. 1998. "Another Vicious Cycle?" *Hospitals and Health Networks* 72 (October 20): 24–28.

Shalowitz, D. 1988. "Hospitals Shift Costs to Cover Costs." *Business Insurance* 22 (February 15): 14.

Sheingold, S. 1986. "Unintended Results of Medicare's National Prospective Payment Rates." *Health Affairs* 5 (Winter): 5–21.

Sheingold, S., and E. Richter. 1992. "Are PPS Payments Adequate? Issues for Updating and Assessing Rates." *Health Care Financing Review* 14 (Winter): 165–175.

Shi, L., and D. Singh. 1998. *Delivering Health Care in America: A Systems Approach.* Gaithersburg, Md.: Jones and Bartlett Publishers.

Sloan, F. 1981. "Regulation and the Rising Cost of Hospital Care." *Review of Economics and Statistics* 13 (November): 479–487.

Sloan, F., M. Morrissey, and J. Valvona. 1988. "Effects of the Medicare Prospective Payment System on Hospital Cost Containments." *Milbank Quarterly* 6: 191–220.

Smith, C. 1986. "Hospital Management Strategies for Fixed-Price Payment." *Health Care Management Review* 11 (Winter): 21–26.

Smith, D. 2002. *Entitlement Politics: Medicare and Medicaid, 1995–2001.* New York: Aldine de Gruyter.

———. 1992. *Paying for Medicare: The Politics of Reform.* New York: Aldine de Gruyter.

Smith, H., and M. Fottler. 1985. *Prospective Payment.* Rockville, Md.: Aspen Publications.

Snow, C. 1997. "Home Health Heats Up: Survey Finds Massive Change at Industry's Door." *Modern Healthcare* 27 (August 18): 28–33.

Social Security Administration. 1995. "Actuarial Status of the Social Security and Medicare Programs." *Social Security Bulletin* 58 (Summer): 58–64.

———. 2005. *Summary Trust Fund Reports: 1995.* www.ssa.gov/history/pdf/1995.pdf (accessed March 25, 2005).

Social Security Boards of Trustees. 1982. *Summary of the 1982 Annual Reports of the Social Security Boards of Trustees.* Washington, D.C.: Social Security Administration and Health Care Financing Administration.

Somers, H., and A. Somers. 1967. *Medicare and the Hospitals.* Washington, D.C.: Brookings Institution Press.

Sorian, R., and J. Feder. 1999. "Whey We Need a Patients' Bill of Rights." *Journal of Health Politics, Policy and Law* 24 (October): 1137–1144.

Sparrow, M. 1996. *License to Steal: Why Fraud Plagues America's Health Care System.* Boulder, Colo.: Westview Press.

Stanton, T. 2001. "Fraud-and-Abuse Enforcement in Medicare: Finding Middle Ground." *Health Affairs* 20 (July/August): 28–42.

Starr, P. 1982. *The Social Transformation of American Medicine.* New York: Basic Books.

Stevens, R. 1989. *In Sickness and in Wealth: American Hospitals in the Twentieth Century.* New York: Basic Books.

Stone, D. 1997. "Bedside Manna: Medicine Turned Upside Down." *American Prospect* (March/April): 42–49.

———. 1980. *The Limits of Professional Power.* Chicago: University of Chicago Press.

———. 1997. *Policy Paradox and Political Reason.* New York: W. W. Norton.

Strunk, B., K. Devers, and R. Hurley. 2001. "Health Plan-Provider Showdowns on the Rise." Issue brief no. 40 (June). Washington, D.C.: Center for Studying Health System Change.

Strunk, B., and J. Reschovsky. 2002. "Kinder and Gentler: Physicians and Managed Care, 1997–2001." Community tracking study no. 5 (November). Washington, D.C.: Center for Studying Health System Change.

Strunk, B., and J. Reschovsky. 2004. "Trends in U.S. Health Insurance Coverage, 2001–2003."

Community tracking study no. 9 (August). Washington, D.C.: Center for Studying Health System Change.

Stuart, B., L. Simoni-Wastila, and D. Chauncey. 2005. "Assessing the Impact of Coverage Gaps in the Medicare Part D Drug Benefit." *Health Affairs* (web exclusive, April 19): W5:167–179.

Sulvetta, M. 1991. "Achieving Cost Control in the Hospital Outpatient Department." *Health Care Financing Review Annual Supplement.*

Swartz, K., 1999. "The Death of Managed Care as We Know It." *Journal of Health Politics, Policy and Law* 24 (October): 1201–1205.

Swenson, P., and S. Greer. 2002. "Foul Weather Friends: Big Business and Health Care Reform in the 1990s in Historical Perspective." *Journal of Health Politics, Policy and Law* 27 (August): 605–638.

Thorpe, K. 1999. "Managed Care as Victim or Villain?" *Journal of Health Politics, Policy and Law* 24 (October): 949–956.

Titlow, K., and E. Emanuel. 1999. "Employer Decisions and the Seeds of Backlash." *Journal of Health Politics, Policy and Law* 24 (October): 941–947.

Tu, H. 2004. "Rising Health Costs, Medical Debt and Chronic Conditions." Issue brief no. 88 (September). Washington, D.C.: Center for Studying Health System Change.

Tyson, L. 2000. "Healing Medicare." *The American Prospect* 11 (February 14): 32–37.

U.S. Census Bureau. 2004. *Income, Poverty and Health Insurance Coverage in the United States: 2003.* Washington, D.C.: GPO.

U.S. Congress. House Committee on Ways and Means, *Summary of Major Provisions of P.L. 89-97, the Social Security Amendments of 1965.* 89th Cong., 1st sess., September 1965.

U.S. Department of Health and Human Services. 1982. *Report to the Congress: Hospital Prospective Payment for Medicare.*

———. 1984. *Report to the Congress: Impact of the Medicare Hospital Prospective Payment System.*

U.S. Department of Health, Education, and Welfare. 1976. *History of the Rising Costs of the Medicare and Medicaid Programs and Attempts to Control These Costs, 1966–1975.* Washington, D.C.: GPO.

U.S. General Accounting Office. 2001. "Civil Fines and Penalties Debt: Review of CMS' Management and Collection Process." GAO-02-211.

———. 1991. *Health Care Spending Control: The Experience of France, Germany and Japan.* GAO/HRD-92-9 (November).

———. 1990. "Health Insurance: Cost Increases Lead to Coverage Limitations and Cost Shifting." (May). Washington, D.C.: GAO.

———. 1997. *Private Health Insurance: Continued Erosion of Coverage Linked to Cost Pressures,* Report to the Chairman, Committee on Labor and Human Resources, U.S. Senate. GAO/HEHS-97-122 (July).

———. 2004. "Medicare Demonstration PPOs: Financial and Other Advantages for Plans, Few Advantages for Beneficiaries." GAO-04-960 (September).

———. 1999. "Medicare Home Health Agencies: Closures Continue, with Little Evidence Beneficiary Access is Impaired." Report to Congress. GAO/HHS-99-120 (May).

U.S. Government Accountability Office. 2004. "Department of Health and Human Services—

Chief Actuary's Communications with Congress." (September 7). www.gao.gov/decisions/appro/302911.pdf (accessed April 26, 2005).

———. 2005. *Federal Employees Health Benefits Program: Competition and Other Factors Linked to Wide Variation in Health Care Prices.* GAO-05-856 (August 15, 2005). Washington, D.C.: GPO.

———. 2004. *Medicare Physician Payments: Concerns about Spending Target System Prompt Interest in Considering Reforms.* Washington, D.C.: GPO.

U.S. Senate. 1970. "Medicare and Medicaid, Problems, Issues, and Alternatives." Staff report, Committee on Finance. 91st Cong., 1st sess.

Vladeck, B. 2005. "Accounting for Future Costs in Medicare." *Health Affairs* (web exclusive, September 26): W5:R94–R96.

———. 1999. "Plenty of Nothing—A Report from the Medicare Commission." *New England Journal of Medicine* 340 (May 13): 1503–1506.

———. 1999. "The Political Economy of Medicare." *Health Affairs* 18 (January/ February): 22–36.

———. 2004. "The Struggle for the Soul of Medicare." *Journal of Law, Medicine, and Ethics* (Fall): 410–415.

Wagner, M. 1989. "No Slowdown in Capital Expenditures: Financial Pressures Not Stopping Hospitals from Expensive Purchases." *Modern Healthcare* 19 (November 17): 50.

Walker, C. 1993. "A Cross-Sectional Analysis of Hospital Profitability." *Journal of Hospital Marketing* 7: 121–138.

Warren, E., T. Sullivan, and M. Jacoby. 2000. "Medical Problems and Bankruptcy Problems." *Norton's Bankruptcy Adviser.* (April). http://ssrn.com/abstract=224581 (accessed March 1, 2005).

Weber, D. 2000. "Managed Care Medical Directors Under Fire." *Physician Executive* (September/October): 12–18.

Weil, T. 1997. "Changes in Physician and Non-Physician Relationships." *Physician Executive* 23 (November/December): 19–24.

———. 2001. *Health Networks: Can They Be the Solution?* Ann Arbor: University of Michigan Press.

Weissenstein, E. 1996. "Changing Tunes: No More 'Whining for Dollars,' by Healthcare Lobbyists in Washington." *Modern Healthcare* 26 (July 22): 30–34.

———. 1995. "Medicare Margins Climb through Cost Shifting." *Modern Healthcare.* 25 (December 18–25): 2.

Wennberg, D., and J. Wennberg. 2003. "Addressing Variations: Is There Hope for the Future?" *Health Affairs* (web exclusive, December 10): W3:614–617. http://content.healthaffairs.org/cgi/content/abstract/hlthaff.var.5.

Wennberg, J., E. Fisher, and J. Skinner. 2003. "Geography and the Debate over Medicare Reform." *Health Affairs.* (web exclusive, October 31): W3:586–602.

Wennberg, J., E. Fisher, T. Stukel, and S. Sharp. 2004. "Use of Medicare Claims Data to Monitor Provider-Specific Performance Among Patients with Severe Chronic Illness." *Health Affairs* (web exclusive, October 7): VAR5–VAR18.

West, H. 1971. "Five Years of Medicare—A Statistical Review." *Social Security Bulletin* 34 (December): 20–25.

Whetsell, G. 1999. "The History and Evolution of Hospital Payment Systems: How Did We Get Here?" *Nursing Administration Quarterly* 23 (Summer): 1–15.

White, C. 2003. "Rehabilitation Therapy in Skilled Nursing Facilities: Effects of Medicare's New Prospective Payment System." *Health Affairs.* 22 (May/June): 214–222.

White, J. 1995. "Budgeting and Health Policymaking." In *Intensive Care: How Congress Shapes Health Policy,* ed. T. Mann and N. Ornstein, 53–69. Washington, D.C.: Brookings Institution Press.

————. 2003. *False Alarm: Why the Greatest Threat to Social Security and Medicare is the Campaign to "Save" Them.* Baltimore: Johns Hopkins University Press.

White, J., R. Hurley, and B. Strunk. 2004. "Getting Along or Going Along? Health Plan-Provider Contract Showdowns Subside." Issue brief no. 74 (January). Washington, D.C.: Center for Studying Health System Change.

White, J., and A. Wildavsky. 1989. *The Deficit and the Public Interest.* Berkeley: University of California Press.

White, W., ed. 2003. *Compelled by Data: John D. Thompson.* New Haven, Conn.: Yale University Press.

Wholey, D., J. Christianson, J. Engberg, and C. Bryce. 1997. "HMO Market Structure and Performance: 1985–1995." *Health Affairs* 16 (November/December): 75–84.

Wickham, J. 1994. "Future Developments: Minimally Invasive Surgery." *British Medical Journal* 308 (January 15): 193–196.

Wiener, J., D. Stevenson, and S. Goldenson. 1998. "Controlling the Supply of Long-Term Care Providers at the State Level." Research report. Washington, D.C.: Urban Institute.

Wilensky, G. 2001. "Medicare Reform—Now is the Time." *New England Journal of Medicine* 345 (August 9): 458–462.

Wilensky, G., and J. Newhouse. 1999. "Medicare: What's Right? What's Wrong? What's Next?" *Health Affairs* 18 (January/February): 92–106.

Williams, D., J. Hadley, and J. Pettengill. 1992. "Profits, Community Role, and Hospital Closure: An Urban and Rural Analysis." *Medical Care* 30 (February): 174–187.

Wooten, J. 2005. *The Employee Retirement Income Security Act of 1974.* Berkeley, Calif.: University of California Press/Milbank Memorial Fund.

World Health Report 2000—Health Systems Improving Performance. Geneva: World Health Organization. www.who.int/whr/2000/en/index.html (accessed October 28, 2005).

Zelman, W., and R. Berenson. 1998. *The Managed Care Blues and How to Cure Them.* Washington, D.C.: Georgetown University Press.

Zwanziger, J., G. Melnick, and A. Bamezai. 2000. "Can Cost Shifting Continue on a Price Competitive Environment?" *Health Economics* 9 (April): 211–225.

diagnosis-related groups (DRGs): annual update, 59; hospital transfers and, 106–7, 150; initial success, 3, 6, 8, 148; New Jersey's experiment, 24–27, 34–37; origin, 24, 31; "outlier" cases, 44–45; patient coding, 49–50; prospective payment proposal, 40–42, 47–48, 57
diagnostic services, 102
diagnostic tests: physician ordering practices for, 48, 54, 143, 146, 148; reimbursement, 89, 154–55
differential pricing, 71–73
disabled population, 2, 136
discharges, hospital: earlier, 52, 54, 98; flat rate payment, 41
discretionary care, 146, 152–53
disproportionate share hospitals (DSH), 60–61
Dobson, Allen, 32, 42, 44, 52, 66, 75
doctor-hospital relationship, 54, 92
doctor-patient relationship, 15, 18, 135, 146
Dole, Bob, 33, 38, 43
"double-dipping," 103
Dowling, William, 21–22
downward-sticky physician fees, 83–84, 148
DRG-creep, 50, 147
Duggan v. Brown, 99

economics: cost shifting, 71–73; inflation, 27, 29, 66; policy decisions, 4–5, 11, 31, 37–38, 118, 141–42, 144; power shift, 7–8, 83–87, 89, 91, 94, 119–21; private sector transformation, 8–9, 92, 118
Economic Stabilization Program (ESP), 19–20
economies of scale, 119, 147
efficiency: DRGs impact, 35–36, 41; improvement strategies, 7, 48, 155–56; PPS impact, 53–55
Eisenberg, John, 117
Ellwood, Paul, 77
Employee Retirement Income Security Act (ERISA) of 1974, 120
employees: hospital reduction, 53, 55, 97–98; in managed care vs. fee-for-service plans, 53, 55, 77–78, 96, 113, 118, 120
employers: cost shifting response, 73–76; downward trend in coverage, 125–26, 132; 1990s market force, 119–20; reform impact, 7–8, 53, 55, 95–96, 118
empowerment, of federal government, 1–4, 7–8, 89, 94
Enthoven, Alain, 137
entitlement, Medicare as, 1–2, 127, 151

entrepreneurs, 151
episodes of care, 146
evidence-based medicine, 99, 153–54
executives. *See* hospital administration
expenditures: Medicare problems with, 16–19, 52–53, 65, 93–94, 115; national, 52–53; ordinary, 140–41, 143; prices vs., 145–47. *See also* costs

"faith-based" initiative, 132
False Claims Act, 104
federal government: empowerment, 1–4, 7–8, 89, 94; regulatory initiatives, 28–31, 38, 127; shutdown, 94; as steward, 155–56. *See also* budget deficit reduction
Federation of American Hospitals (FAH), 16, 42, 44, 51, 73
fee-for-service reimbursement, 8, 14–16, 18; continuation, 145–46; fixed budgets, 92; managed care vs., 77–79, 108, 120, 123–24, 132
fee schedules, physician, 81–82, 85; difficulties with, 91–92; distortions, 148–49; Medicare's, 15, 87–89, 144–45; national standard, 3, 8, 85; RBRVS, 87–92
Feinstein, Patrice, 33
Fetter, Robert, 5–6, 23–24
financial health, hospitals': DRGs impact, 35–36, 41; managed care impact, 97–98, 101, 110–11, 138; Medicare's vs., 37–40, 42–43, 57, 133; 1990s backlash, 114–17, 121, 124; PPS impact, 49–52, 141
financial incentives: for employers, 96; realignment of, 6, 37, 46, 48, 110, 150
financial information, hospital: standardized, 7, 15–16, 23; withholding of, 57–58
financial interests, technology-related, 55, 151–52
financial power, shift of, 7–8, 11–12, 89, 94, 119–22
financial risk: hospitals' management of, 72, 149–50; in managed care, 79, 96, 127
Finley, Joanne, 25–27, 34–35
fiscal intermediaries, 99
fiscal policy, payment policy vs., 11–12, 48–49, 62, 94, 110–11, 133, 141, 151
Fisher v. United States, 140–41
fixed budget, difficulties with, 92
fixed costs, hospitals', 72
flat rate payment, per discharge, 41
"focused factories," 147
for-profit providers, 25, 36, 44, 54, 72; of managed care, 78–79, 95, 102, 110

RICK MAYES, PH.D., is an assistant professor of public policy in the Department of Political Science at the University of Richmond, as well as a faculty research fellow at the Petris Center on Healthcare Markets and Consumer Welfare at the University of California, Berkeley. He received his Ph.D. in political science from the University of Virginia and completed an NIMH postdoctoral traineeship at the UC Berkeley School of Public Health. In the early 1990s, he worked on Medicaid policy in the White House for George Bush Sr., and thereafter he worked on health care reform and Medicare policy at the American Association of Retired Persons (AARP) during the Clinton administration. His writings have appeared in *Health Affairs*, the *Journal of Health Law*, the *Journal of Health Care Law and Policy*, *Health Law Review*, the *Journal of the History of Medicine and Allied Sciences*, the *Journal of Policy History*, the *Journal of Health Economics, Policy, and Law*, *Applied Health Economics and Health Policy*, and the *Journal of the History of Behavioral Sciences*. He is also the author of *Universal Coverage: The Elusive Quest for National Health Insurance* (University of Michigan Press, 2005).

ROBERT A. BERENSON, M.D., is a senior fellow at the Urban Institute. He is an expert in health care policy, particularly Medicare, with experience practicing medicine, serving in senior positions in two presidential administrations, and helping organize and manage a successful preferred provider organization. Dr. Berenson received his M.D. from the Mount Sinai School of Medicine in New York City and served as Robert Wood Johnson Clinical Scholar at the White House from 1977 to 1979. From 1998 to 2000, he was in charge of Medicare payment policy and managed care contracting in the Health Care Financing Administration (now the Centers for Medicare and Medicaid Services). In the Carter administration, he served as an assistant director of the Domestic Policy Staff. He was also national program director of IMPACS (Improving Malpractice Prevention and Compensation Systems), a grant program funded by the Robert Wood Johnson Foundation, from 1994 to 1998. Dr. Berenson is a board-certified internist who practiced for twelve years in a Washington, D.C., group practice and is a Fellow of the American College of Physicians. His writings have appeared in the *New England Journal of Medicine*, *Medical Care*, *Health Affairs*, the *Annals of Internal Medicine*, *Health Services Research*, *Medical Economics*, *Law and Contemporary Problems*, *Health Services Research*, *American Journal of Law and Medicine*, the *New Republic*, and the *New York Times*. He is also the co-author of *The Managed Care Blues and How to Cure Them* (Georgetown University Press, 1998).